AF365182

Biostatistics and Computer Applications

Biostatistics and Computer Applications

Dr. G. Nageswara Rao, *PhD*
Professor and University Head (Retd.),
Department of Statistics and Mathematics,
Acharya N.G. Ranga Agricultural University,
Hyderabad.

Dr. N.K. Tiwari
Former Scientist, (MPCST, Bhopal)
Director,
Rukmani Devi Institute of Science and Technology,
Bhopal (M.P.).

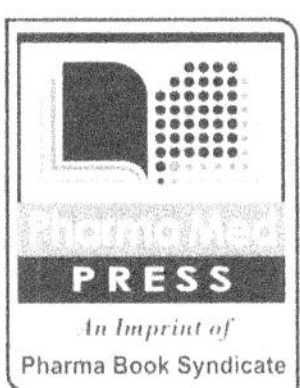

PharmaMed Press
An imprint of Pharma Book Syndicate

A unit of **BSP Books Pvt., Ltd.**

4-4-309/316, Giriraj Lane,
Sultan Bazar, Hyderabad - 500 095.

Published by

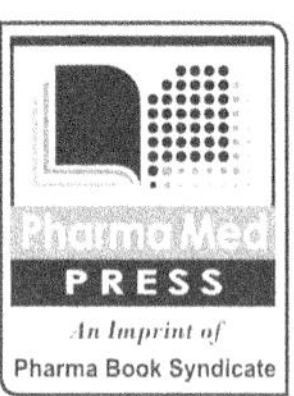

PharmaMed Press
An imprint of Pharma Book Syndicate

A unit of BSP Books Pvt., Ltd.

4-4-309/316, Giriraj Lane, Sultan Bazar, Hyderabad - 500 095.
Phone: 040-23445605, 23445688; Fax: 91+40-23445611
E-mail: info@pharmamedpress.com

ISBN : 978-93-52300-72-3 (HB)

Preface

The combination of Biostatistics and computer are very much useful for bio-sciences and bio-informatic fields. The book provides both concepts in synoptic view.

The first part of the book includes 12 chapters. They include chapters on basic concepts and sampling methods, probability and distributions, correlation and regression, Chi-Square test, analysis of variance, experimental designs and statistical quality control.

The second part of the book provides a detailed yet easy to understand description of the computer fundamentals. Each and every aspect is presented very clearly and logically. This parts of book includes 11 chapters from chapter 13 to 23. They include chapters on computer and its application histroy of computer, type of computers, number system, system concept fundamental of operating system, computer languages, networking concept, database management, C programming and application of computers in Pharmaceutical and clinical studies.

All the chapters are written in a lucid manner so that the students can easily understand without any difficulty. This book is also intended to serve as a textbook for pharmacy, biology, biotechnology, information technology, computer applications, medicine, home science etc., students as a part of their degree or PG degree programme.

We are grateful to the publishers, PharmaMed Press for the careful processing of the manuscript, both at editorial and production stages. We will be glad to receive comments and suggestions for improving the contents of the book.

- **Authors**

Contents

PART - A
Biostatistics

Chapter 1

Introduction

Chapter 2

Collection of Data

Chapter 3

Data Organization

Chapter 4

Dispersion and Standard Deviation

Chapter 5

Skewness and Kurtosis

Chapter 6

Probability and Distributions

Chapter 7

Correlation and Regression

Chapter 8

Tests of Hypotheses

Chapter 9

Chi-Square Test

Chapter 10

Analysis of Variance

Chapter 11

Experimental Designs

Chapter 12

Statistical Quality Control

PART - B
Computer Applications

Chapter 13

Introduction to Computers

Chapter 14

History of Computers

Chapter 15

Classifications of Computers

Chapter 16

The System Concept

Chapter 17

Fundamentals of Operating System

Chapter 18

Computer Languages

Chapter 19

Concept of Programming

Chapter 20

Computer Networks

Chapter 21

Database Management

Chapter 22

C Programming Language

Chapter 23

Applications of Computers in Pharmaceutical and Clinical Studies

Part - A
Biostatistics

CHAPTER 1

Introduction

1.1 Introduction

In recent days Statistical Methods have been applied to different branches of sciences such as Biology, Agriculture, Medicine, etc., besides social sciences such as Economics, Sociology, Anthropology and technical subjects like Engineering, etc., in order to draw proper, valid conclusions from the research investigation, experiment and survey conducted. In most of the published research articles also we find lot of statistical treatment to the data collected which brings weightage and importance to the research article. Statistical analysis of data in a research investigation gives more validity, consistency and leads to generalization of the conclusions obtained from a sample. Statistical Methods applied in Genetics is well known.

The word 'Statistics' has been derived from a Latin word which means 'state' which means 'politically organized people', i.e., Government. Since Governments or kings in olden days used to collect relevant data on births and deaths, tax collection, defence personnel, import and export of goods, etc., 'Statistics' was identified with 'state' or Government. The word 'state' became 'statistics'.

'Statistics' word can be used as 'singular' or 'plural'. Statistics, when it is used as singular, is a science which deals with functions such as (i) Collection of data (ii) Classification of data (iii) Analysis of data, and (iv) Interpretation of data. Here data refers to information collected from the research experiment conducted in the laboratory, field or survey conducted in a village, district, state or country. Statistics when it is used in plural sense, refers to mere 'facts' and 'figures', e.g., the data or figures published in journals such as 'Economic Times', 'Financial Express'. Agricultural situation in India, demographic statistics, etc., are called statistics when it is used in plural sense. However, we deal in this book statistics used in singular sense.

Statistics has to be handled carefully since if it is used properly and appropriately it gives valid and accurate conclusions. If it is not properly used in cases such as (i) data are not reliable (ii) computing spurious correlations between variables, and

(iii) generalizing from a small sample to a large area or population without considering sampling errors involved.

The reliable data is basic necessity for application of statistical techniques just as strong foundation for multistoreyed building.

If it is ensured that data is reliable and is properly handled by a 'skilled statistician' the mistrust of statistics will disappear and, in place of it, precise and exact revelation of data will come up for reasonable conclusions.

CHAPTER 2

Collection of Data

2.1 Introduction

The data are of two kinds : (i) Primary data and (ii) Secondary data.

Primary data are based on primary source of information and secondary data are based on secondary source of information. When data are generated or collected for the first time it is called primary source and if the data are not obtained for the first time then it is called secondary source.

2.1.1 Methods of Collection of Primary data

    (i)   By the investigator himself / herself

    (ii)   By questionnaire method

    (iii) By conducting large-scale survey

    (iv) By telephone method

    (v)   By videoconference method

(i) *Investigator himself/herself*

In this method the investigator himself/herself prepares the experiment with the help of his or her guide and records the observations in the laboratory. For example, a student of pharmacy collects or records data on the experiment conducted in the laboratory with regard to a drug at different potencies or drugs at different potencies with respect to their effect on small animals like mice, rats or patients. Also, a student of pharmacy prepares list of questions with the help of guide and conducts survey in a village or locality with regard to prevelance of diseases like malaria, dengue, chicken pox etc., and collects information. This method is being adopted by individual investigators who submit theses for Masters and Doctoral degrees in pharmacy, medicine and biological sciences etc.

(ii) *By questionnaire method*

In this method different questions are prepared and arranged in logical sequence related to objective of survey and got approved by the experts in the area of investigation. These questionnaries will be sent to the respondents by post and filled questionnares will also be obtained by post by the investigatior. The questions in the questionnaire should be of objective type that elicit answers such as 'Yes' or 'No' or multiple choice, fill up the blanks etc. The questions should be simple and understandable. No personal or privacy questions should be included. Some incentives like gifts etc., are offered to respondents to obtain filled in questionnaires in time and in complete form to the investigator. The respondents should be educated and feel responsible in sending back the filled questionnaire realizing the importance of survey. The advantage of this method of collecting data is that the information can be obtained quickly with minimum expenditure. The drawback of this method is some questionnaires would be incomplete and some filled in questionnaires will not be sent back by respondents.

(iii) *By conducting large-scale survey*

Data also will be collected through large-scale surveys through schedule. Schedule is prepared by the chief investigator with the assistance of several experts based on objectives of survey. The field investigators will be employed and they will be trained with respect to statistical methodology including sampling method adopted, importance of survey, different concepts and implications of informations sought in schedule, mode of filling the schedule and skill of conducting interviews with the respondents etc. The field investigators either fill in the schedules themselves or get filled by the respondents. These filled in schedules will be submitted to chief investigator for further statistical analysis.

This method of collecting data requires more time and involves expenditure since wide range of information covering large area is involved. However, the conclusions drawn from this survey will be useful for policy-makers for taking appropriate decisions at the administrative level.

This method of collecting data is being adopted by Government of India while conducting decennial census in India and also large-scale surveys on different aspects such as Health, Education, Industries, Transport, Communication, Imports and Exports of goods and Raw material, Agriculture, Irrigation, Power, Roads, Mines etc., through National Sample Survey Organization (NSSO), Department of statistics. NSSO conducts surveys every year or twice in a year depending upon the need and urgency of data required by the policy-makers. For example if the policy-maker needs data on AIDS affected area, people, locations, age group of people affected, economic levels, preventive measures taken, availability of manpower, availability of printed material etc., a large-scale survey will be conducted for taking policy decisions by NSSO. Similarly State Governments are conducting surveys independently and also coordinating with NSSO in countrywide surveys.

(iv) *By telephone method*

Now-a-days surveys are also conducted by collecting information through telephone. In this method the respondents are expected to own telephones. By this method the information can be obtained quickly and with greater accuracy. The analysis of the data can be done in less time and with less expenditure. However large information cannot be collected and detailed figures and data cannot be obtained easily by this method. Some proxy persons also will be responding and wrong information also will be supplied by them.

(v) *By videoconference method*

The latest method of collecting data is by videoconference method. On this method we can collect information quickly, accurately and proxy response can be avoided as we can see the persons giving data. This method requires large network of online computer systems for the respondents. This method can be adopted where the respondents are heads of offices etc.

2.2 Basic Concepts

Data: The numbers or figures are called data. The numbers may come from 'measurement' or from 'counting'. A patient's temperatures in Fahrenheit at different timings may be called data. Also, the number of patients admitted on a particular day is called data.

2.2.1 Variable

The characteristic which varies is called variable. The height, weight, blood pressure, heart rate vary with individuals. These are called variables.

2.2.2 Quantitative Variable

The variable which can be quantified is called quantitative variable. For example height, weight, volume, diastolic blood pressure, age, income etc., can be measured precisely. Therefore, they are called quantitative variables.

2.2.3 Qualitative Variable

The variable which cannot be quantified or measured is called qualitative variable. For example, sick person, short person, intelligent person, progressive person etc., are qualitative variables. However, we can count the persons or objects having qualitative characteristics. These are called 'frequencies'.

Random Variable: The variable that occurs by chance or without predictions is called Random Variable. Rainfall, Temperature, Relative humidity, adult height at maturity cannot be predicted in advance and therefore they are called random variables.

2.2.4 Discrete Variable

A variable which can take fixed number of values is known as discrete variable. In other words there will be definite gap between any two values. The number of beds available in hospital, the number of patients admitted in a hospital on particular day, the number of decayed teeth per child in an elementary school etc., are examples of discrete variable.

2.2.5 Continuous Variable

A variable which can assume any value between two fixed limits is known as continuous variable. Height, weight, arm circumference, skull circumference etc., of individuals are examples of continuous variable.

2.2.6 Population

A large group of values of variable is called population or statistical population. For example, heights of patients in the hospital, body temperatures in Fahrenheit of all patients in hospital, weights of all patients in hospital are called populations. Population does not necessary mean only human or animal population.

2.2.7 Sample

A part of a population is called sample. Suppose we take blood sugar content for pre and post-lunch from few patients out of total patients available, then it is called sample data.

2.3 Measurement

Measurement may be defined as assigning numerical value to objects or events such that numerical values follow certain mathematical laws in physical and biological sciences. However, this is not always possible, especially when we deal with qualitative characters such as intelligence, colour, shape etc., in behavioural sciences. The measurement can be done in four stages, (i) Nominal (ii) Ordinal (iii) Interval, and (iv) Ratio.

2.3.1 Nominal Scale

This is the lowest scale of measurement. When nomenclature is used to identify the groups, the measurement is done at nominal scale. For example, blood groups among individuals. Diabetic – Non-diabetic, Healthy - Malnutrition children, Married-un married etc.

If numbers are allotted to Cricket team then they are said to be classified under nominal scale. These numbers only help in identifying the players. For example, if a particular player is allotted 9th number and another player 8th number that does not mean that 9th number player is superior to 8th number player. Further, average of the numbers of whole team will not give any meaning and it cannot be compared with the average of numbers of other team or group. No parametric tests like t-test, z-test, Analysis of variance etc., can be applied for analyzing the data based on nominal scale. However, chi-square test and other Non–parametric tests can be applied for the data measured on nominal scale. In sample surveys, where measurable data is not possible, Nominal scale of measurement is being used for collecting information from respondents.

2.3.2 Ordinal Scale

In nominal scaling the objects (observations) in a group are not much different from each other but they can be ranked according to some criterion then they are said to be measured on an ordinal scale. For example, estimation of malnutrition in children can be measured as very much improved> average > below average.

2.3.3 Interval Scale

If the distance between two values in ordinal scale can be measured then interval scaling is achieved. This scale is more sophisticated than 'ordinal scale'. The temperature is usually measured (Fahrenheit or celsius) in interval scale. Here the unit of measurement is the degree and the point of comparison is the arbitrarily chosen 'Zero degrees" which does not indicate lack of heat. The interval scale is used for measurement data unlike 'Nominal' and 'Ordinal' scales.

2.3.4 Ratio Scale

An interval scale with true zero point is called 'Ratio scale'. This is the highest level of measurement. Height, weight, length etc., variables make use of ratio scale.

2.4 Sampling

The method of drawing a sample from population is called sampling. In order to make a valid inference about population a sample is drawn. There are several methods available in literature for different situations to estimate the population characteristic with minimum errors. These methods were developed based on probability theory. These methods involve drawing samples at random at one stage or order.

The following are some of the sampling methods used. These methods are developed based on the nature of population, cost, time and objectives of survey.

2.4.1   Simple Random Sampling

In this method if a sample size 'n' is drawn from a population size 'N' then every possible sample out of $\binom{N}{n}$ possible samples will have equal chance of being selected as a sample.

Selection of a random sample

List out all the units in the population serially from 1 to N. This list is called sampling frame. Then darw a sample of 'n' units from this list using random number tables. The random number tables are available from text books of statistical theory, such as Fisher and Yates (1948) Snedecor and Cochran (1968). For example if N 150 and n=20 then select a page of random numbers and select adjacent three columns starting from any column since N = 150 which is a three-digit figure. Then go on selecting numbers which are less than or equal to 150 till we get 20 distinct numbers. If first three columns are exhausted then next three columns will be considered, and so on, in that page of random numbers. By this method we can estimate the population mean, standard error and confidence limits for population mean. In this method the population is assumed to be uniform or homogenous as far as possible.

A sample is drawn in such a way that one number is drawn from the list of population of units by random method and that number is noted and replaced back into the list of population of units and another number is drawn from the same list and that number is noted and so on. If the same number is repeated and it will not be taken into consideration for the sample, The sampling process is continued till all distinctive units are included in the sample. In this method all units will have equal probability of selection at each stage of drawing sample. Any number of samples can be drawn from the sampling frame if repeated samples are accepted.

Simple Random Sampling without Replacement (SRSWOR)

In this method a sample is drawn in such a way that every number is drawn from the sampling frame and is not replaced back. In this way all the numbers in the sample drawn will be distinct and no repetition of numbers occur. However, the probability of drawing number at each stage will be different. For example, if there are 10 numbers from which 4 numbers are it be drawn. The probability of drawing 1st number is 1/10, second number is 1/9 and so on. If there are 'N' units in the population and 'n' units in the sample, then there will be NC_n distinct samples in all.

Lottery Method of Sampling

In this method sampling can be drawn from the population using Lottery method. Here simple random sampling method without replacement is followed. For example; if there are 100 houses which are to be allotted to 200 customers then lottery method is followed. All the customers who have applied for allotment of house are listed from

1 to 200. These numbers are painted on metal tokens and put in a metal vessel specially prepared for the purpose. This vessel is rotated manually or mechanically so that all the tokens in the vessel are mixed thoroughly so that no number could get advantage and no number could be at disadvantage stage and every number will have equal probability of being selected in the sample. After several rounds of rotation of vessel, one token is drawn at random without looking inside into the vessel. That number customer is allotted 1st house and that number is kept out from the vessel. Again vessel will be rotated as same number of times as in the first draw another token is drawn from the vessel in the same way as 1st token and that number person is allotted 2nd house. In the way all 100 houses are allotted to 100 applicants out of 200 applicants. Similarly, state government lotteries are conducted for awarding 1st, 2nd, etc. prizes for the lottery ticket owners.

Accuracy: If the data are not accurate the conclusions drawn from sample have no relevance or reliability. If the enumerator or respondent gave false information about age, income, land holdings etc. then the estimates obtained from such data will give wrong conclusions about the population. Even editing of schedules, questionnaires will not prevent such inaccuracies of data. Proper supervision and cross checking and in certain surveys third party survey only can provide accurate information from the respondents.

Accuracy of Measurement: Accuracy of measurement depends on precision required, the tools available for measurement and skill of the investigator undertaking survey. Though absolute accuracy is neither possible nor desired in surveys, a reasonable degree of accuracy is needed. For example, monthly income of a person should be rounded to the nearest ten of rupees as has been done in Income tax returns and age to the nearest years.

Precision: Precision is the product of tabulated value of z or t and standard error. For example, 95 per cent level is required for estimating the confidence interval in which population mean will lie then z (tabulated) value is taken as 1.96 and which is multiplied by standard error. The confidence interval will increase if the precision is to be increased. Since z (tabulated) value will increase if the confidence level increases. If 99 per cent level is required z (tabulated) value is 2.58. similarly in small samples t (tabulated) value will increase with the increase in confidence level. For example, if the estimate is Rs 200 and the precision desired is $\pm$ 2%. Then the true value will be not less than 196 and not more than 204. The range is Rs 196 to 204 within which the true value will lie.

Standard Error: It is defined as the standard deviation of the sampling distribution of characteristic such as mean, standard deviation etc.

If x follows normal distribution with mean, μ and standard deviation, σ then $\bar{x}$, the mean which is based on 'n' observations also follows normal distribution with mean,

μ and standard deviation, $\dfrac{\sigma}{\sqrt{n}}$. This S.D. of mean $\bar{x}$, i.e. $\dfrac{\sigma}{\sqrt{n}}$ is called standard error of mean.

$\dfrac{\bar{x} - \mu}{\dfrac{\sigma}{\sqrt{n}}}$ follows normal distribution with mean as zero and standard deviation as one

For example, if $\sigma = 15$ and $n = 9$ then standard error of mean is

$$\frac{\sigma}{\sqrt{n}} = \frac{15}{\sqrt{9}} = \frac{15}{3} = 5$$

The standard error of mean is used in finding out confidence interval of population mean and in test of hypotheses such as z – test, t – test etc.

Confidence Interval: It is the range of limits in which population parameter such as mean will lie. For example, the confidence limits of population mean are obtained as

$$\bar{x} \pm 1.96 \times \frac{\sigma}{\sqrt{n}}.$$

Where $\bar{x}$ = mean, 1.96 is the tabulated value of normal distribution at 5 per cent level of significance (95 per cent confidence level) and $\dfrac{\sigma}{\sqrt{n}}$ is the standard error of mean, $\bar{x} + 1.96\,\dfrac{\sigma}{\sqrt{n}}$ is the upper limit and $\bar{x} - 1.96\,\dfrac{\sigma}{\sqrt{n}}$ is the lower limit and within these two limits the population mean will lie. The difference between upper and lower limits is called confidence interval. The lower and upper limits are called confidence limits and which are also called as fiducial limits.

For example, if $\bar{x} = 10$, $\sigma = 2$ and $n = 4$ then the upper confidence limit is $10 + 1.96 \times \dfrac{2}{\sqrt{4}} = 10 + 1.96 = 11.96$ and lower confidence limit is

$10 - 1.96 \times \dfrac{2}{\sqrt{4}} = 9.04$ and confidence interval is $11.96 - 9.04 = 2.92$.

2.4.2 Non-random Sampling

If the selection of sample is not done based on random numbers then it is called non-random sampling. The method based on non-random sampling procedure is called non-random sampling method. This method sometimes is also called as purposive sampling method. Case studies highlighting the 'sucess' or 'failure' stories are examples of non-random sampling methods. For example, if we want to highlight the prevalence of AIDS disease in society, the individuals suffering from AIDS disease will be selected for study and they will narrate the full history about them so that other individuals in society will be benefited. The drawback of this method is we cannot generalize the estimates based on this sample to population.

2.4.3　Advantages of Sampling Techniques

(i)　The cost of the survey will be reduced as we are studying a part of the whole population.

(ii)　The time involved in studying the sample would be much less compared to population or census.

(iii)　Sometimes sampling is a must where we cannot afford the study of whole population. For example, for examining of blood from patients we can only take small sample.

(iv)　Accurate results can be obtained from sampling. For example, the instruments of survey like questionnaire and schedule can be filled up accurately, with reliable and accurate data for sample than population.

(v)　Sampling is must when population is very large.

Disadvantages of Sampling Techniques

(i)　The complete list of units in the population i.e., sampling frame may not be available everytime.

(ii)　If the sample is not drawn based on random number tables then the estimates based on sample may not be representative of the population and therefore cannot be generalized.

(iii)　Sampling is not useful and also gives less accurate results when the population is very small. For example, studying the patients affected with rare disease requires to study all patients.

(iv)　Personal bias and prejudice in drawing sample may affect the validity and reliability of the estimate obtained from sample.

2.4.4　Stratified Random Sampling

In this method the population is divided into different homogeneous groups known as strata and a simple random sample is selected from each of the strata. This method is applied when population is heterogeneous with respect to a variable or characteristic under study. By doing so we can estimate the population mean more efficiently in the sense that with less standard error compared to simple random sampling method. In simple random sampling if the size of the sample is increased the estimate of standard error can be decreased. But it is not always possible to increase the size of the sample due to lack of time and money or financial resources. In such situation stratified random sampling method is more appropriate. For example, if the patients are heterogeneous with respect to heart disease then they will be sub divided into groups such as children, middle age and old age. Then the survey can be conducted using stratified random sampling method. Separate sample of patients will be selected from each group and observations will be recorded and the estimate of population mean, standard error and confidence limits for the population can be obtained.

Proportional Allocation of Sample

If sample size is selected for each stratum based on the size of the stratum in the population, then it is called proportional allocation. If N_i is the size of i-th stratum in the population where $\sum_{i=1}^{K} N_i = N$, the total population and If n is the size of the sample in the i-th stratum where $\sum_{i=1}^{K} n_i = n$ is the total sample.

If $\dfrac{n_i}{n} = \dfrac{N_i}{N}$ = then $n_i = n \times \dfrac{N_i}{N}$ for **i** = 1, 2, ...k. If allotment of sample is done in this way then it is called proportional allocation.

For example, there are 50 children, 100 middle aged and 150 old aged patients are available in hospital who are suffering with heart disease. Suppose 30 patients are to be selected based on proportional allocation, the number of children to be selected is $30 \times \dfrac{50}{300} = 5$ (where 300 = 50+100+ 150 = total patients in the hospital).

No. of middle aged patients to be selected is $30 \times \dfrac{100}{300} = 10$

No. of old aged patients to be selected is $30 \times \dfrac{150}{300} = 15$

Total sample = 5+10+15 = 30.

The estimate of standard error based on proportional allocation is less than or equal to the estimate based on non-proportional allocation.

Merits and Demerits of stratified random sampling

Merits

(i) This method ensures representation from each group of the population. Therefore the estimate based on this sampling method is better representative of population mean or characteristic.

(ii) The estimate based on stratified random sampling is more efficient than the estimate based on simple random sampling method.

Demerits

(i) If stratification is not done based on the important characteristic to be studied then the estimate based on this method may not yield efficient one compared to simple random sampling.

2.4.5 Systematic Sampling

In this method if one unit is selected at random the other units will be selected automatically. For example in order to estimate the prevalence of eye disease in school going children, a survey based on systematic sampling method will be done in a school consisting of 1000 children. If we want to select 100 children for check up one child out of 10 children by selecting every 10th children i.e., $\dfrac{1000}{100} = 10$. If first child is 7th one out of 1st 10, then second child is 17th, third child is 27th etc. The last child number is 997.

In general if N be the size of population and n be the size of the sample such that N = nk, where k is a positive integer or sampling interval. If one unit be selected at random out of k units and the remaining (n – 1) units will be selected at equally spaced intervals of k units. If 4th unit is selected out of k units at random then the remaining units in the sample are k+4, 2k+4, ... (n – 1) k+4. This could be well understood from the Table 2.1.

Table 2.1

1	2	3		---	k
k + 1	k + 2	k + 3	k + 4		2k
2k + 1	2k + 2	2k + 3	2k + 4		3k
.	.	.	.		.
.	.	.	.		.
.	.	.	.		nk.
(n – 1)k + 1	(n – 1)k + 2	(n – 1)k + 3	(n – 1)k + 4		

From Table 2.1 it can be observed that each column will form a sample.

Merits and Demerits of Systematic Sampling

Merits

  (i) The method of drawing sample is relatively easy and simple since only one unit is drawn at random.

  (ii) This method is applicable in forest surveys for estimation of forest products such as volume of timber, amount of tamarind, honey etc. This method is useful for estimation of marine and inland fish population etc. This method is also useful in estimation of prevalence of viral diseases like malaria, dengue etc.

Demerits

  (i) The total population may not be multiple of sample i.e., k may not always be positive integer.

  (ii) The estimate sometimes may be bias one.

2.4.6 Cluster Sampling

In this method the population is divided into sub-groups called clusters. A sample of clusters is drawn at random from the entire list of clusters and then all the units in all the selected clusters will be studied.

For example, a survey is to be conducted to study the prevalence of diabetes in individuals in families, a sample of families will be selected at random and all members in selected families will be checked up with respect to prevalence of diabetes. Here families are considered as clusters and locality or village as population and units are family members.

Merits and Demerits of Cluster Sampling

Merits

    (i) This method is convenient whenever the list of units (sampling frame) is not available and list of clusters is available.

    (ii) The cost of survey will be less since the units in the clusters are located at the same place.

Demerits

    (i) This method is less efficient whenever the correlation between individual units in the cluster is positive compared to sampling of units directly from the population.

Non - Random Sampling Methods

2.4.7 Purposive Sampling

In this method the selection of units in the sample is not based on random numbers. The selection of units is based on the judgement of investigator. Therefore this method is also called as judgement sampling. The investigator selects units in the sample which he or she thinks represents the population. However, this method depends upon the experience and expertise of the investigator. Case studies conducted highlighting the success or failure stories of any aspect of life are the examples of purposive sampling. For example the incidence of AIDS disease is to be highlighted. The individuals suffering from AIDS disease are selected for the study and they narrate the entire history about them with respect to their socio-economic background, in what way they were attacked with the disease etc., so that others in the society can be benefited by taking preventive measures.

Merits and Demerits of Purposive Sampling

Merits

    (i) The method of drawing sample is easy .

    (ii) The representative units can be selected to highlight the objectives of survey.

(iii) The analysis could be simple.

(iv) The method can be implemented with limited budget and time.

Demerits

   (i) The selection of units is based upon the judgement of investigator and hence may not always be representative.

 (ii) It is not possible to generalize from sample to population.

(iii) The error involved in the sampling cannot be calculated.

2.4.8   Convenience Sampling

As the name indicates the method of sampling is based on convenience of the investigator for carrying out the study. For example, in order to find the prevalence of high B.P. in villages in a district, the villages which are nearer to the headquarters and accessible by road transport are selected. This method gives the estimate of the population but it may be biassed one. However, the method of sampling and collection of data is easy and convenient and therefore can be implemented without any difficulty.

2.4.9   Quota Sampling

In this method a sample number of units is fixed for each category based on characteristic in the sample. For example, for estimating the prevalence of diabetes in the population a fixed number of children, middle aged and old age people in male and female population is selected and studied. The selection of individuals in each category of people is based on judgement of investigator. Here the sample size is fixed beforehand irrespective of size of the population. The method involves fixed expenditure and fixed time. The estimates of the characteristics can be arrived at within fixed time. For example, the exit poll results are obtained adopting this method by different agencies in order to predict the results of different political parties in less time with limited expenditure.

2.4.10   Sampling Errors

The errors occurring through adoption of sampling method for estimating the population characteristic are called sampling errors. In other words the difference between estimate based on sample and the estimate obtained by studying entire population is termed as sampling error. Suppose samples of same size are drawn at random from the population and their means are computed. These means are different among themselves and they are different from population mean unless the units in the population are exactly same. The standard deviation of the sampling distribution of means is called standard error of mean. This is called 'sampling error'. These errors occur even when the estimate is 'unbiased'.

The sampling error can be reduced by increasing the size of sample. However, it is not possible to increase the size of the sample always as it is directly related to increase in expenditure and time involved in completing the survey. In census, all units are studied in the population and hence there will be no sampling error.

2.4.11 Non-Sampling Errors

The errors occurring in surveys other than due to sampling are called non-sampling errors. These might occur through (i) observational errors and (ii) incomplete samples.

(i) *Observational Errors*

The investigator or enumerator may commit mistake in recording observations due to (a) personal bias (b) improper knowledge of the questions in schedule (c) improper understanding of the response from respondent and (d) improper recording of the observation supplied by third person.

(ii) *Incomplete Samples*

The non-sampling errors also occur due to incomplete schedules furnished by field investigators or enumerators or false type of information provided by respondents or investigators. If the information is not available for complete sample then the estimates based on incomplete sample are biased. Further the cost of the survey would be increased if information is to be collected again on the incomplete sample.

Choice of Sampling Methods

The choice of sampling methods depends upon many factors such as size of population, availability of sampling frame, nature of population such as heterogeneity or homogeneity, administrative setup, time and money at one's disposal, aims and objectives of survey etc. For example, if generalization to the population is not necessary and quick reliable estimates are needed, then purposive or judgment sampling may be adopted. If the population is of homogeneous nature with respect to characteristic under consideration then simple random sampling may give better results for generalization. If the population is heterogeneous with respect to characteristic or due to administration then stratified random sampling method may be suitable. If the sampling frame is available for clusters instead of individual units due to administrative set up then cluster sampling method may be more appropriate. If the units in the population are very large and they are arranged or located in a manner like rows or columns then systematic sampling may be suitable. Whatever the method of sampling adopted if the size of the sample increases the precision of the estimate increases.

2.4.12 Size of the Sample

Though it is said that if the size of the sample increases the precision of the estimate increases, it is not always necessary to increase the sample size when the population is perfectly uniform. A drop of blood in human body is sufficient for blood analysis. When the population is homogeneous with respect to characteristic under consideration, small sample is sufficient. When the population is large and heterogeneous a large sample will be necessary. However, the decision with respect to size of sample depends on (i) aims and objectives of survey (ii) area to be covered (iii) time involved (iv) expenditure involved (v) precision required for the estimates (vi) continuous survey or one-time survey (vii) availability of skilled and semi skilled personnel (viii) to whom the results are to be submitted and (ix) nature of population.

2.4.13   Determination of Sample Size

The sample size can be determined if the value of standard deviation in the population is known beforehand.

In tests of hypothesis the one-sample Standard Normal Deviate (SND) test is given as

$$Z = \frac{\left|\overline{X} - \mu\right|}{\dfrac{\sigma}{\sqrt{n}}} \qquad\qquad .....(2.1)$$

where $\overline{X}$ = sample mean, μ = population mean, σ = standard deviation of population, n = size of sample and Z = standard normal deviate value.

From (2.1) we can have

$$Z\,\frac{\sigma}{\sqrt{n}} = \left|\overline{X} - \mu\right| \qquad\qquad .....(2.2)$$

$$\frac{Z\sigma}{\left|\overline{X} - \mu\right|} = \sqrt{n} \qquad\qquad .....(2.3)$$

$$n = \frac{(Z\sigma)^2}{\left(\overline{X} - \mu\right)^2} \qquad\qquad .....(2.4)$$

Z (tabulated) value at 5 percent level of significance is 1.96, and at 1 percent level of significance it is 2.58. If $(\overline{X} - \mu)$ is to be assumed as 10 or 15 or 20 and a value is known, then sample size 'n' can be determined. Sometimes 'σ' value can be assumed from the value obtained from previous survey.

This method is generally adopted for large scale surveys sponsored by Government of India or State Governments. In general, if the population is small 10 percent of the population is taken as sample size. The population size increases the percent sampling, decreases depending upon the time and financial resources.

CHAPTER 3

Data Organization

3.1 Introduction

When the data is collected then data has to be organized in such a way that the important information contained in the data can be understood by the user. Data has to be organized in an orderly way. For example, the number of people suffering from AIDS, malaria, diabetes, high blood pressure, cancer, heart diseases can be arranged in an alphabetical way or nature of disease (Table 3.1).

Table 3.1

Disease	People (millions)
AIDS	2
Cancer	10
Diabetes	22
Heart Diseases	35
High B.P	42
Malaria	14

Similarly the persons can be classified according to blood group like A, B, O, AB, A^+, etc.

If the data pertains to weight, height, age, blood sugar, high B.P. etc., they can be arranged in ascending order starting from lowest value to highest value. If the data is large it can be classified according to groups or classes. For example, the age of inpatients in hospital can be presented as in Table 3.2.

Table 3.2

Age (years)	Patients
15-24	6
25-34	20
35-44	35
45-54	41
55-64	43
65-74	10

The above presentation in the table is called frequency distribution. The number of patients in each group is called frequency and the groups are called classes. The difference between upper and lower limits of class is called interval. Usually the number of classes will be formed ranging from 6 to 15 depending upon data. The class interval will be arrived at by taking ratio of the difference between highest and lowest values of data and the number of classes required. For example, the highest value is 74 and lowest value is 15 and we require 6 classes, then the class interval is $\frac{74-15}{6} = \frac{59}{6}$ = 9.8 (approximately rounded off to 10). This can be observed from Table 3.2.

3.1.1 Inclusive Method of Grouping

If both upper and lower limits are included in the same class or group then it is called inclusive method of grouping. The data in Table 3.2 is an example of inclusive method of grouping.

3.1.2 Exclusive Method of Grouping

If upper limits in each class are excluded and included in next higher class then it is called exclusive method of grouping.

For example, Table 3.2 can be modified and presented as in Table 3.3

Table 3.3

Age (years)	Patients
15-25	5
25-35	21
35-45	31
45-55	45
55-65	40
65-75	13

In first group if a patient has age 25 years then he/she will be included in the next higher group, i.e., 25-35 but not in 15-25. The average of the lower and upper limits of class is called mid-value or mid-point of the class. The number of patients in Table 3.2 or Table 3.3 is called 'frequency' and the tables are called frequency distributions. If inclusive method of grouping is given then it can be modified to exclusive method of grouping by taking average of the upper limit of the class and lower limit of the next higher class. From Table 3.2 the modified exclusive method of grouping is given in Table 3.4.

Table 3.4

Age	Patients
14.5 - 24.5	6
24.5 - 34.5	20
34.5 - 44.5	32
44.5 - 54.4	44
54.5 - 64.5	43
64.5 - 74.5	10

In general the data of continuous variable is represented by exclusive method of grouping, which is convenient for further processing of data like computing arithmetic mean, standard deviation etc.

3.2   Diagrammatic Representation

The representation of data with the help of diagram is called diagrammatic representation.

3.2.1   One-Dimensional Diagram

3.2.1(a) One-Dimensional Diagram or Bar Diagram

In this diagram, the height of each bar is directly proportional to the magnitude of the variable. The width of each bar and the space between bars should be same.

Example

The production of Anti-rabies serum boxes for dog bite in the country for different years can be presented by bar diagram, given the data in Table 3.5.

Table 3.5

Year	No. of boxes (1000)
1998	12
1999	15
2000	22
2001	25
2002	30

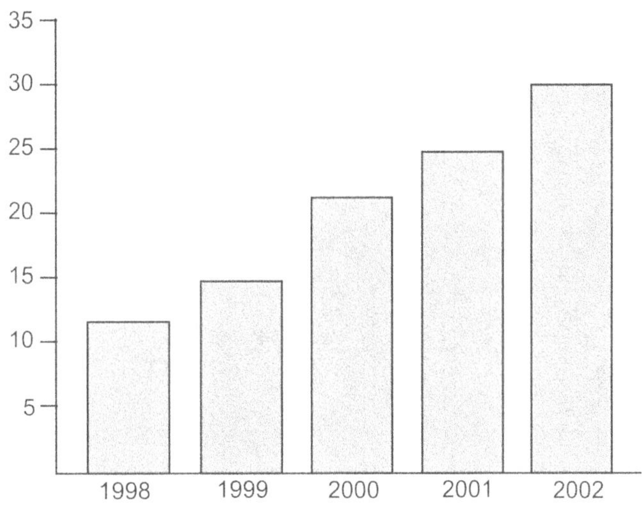

Fig. 3.1 Bar diagram.

The bars can be coloured with the same colour for appealing to eye. The width of the bar can be chosen as per our choice depending upon the availability of space in the chart.

3.2.1(b)   *Divided Bar Diagram or Component Bar Diagram*

In this diagram, the heights of the component parts of the bar are directly proportional to the magnitude of the constituent parts of the variable. Here also the width of the bars and the space between bars should be same. This diagram would not be much of advantage if the component parts are more than three as they will become clumsy.

Example

The number of category of people who were administered anti-rabies serum in one year in a particular city can be depicted by the following diagram.

Table 3.6

People (100)

Year	Children	Middle aged	Old	Total
1998	4	10	6	20
1999	5	12	8	25
2000	9	16	10	35
2001	12	18	14	44
2002	16	24	18	58

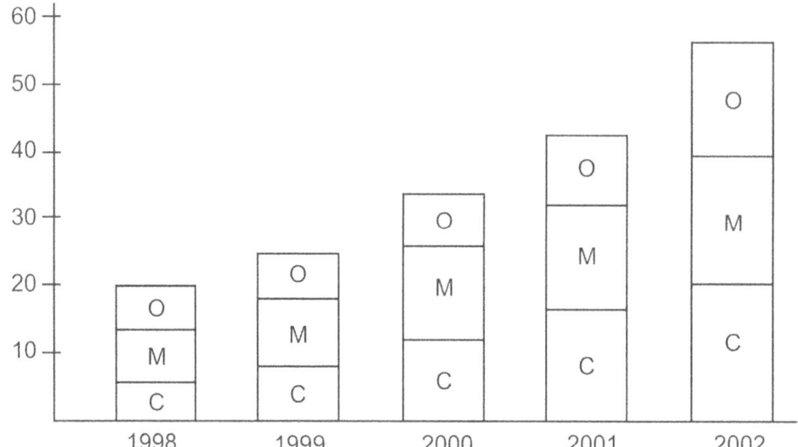

Fig. 3.2   Divided bar diagram.

C = Children, M = Middle aged, O = Old.

In this diagram overall comparison of persons who were administered anti-rabies serum can be done for different years but also comparison between categories such as children, middle aged and old also can be done simultaneously.

3.2.1(c) Percentage Bar Diagram

In this diagram the length of the bars will be same as the magnitude. Each magnitude of the variable is made equal to 100.

Example

The data in Table 3.6 is presented here for presentation of percentage bar diagram (Fig. 3.3).

Table 3.6

Year	Children	People Middle aged	old	Total
1998	20	50	30	100
1999	20	48	32	100
2000	26	46	28	100
2001	27	41	32	100
2002	28	41	31	100

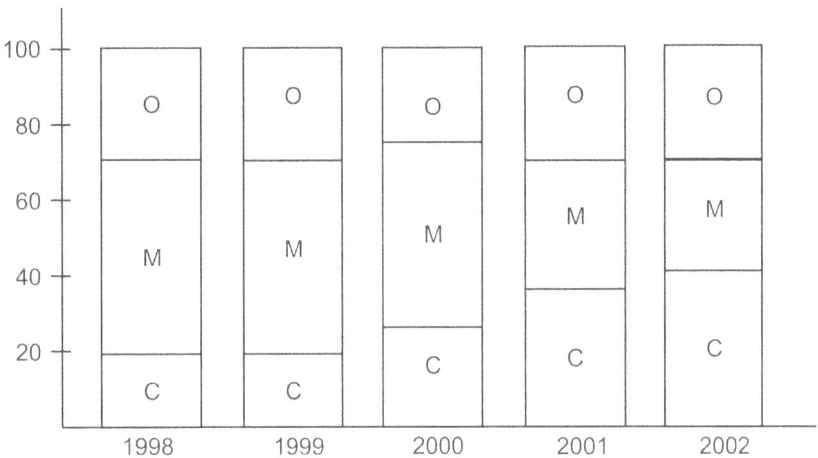

Fig. 3.3 Percentage bar diagram.

3.2.1(d) Multiple Bar Diagram

In this diagram more than one bar will be attached to each other. These attached bars represent the related variables. For example, the number of persons who were administered anti-rabies injection is to be represented by male and female in different years. Multiple bar diagram can be represented as follows :

Table 3.7

Year	Male (100)	Female (100)
1998	14	6
1999	18	7
2000	22	14
2001	20	10
2002	25	12

The data in Table 3.7 can be represented in multiple bar diagram in Fig. 3.4.

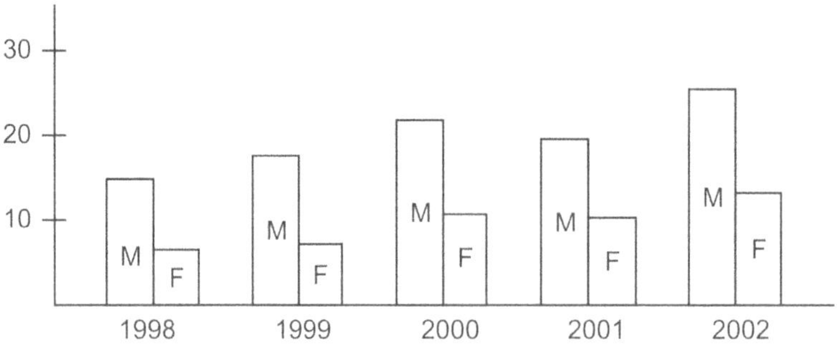

Fig. 3.4 Multiple bar diagram.

M = male; F = female

3.2.2   Two-Dimensional Diagrams

3.2.2(a) Rectangles

In one-dimensional diagrams height of bars are only compared. In two-dimensional diagrams both height and width of bars are to be considered. In other words, height × width = area of bars or rectangles are to be compared with respect to characteristic under consideration. Rectangles will represent two-dimensional diagrams.

Example

The following data represents the number of persons suffered by burns in hospital with respect to percentage of skin burnt (Table 3.8).

Table 3.8

Area (percent)	No. of Persons
0-20	24
20-40	18
40-60	10
60-80	6
80-100	2

The data in Table 3.8 can be represented by rectangles.

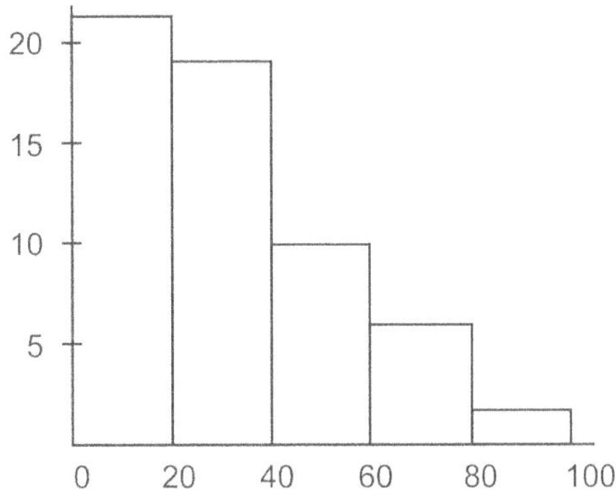

Fig. 3.5 Rectangles.

In Fig. 3.5 the area of the rectangles represents the total area of skin burnt by taking all persons together for different years. This will indicate the extent of plastic surgery required for the skin damaged to the persons.

3.2.2(b) Squares

In this diagram if the height and width of bars are equal then bar diagram becomes squares. For example, if persons suffering from two variables (blood sugar and high B.P),are considered simultaneously in the hospital for different years then squares can be used as two-dimensional diagrams for comparison.

3.2.2(c) Pie Diagram

In this diagram circle instead of rectangle or square will be used. This diagram is useful when the component parts of the variable are more than three. The areas of different sectors of a circle are directly proportional to the magnitudes of component of the variable.

Example

The following are the amounts allocated in a year by State Medical Department to prevent diseases like polio, cholera, malaria, AIDS, T.B., and presented in Table 3.9 and represented the data by Pie-diagram (Fig. 3.6).

Table 3.9

Item	Amount (Rs lakhs)	Sector angle
AIDS	23	$360° \times \dfrac{23}{60} = 138$
Cholera	8	$360° \times \dfrac{8}{60} = 48$
Malaria	6	$360° \times \dfrac{6}{60} = 36$
Polio	10	$360° \times \dfrac{10}{60} = 60$
T.B.	13	$360° \times \dfrac{13}{60} = 78$
Total	60	360

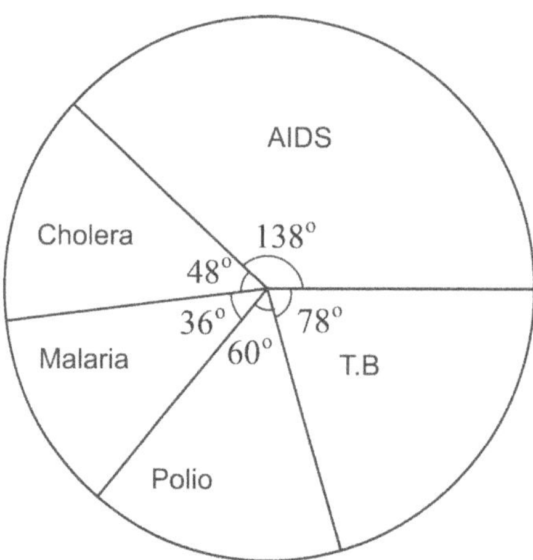

Fig. 3.6 Pie Diagram.

If the expenditure for different years are to be presented then circles or pie diagrams are to be drawn as many as the number of years. It may be noted that from the Fig. 3.6 the maximum amount of funds were allocated to AIDS followed by T.B, etc.

3.3   Three-Dimensional Diagrams

3.3.1   Pictograms

These are also called pictorial charts. In this diagram the volume of picture is directly proportional to the magnitude of the variable.

These diagrams are useful when the range of values is very large. In other words if the range is very large it is difficult to represent by bars. For example the production of polio vaccine can be represented by picture of bottle or drum in different years. The production of vitamins can be represented by boxes containing small bottles containing tablets. Here the volumes of boxes are directly proportional to the magnitudes of the variable.

Advantages and Disadvantages of Diagrammatic Representation

Advantages

A diagram is more appealing to eye than mere numerical data. It is easy for making comparisons within a shortest time even by a layman and also for VIPs with whom limited time will be available at their disposal.

Disadvantages

The main disadvantage of this representation is that it only gives rough idea of the variable but not exact value. No further analysis can be done with the diagrams. Also when the number of items are more then it will be clumsy and confusing for drawing comparisons.

Exercises

1. Represent the following data on incidence of AIDS in a State in India by bar diagram.

Year	Population (100)
1998	12
1999	18
2000	24
2001	25
2002	31
2003	32

2. The following data gives the production of foodgrains in different years in India. Represent by bar diagram.

Year	Food Production (million tons)
1999	214
2000	218
2001	228
2002	210
2003	230
2004	234

3. The following is the data on incidence of diabetes in different age groups of population in different years of a State in India. Represent the data by divided or component bar diagram and also by percentage bar diagram.

Year	Children (1000)	Middle aged (1000)	Old (1000)
2000	4	12	18
2001	5	13	20
2002	8	18	25
2003	9	20	27
2004	10	24	30
2005	11	30	36

4. The following is the data on patients treated for leprosy in a leprosy rehabilitation centre in a State for male and female patients.

Year	Male (100)	Female (100)
2001	38	14
2002	44	16
2003	49	26
2004	55	30
2005	40	20

Represent the above data by a multiple bar diagram.

5. The following are the amounts allotted to different categories of hospitals for treating patients by a State Government in different years.

Year	Amount (lakhs)		
	P	D	T
2001	28	24	20
2002	36	30	24
2003	42	36	30
2004	56	40	35
2005	64	50	40

P = primary health centre, D district and mandal hospitals and T = Teaching hospitals. Represent the above data by divided bar diagram and also percentage bar diagram.

6. The following is the data on amounts (Rs. In lakhs) spent on purchasing different items by a teaching hospital in a State for one year.

Item	Amount (Rs. In lakhs)
Vaccines	4
Antibiotics	12
Vitamins	6
Surgery items	18
Injections	20
Blood of different groups	10

Represent the above data by pie diagram.

7. The following is the data on number of male and female births occurred in a maternity hospital in a city in different years. Represent the data by multiple bar diagram.

Year	Male	Female
2002	120	110
2003	160	165
2004	150	156
2005	138	144
2006	130	120

CHAPTER 4

Dispersion and Standard Deviation

4.1 Introduction

Measure of location or central tendency will give the central or representative value of the data. The measures of central tendency are also known as measures of location or averages. It is always advisable to represent group of data by a single observation provided it does not loose any important information contained in the data and brings out every important information from it. This single observation or value is called as 'central tendency'. The different methods used for finding central tendency values are called measures of central tendency. The different measures of central tendency are 1. Arithmetic Mean 2. Median 3. Mode. 4. Geometric Mean and 5. Harmonic Mean. Here the first three measures; Arithmetic Mean, Median and Mode are dealt in this book.

4.2 Arithmetic Mean

It is most important measure of central tendency. It is defined as the sum of the observations divided by its number.

4.2(a) Variate Values or Individual Observations

If x_1, x_2, ..., x_n be 'n' observations, then the arithmetic Mean (A.M.) is give as;

$$\text{A.M.,} \quad \bar{x} = \frac{x_1 + x_2 + \dots + x_n}{n} = \sum_{i=1}^{n} \frac{x_i}{n}$$

where 'Σ' indicates summation of observations from x_1 to x_n.

Example: The following are the weights (kg) of 10 children admitted in a hospital. Find the mean weight of children

$$6, 8, 3, 5, 4, 7, 6, 10, 4, 7$$

$$\bar{x} = \frac{6+8+...+7}{10} = \frac{60}{10} = 6 \text{ kg}.$$

The mean weight of child is 6 kg.

4.2(b) *Discrete Distribution / Frequency Distribution*

If $f_1, f_2, ..., f_n$ be 'n' frequencies corresponding to the variate values $x_1, x_2, ...x_n$ respectively then the Arithmetic Mean is given as

$$\bar{x} = \frac{f_1 x_1 + f_2 x_2 + ... + f_n x_n}{f_1 + f_2 + ... + t_n} = \frac{\sum_{i=1}^{n} f_i x_i}{\sum_{i=1}^{n} f_i}$$

$$= \frac{\sum_{i=1}^{n} f_i x_i}{N} \text{ where } N = \sum_{i=1}^{n} f_i$$

Where 'N' is called the total frequency.

Example: The following are the distribution of weights (kg) of children in an hospital. Find Arithmetic Mean weight of children.

Weight (kg)	3	5	6	8	10
Children	10	16	12	9	3

Table 4.1

S.No	Weight(x_i) (kg)	Children (f_i)	$f_i x_i$
1	3	10	30
2	5	16	80
3	6	12	72
4	8	9	72
5	10	3	30
Total		50	284

$$\bar{x} = \frac{\Sigma f_i x_i}{N} = \frac{284}{50} = 5.68 \text{ Kg}.$$

Here $N = \Sigma f_i = 50$

The mean weight of children in hospital is 5.68 kg.

4.2(c) Grouped Frequency Distribution

If f_1, f_2,...,f_n be 'n' frequencies corresponding to the mid values of the classes $x_1, x_2,...x_n$ respectively then Arithmetic Mean is given as;

$$\text{A.M.,} \quad \bar{x} = \frac{\sum_{i=1}^{n} f_i x_i}{\sum_{i=1}^{n} f_c} = \frac{\sum_{i=1}^{n} f_i x_i}{N} \quad \text{where } N = \sum_{i=1}^{n} f_i$$

Example: The following is the distribution of weights (Kg) of children in an hospital.

Weight (kg)	2 – 4	4 – 6	6 – 8	8 – 10	10 -12
Children	3	6	10	7	4

Table 4.2

Weight (Kg)	Children (f_i)	Mid–Value (x_i)	$f_i\, x_i$
2 – 4	3	3	9
4 – 6	6	5	30
6 – 8	10	7	70
8 – 10	7	9	63
10 -12	4	11	44
	30		216

$$\text{A.M.,} \quad \bar{x} = \frac{216}{30} = 7.2$$

The mean weight of children in the hospital is 7.2 Kg.

4.2(d) Characteristics of a Satisfactory Average

The different characteristics of a satisfactory average are listed here in order to identify the best average among available averages.

(i)   It should have well defined formula.

(ii) It should be based on all observations.

(iii) It should be comprehensible.

(iv) It should be least effected by sampling fluctuations

(v)   It should be easily computed.

(vi) It should have further applications in statistical tests.

4.2(e) Merits of Arithmetic Mean

(i) It possesses all the characteristics of satisfactory average

(ii) It possesses two algebraic properties such as;

    (a) The algebraic sum of the deviations taken from A.M. is zero

$$\text{i.e. } \sum_{i=1}^{n}(x_i - \overline{x}) = 0$$

    (b) If $\overline{x}_1$, be the mean of n_1 observations, $\overline{x}_2$ be the mean of n_2 observations,..., $\overline{x}_k$ be the mean of n_k observations then $\overline{x}$, the mean of 'n' observation where $n = n_1 + n_2 + ... + n_k$ is

$$\overline{x} = \frac{n_1\overline{x}_1 + n_2\overline{x}_2 + ... + n_k\overline{x}_k}{n_1 + n_2 + ... + n_n}$$

4.2(f) Demerits of Arithmetic Mean

(i) It may not be identified with any one of the observations from which it is calculated

(ii) It gives more weightage to extreme items whenever they are present.

(iii) It is difficult to compute when the extreme classes are not well defined in grouped frequency distribution.

4.3 Median

It is defined as that value of the variate below which half of the values will lie and above which the remaining half will lie when the values are arranged in ascending order of magnitude.

4.3(a) Variate Values or Individual Observations

Example: Find the Median height (cm) of 10 patients in an hospital

158, 140, 138, 160, 182, 171, 174, 139, 184, 176. The heights are arranged in ascending order of magnitude as;

S.No.	1	2	3	4	5	6	7	8	9	10
Height	138	139	140	158	160	171	174	176	182	184

$$\text{Median No.} = \frac{n+1}{2} \text{ where } n = \text{number of observations}$$

$$\text{Median No} = \frac{10+1}{2} = 5.5$$

$$\text{Median} = 5^{th} \text{ value} + 0.5 (6^{th} \text{ value} - 5^{th} \text{ value})$$

$$= 160 + 0.5 (171 - 160) = 165.5$$

This method of computation can be adopted even when n is odd or even number of observations.

4.3(b) Discrete Distribution / Frequency Distribution

Example: The following is the distribution of heights (cm) of patients in a hospital

Height (cm)	Patients
148	3
152	10
140	24
175	16
169	9
180	11

In order to find the median number the above frequency distribution is rearranged in ascending order of magnitude as follows;

Table 4.3

Height (cm)	Potentials	Cum. Freq.
140	24	24
148	3	27
152	10	37
169	9	46
175	16	62
180	11	73
	73	

$$\text{Median No.} = \frac{n+1}{2}$$

Where $N = \Sigma f_i$ = Total frequency

$$\text{Median No.} = \frac{73+1}{2} = 37$$

The median height of the patient corresponds to the 37th person when the heights are arranged in ascending order of magnitude. Here 37th person height is 152cm and which is the median height.

4.3(c) Grouped Frequency Distribution

if f_1, f_2,…,f_n be 'n' frequencies corresponding to the mid-values of the classes x_1, x_2,…,x_n respectively then Median is obtained by the formula as;

$$\text{Median} = l + \frac{\left(\dfrac{N+1}{2} - m\right)c}{f}$$

Where l = lower limit of the median class, $\dfrac{N+1}{2}$ = median number, m = cumulative frequency just before the median class, f = frequency of the median class and c = class interval of the median class and 'median class' is that class wherein median No, $\dfrac{N+1}{2}$ exists.

Example: The following is the distribution of heights of patients in an hospital. Find the median height.

Table 4.4

Height (cm)	Patients	Cum. Freq.
140 – 150	8	8
150 – 160	16	24
160 – 170	27	51
170 – 180	13	64
180 – 190	7	71

$$\text{Median No} = \frac{N+1}{2} = \frac{71+1}{2} = 36$$

Here $N = \Sigma f_i = 71$ = Total frequency

$$\text{Median} = l + \frac{\left(\dfrac{N+1}{2} - m\right)c}{f}$$

Here '36' lines between 24 and 51 in cum. frequency column. From 27th person to 51st person the class of heights is $160 - 170$ and which is the median class.

Therefore

$$l = 160, \quad \frac{N+1}{2} = 36, \quad m = 24, \quad f = 27, \quad c = 10$$

$$\text{Median} = 160 + \frac{(36-24)10}{27} = 164.44 \text{ cm}$$

The Median height of patients is 164.44 cm

4.3(d) Merits of Median

(i)   It can be computed even when extreme classes are not well defined.

(ii) It can be located easily on frequency curve by taking $\frac{n+1}{2}$ on y - axis.

(iii) It can be useful whenever the income tax limits are to be increased or decreased for assessing income tax by the Government.

(iv) It is having one important property i.e. the sum of the absolute values of the deviations is least when the deviations are measured from median.

43(e) Demerits

(i)   It is not based on all the observations.

(ii) It is not widely used in practice

4.4 Mode

Mode is that value of the variate which occurs most frequently.

4.4(a) Variate Values or Individual Observations

Example: Find the modal height (cm.) of the ten persons

$$164, 176, 184, 178, 184, 190, 171, 184, 179, 180$$

In the above 184 is repeated 3 times where as other values are repeated each only once. Hence Modal height is 184 cm.

4.4(b) Discrete Distribution / Frequency Distribution

If $f_1, f_2, \ldots, f_n$ a are 'n' frequencies corresponding to the variate values $x_1, x_2, \ldots x_n$ respectively then mode is given as the variate value which has the highest frequency.

If f_i is the highest value among f_i for $i = 1, 2, \ldots, n$ then x_i is the modal value.

Example:

Height(cm)	174	179	182	185	190	195
Frequency	6	8	10	18	9	4

In the above distribution, 185 has the highest frequency '18'and hence 185 cm is the modal height.

4.4(c) Grouped Frequency Distribution

If f_1, f_2, ..., f_n. be n frequencies corresponding to the mid-values of the classes $x_1, x_2, \ldots x_n$. respectively then 'Mode' is given by the formula.

$$\text{Mode} = l + \frac{(f - f_1) c}{2f - f_1 - f_2}$$

Where l = lower limit of the modal class, f = frequency of the Modal class, f_i = frequency just before the modal class, f_2 = frequency just after the modal class and c = class interval of the modal class and modal class is that class wherein maximum frequency exits.

Example: The following is the distribution of heights of patients in an hospital.

Height (cm)	170 -174	174 – 178	178 – 182	182 – 186	186 – 190
Patients	8	14	20	16	5

From the above distribution, it can be observed that 178 – 182 group is having highest frequency '20' and therefore it is the modal class.

$$\text{Mode} = l + \frac{(f - f_1) c}{2f - f_1 - f_2}$$

Here l = 178, f = 20, f_1 =14, f_2 = 16, c = 4

$$\text{Mode} = 178 + \frac{(20 - 14) 4}{2 \times 20 - 14 - 16} = 178 + \frac{24}{10}$$

$$= 178 + 2.4 = 180.4$$

The modal height of the Patients is 180.4 cm

4.4(d) Merits of Mode

(i) It can be easily located on frequency curve

(ii) It can be calculated even when extreme classes are not well defined

(iii) It is used mostly in business where an item which is preferred by maximum number of customers

4.4(e) *Demerits of Mode*

(i)   It is not based on all the observations

(ii) It is not having algebraic properties

(iii) It is not stable since different methods of forming class intervals would lead to different modal values.

4.5   Measures of Dispersion

Measure of dispersion will give the variation or spread of the data. In most of the medical analysis the range or lowest and highest values of different parameters are presented. For example, for a person the blood sugar should be between lowest and highest values for fasting, post-lunch and random stages of patient. Similarly high B.P., low B.P., have lowest and highest values in which a person's B.P., should lie to be normal person. Similarly lowest and highest daily temperatures are recorded to have an idea about the place for human habitation. All these examples emphasize the importance of spread or variation in the data and more so in medical data.

Sometimes the means of different series of data may be same but dispersion may be different. Also sometimes dispersion of different series of data may be equal but means may be different. This can be observed from the following Fig. 4.1 and Fig. 4.2, respectively.

From Fig. 4.1 it can be seen that mean is same for all the three curves but dispersion or spread of the curves is different. In Fig. 4.2, the spread or dispersion of the three curves is same but means are different. Therefore, for identifying data dispersion of data for different variables central tendency value is equally important.

The different measures of dispersion are (i) Range, (ii) Quartile deviation (iii) Mean deviation and (iv) Standard deviation.

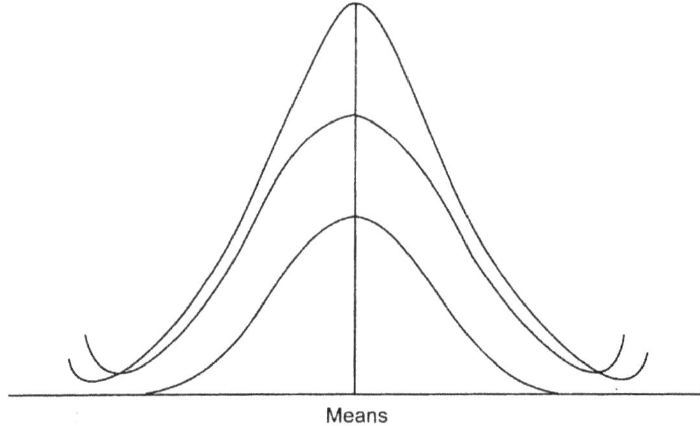

Fig. 4.1

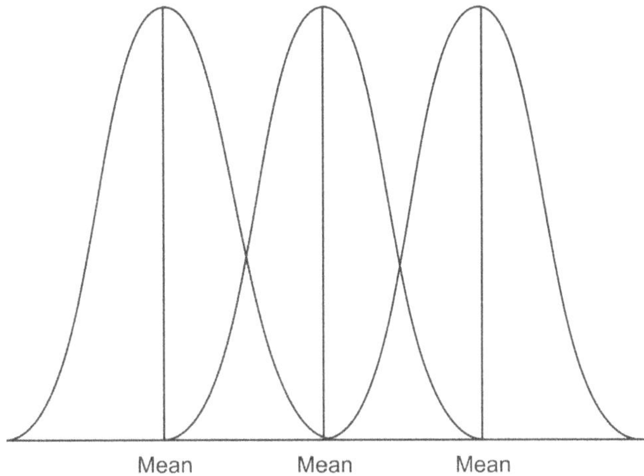

Fig. 4.2

4.5.1   Range

It is defined as the difference between the highest and lowest values of data.

For example, in the diagnostic analysis of human body the lowest and highest values of parameters are specified such as high and low B.P., blood sugar etc.

Quartile deviation and **mean deviation** are not generally used in practice and hence are not dealt with in detail here.

4.5.2   Standard Deviation

It is most important measure of dispersion just as arithmetic mean in measures of central tendency. It is defined as the positive square root of the mean of squares of deviations taken from arithmetic mean.

4.5.2(a)   Variate Values or Individual Observations

Let x_1, x_2,...x_n be n variate values of a characteristic, then standard deviation (S.D.) is given by the formula

$$\sigma = \sqrt{\frac{1}{n}\Sigma(x_i - \bar{x})^2}$$

where $\bar{x}$ = A.M.

variance = σ^2

The above formula can be simplified as

$$\sigma = \sqrt{\frac{1}{n}\left[\Sigma x_i^2 - \frac{(\Sigma x_i)^2}{n}\right]}$$

Variance

The square of standard deviation is called variance.

$$\text{Variance} = \sigma^2$$

Example

The following are the ages (years) of 10 children admitted in a hospital on a particular day. Compute the mean and standard deviation of ages.

10, 3, 8, 7, 11, 2, 1, 5, 14, 9

Table 4.5

S.No.	Age (x_i)	$(x_i - \bar{x})$	$(x_i - \bar{x})^2$	x_i^2
1	10	3	9	100
2	3	-4	16	9
3	8	1	1	64
4	7	0	0	49
5	11	4	16	121
6	2	-5	25	4
7	1	-6	36	1
8	5	-2	4	25
9	14	7	49	196
10	9	2	4	81
Total	70		160	650

$$\text{Mean } \bar{x} = \frac{\Sigma x_i}{n} = \frac{70}{10} = 7, \text{ where } n = 10$$

$$\Sigma(x_i - \bar{x})^2 = 160$$

$$\sigma = \sqrt{\frac{160}{10}} = \sqrt{16} = 4$$

Alternatively, we have

$$\Sigma x_i = 70, \qquad \Sigma x_i^2 = 650$$

$$\sigma = \sqrt{\frac{1}{10}\left[650 - \frac{(70)^2}{10}\right]} = \sqrt{\frac{1}{10}[650 - 490]}$$

$$= \sqrt{\frac{160}{10}} = \sqrt{16} = 4$$

The mean of age of child is 7, standard deviation is 4 and variance is 16.

4.5.2(b) Discrete Distribution

Let f_1, f_2, ...f_n be n frequencies corresponding to the variate values x_1, x_2, ...,x_n respectively. Then the mean, standard deviation and variance formulae are given as

$$\text{Mean} = \frac{\Sigma f_i x_i}{\Sigma f_i} = \frac{\Sigma f_i x_i}{N}, \quad \text{where } N = \Sigma f_i.$$

$$\text{Standard deviation } \sigma = \sqrt{\frac{1}{N}\Sigma f_i\left(x_i - \bar{x}\right)^2}$$

$$\text{Variance} = \sigma^2$$

Alternatively,

$$\sigma = \sqrt{\frac{1}{N}\Sigma f_i x_i^2 - \frac{\left(\Sigma f_i x_i\right)^2}{N}}$$

$$\text{Variance} = \sigma^2$$

Example

The following are the distribution of ages of outpatients in a district hospital on a particular day. Find the mean age, standard deviation and variance.

Table 4.6

Age (years) (x_i)	Patients (f_i)	$f_i\,x_i$	$f_i\,x_i^2$	$(x_i - \bar{x})$	$f_i\,(x_i - \bar{x})^2$
12	3	36	432	-28	2352
18	5	90	1620	-22	2420
23	4	92	2116	-17	1156
38	10	380	14440	-2	40
46	7	322	14812	6	252
52	2	104	5408	12	288
64	9	576	36864	24	5184
	40	1600	75692		11692

$$\text{Mean} \quad \bar{x} = \frac{\Sigma f_i x_i}{\Sigma f_i} = \frac{1600}{40} = 40 \text{ years}$$

$$\text{S.D. } \sigma = \sqrt{\frac{1}{N}\Sigma f_i\left(x_i - \bar{x}\right)^2}$$

$$= \sqrt{\frac{11692}{40}} = \sqrt{292.3} = 17.10$$

(Round off to second decimal place)

$$\text{Variance } \sigma^2 = 292.3$$

Alternatively,

$$\text{S.D. } \sigma = \sqrt{\frac{1}{N}\left[f_i x_i^2 - \frac{\left(\Sigma f_i x_i\right)^2}{N}\right]}$$

$$= \sqrt{\frac{1}{40}\left[75692 - \frac{(1600)^2}{40}\right]}$$

$$= \sqrt{\frac{1}{40}\left[75692 - 64000\right]}$$

$$= \sqrt{292.3} = 17.10 \text{ years}$$

$$\text{Variance} = 292.3 \text{ (years)}^2$$

4.5.2(c) Grouped Frequency Distribution

Let f_1, f_2, ..., f_n be frequencies corresponding to the mid-values of the classes x_1, x_2...,x_n respectively. Then the Mean, Standard Deviation and Variance are given by the following as

$$\text{Mean} = \frac{\Sigma f_i x_i}{\Sigma f_i} = \frac{\Sigma f_i x_i}{N} \qquad \text{where N} = \Sigma f_i$$

$$\text{Standard Deviation } \sigma = \sqrt{\frac{1}{N}\Sigma f_i \left(x_i - \bar{x}\right)^2}$$

$$\text{Variance} = \sigma^2$$

Alternatively,

$$\text{Standard Deviation } \sigma = \sqrt{\frac{1}{N}\Sigma f_i x_i^2 - \frac{\left(\Sigma f_i x_i\right)^2}{N}}$$

$$\text{Variance} = \sigma^2$$

Example

The following is the distribution of inpatients according to age groups in a teaching hospital. Compute mean age, standard deviation and variance.

Table 4.3

Age (years)	Patients (f_i)	Mid-value (x_i)	$f_i x_i$	$f_i x_i^2$	$(x_i - \bar{x})$	$f_i (x_i - \bar{x})^2$
10-20	4	15	60	900	-30	3600
20-30	12	25	300	7500	-20	4800
30-40	18	35	630	22050	-10	1800
40-50	24	45	1080	48600	0	0
50-60	30	55	1650	90750	10	3000
60-70	12	65	780	50700	20	4800
	100		4500	220500		18000

$$\text{Mean } \bar{x} = \frac{\Sigma f_i x_i}{\Sigma f_i} = \frac{4500}{100} = 45 \text{ years.}$$

$$\text{Standard Deviation, } \sigma = \sqrt{\frac{1}{N}\Sigma f_i (x_i - \bar{x})^2}$$

$$= \sqrt{\frac{18000}{100}} = \sqrt{180} = 13.42 \text{ years}$$

(Rounded off to second decimal place)

$$\text{Variance } \sigma^2 = 180 \text{ (years)}^2$$

Alternatively,

$$\text{Standard Deviation } \sigma = \sqrt{\frac{1}{N}\Sigma f_i x_i^2 - \frac{(\Sigma f_i x_i)^2}{N}}$$

$$= \sqrt{\frac{1}{100}\left[220500 - \frac{(4500)^2}{100}\right]}$$

$$= \sqrt{\frac{1}{100}[220500 - 202500]} = \sqrt{\frac{18000}{100}}$$

$$\sigma = \sqrt{180} = 13.42 \text{ years}$$

$$\text{Variance} = 180 \text{ (years)}^2$$

Merits

(i)   It is useful in knowing the variation in data.

(ii)   It is used in further statistical analysis like tests of hypotheses, normal distribution, coefficient of variation, sampling methods, quality control etc.

(iii)   It has got well defined formula.

(iv)   It is based upon all the observations.

Demerits

(i)   It is difficult to compute compared to other measures of dispersion.

(ii)   It is difficult to comprehend.

4.5.3   Coefficient of variation

It is a relative measure of dispersion. Sometimes it is useful and necessary to know the variation of series of data relative to an average. Coefficient of variation can be used as a measure of consistency. If less is the coefficient of variation (C.V.) the more is the consistency and vice-versa. For example, if two drugs are to be compared with respect to their performance in giving relief to patients of Typhoid the one which is having less C.V. is considered as more consistent. C.V. also can be used for comparing more than two series of data.

$$\text{C.V.} = \frac{\text{S.D.}}{\text{Mean}} \times 100$$

Example

The following is the data on *number* of days taken by 6 patients each to come to normal temperature by administering two drugs who were suffering with typhoid.

Table 4.8

Patient (days)

Drug	1	2	3	4	5	6
A	6	4	8	10	9	5
B	9	4	6	13	12	4

Table 4.9

S.No.	Drug A (x_{1i})	$(x_{1i} - \bar{x}_1)$	$(x_{1i} - \bar{x}_1)^2$	Drug B (x_{2i})	$(x_{2i} - \bar{x}_2)$	$(x_{2i} - \bar{x}_2)^2$
1	6	-1	1	9	1	1
2	4	-3	9	4	-4	16
3	8	1	1	6	-2	4
4	10	3	9	13	5	25
5	9	2	4	12	4	16
6	5	-2	4	4	-4	16
Total	42		28	48		78

Drug A

Mean, $\qquad \bar{x}_1 = \dfrac{42}{6} = 7$

$$\text{S.D. } \sigma = \sqrt{\dfrac{1}{n}\Sigma\left(x_{1i} - \bar{x}_1\right)^2}$$

$$= \sqrt{\dfrac{28}{6}} = \sqrt{4.67} = 2.16$$

$$\text{C.V.} = \dfrac{2.16}{7} \times 100 = 30.86\%$$

Drug B

$$\text{Mean } \bar{x}_2 = \dfrac{48}{6} = 8$$

$$\text{S.D.} \sigma = \sqrt{\dfrac{1}{n}\Sigma\left(x_{2i} - \bar{x}_2\right)^2}$$

$$= \sqrt{\dfrac{78}{6}} = \sqrt{13} = 3.61$$

$$\text{C.V.} = \dfrac{3.61}{8} \times 100 = 45.13\%$$

The C.V. of drug A is less than C.V. of drug B and hence drug A is more consistent than drug B.

4.5.4 Standard error of mean

It is not always possible to study the population due to lack of time and money. Hence a part of the population called sample will be drawn from the population to draw inference about population. This sample should be representative of the population. This can be ensured by drawing the sample at random.

The mean of the sample need not be equal to population mean. The difference between sample mean and population mean is called sampling error. Suppose if we take all possible samples and calculate their means. The mean of all the means of samples of equal size is an estimate of the population mean. Standard deviation of means of all these samples is known as 'standard error of means'.

Since it is not possible to study all the samples, a single sample is to be studied.

The standard error of mean (S.E.) based on single sample of observations x_1, $x_2, \ldots x_n$ is given as

$$\text{S.E. } (\bar{x}) = \dfrac{\sigma}{\sqrt{n}}$$

where σ = population S.D., n = size of sample.

If σ is not known then it is estimated from sample of observations as follows.

Case (i)   If n is large sample (n > 30)

$$\text{S.E.} \left(\overline{x}\right) = \frac{S}{\sqrt{n}} \quad , \quad \text{where} = S = \sqrt{\frac{1}{n}\Sigma(x_i - \overline{x})^2}$$

Case (ii)   If n is small sample (n $\leq$ 30)

$$\text{S.E.} \left(\overline{x}\right) = \frac{s}{\sqrt{n}} \quad , \quad \text{where } s = \sqrt{\frac{1}{n-1}\Sigma(x_i - \overline{x})^2}$$

Exercises

1. Find the mean, standard deviation, variance and coefficient of variation and standard error of mean of the following data on random blood sugar (mg) of 10 individuals recorded in hospital.

    112, 118, 150, 170, 132, 128, 140, 110, 175, 125

2. Find the Mean, Median and Mode for the following distribution.

No. of days absent	No. of Students
More than 40	18
More than 30	30
More than 25	45
More than 15	48
More than 10	52
More than 5	60
More than 0	90

3. Compute Mea, Median and Mode for the following distribution of heights of patients in hospital.

Heights (cm)	170	173	180	184	160	169	189
Patients	3	10	11	5	13	14	6

4. Calculate Mean, Median and Mode for the following ages (years) of Patients in a hospital.

Age (years)	50-54	40-44	54-58	44-50	58-60
Patients	18	10	16	12	6

5. Find the mean, standard deviation, variance and coefficient of variation and standard error of mean of the following data on random blood sugar (mg) of 10 individuals recorded in hospital

    112, 118, 150, 170, 132, 128, 140, 110, 175, 125

7. Compute mean, standard deviation, variance, coefficient of variation and standard error of mean for the distribution of percentage iron content in leafy vegetable samples.

Percent iron content	0-5	5-10	10-15	15-20	20-25
Samples	16	10	8	5	1

8. The following is the distribution of weights (kgs) of patients admitted in a month in a district hospital. Compute mean, S.D. variance, C.V, and S.E of mean.

Weight (kgs)	20-30	30-40	40-50	50-60	60-70
Patients	4	10	26	18	22

9. The following are the days taken for recovery of two groups of patients suffering from 'Malaria' by administering drug A and drug B.

Drug	Patients					
A	6	14	10	5	7	12
B	10	5	14	9	3	7

Find which drug is more consistent.

10. Compute standard deviation, coefficient of variation and standard error of mean given the following distribution of black gram samples collected from different farms with respect to protein content (percentage).

Protein (%)	0-3	3-6	6-9	9-12	12-15	15-18
Samples	10	18	20	6	5	11

11. The following are scores of two batsmen A and B in a series of innings of cricket match.

A	12	115	6	73	7	19	119	36	84	29
B	47	12	16	42	4	51	37	48	13	0

Who is the better score getter and who is more consistent?

12. The scores obtained by two batsmen A and B in 10 matches of cricket are given below

A	30	44	66	62	60	34	80	46	20	38
B	34	46	70	38	55	48	60	34	45	30

Calculate the mean, the standard deviation and the coefficient of variation for each batsman. Determine who is better scorer and who is more consistent.

CHAPTER 5

Skewness and Kurtosis

5.1 Moments

Let x_1, x_2, ..., x be n observations on a characteristic then k-th central moment or k-th moment is defined as

$$\mu_k = \frac{1}{n}\Sigma(x_i - \overline{x})^k,$$

where $\overline{x}$ = Arithmetic mean

If $\qquad$ k = 1, $\quad \mu_1 = \dfrac{1}{n}\Sigma(x_i - \overline{x}) = 0$

$\qquad\qquad$ k = 2, $\quad \mu_2 = \dfrac{1}{n}\Sigma(x_i - \overline{x})^2 =$ Variance

$\qquad\qquad$ k = 3, $\quad \mu_3 = \dfrac{1}{n}\Sigma(x_i - \overline{x})^3$

$\qquad\qquad$ k = 4, $\quad \mu_4 = \dfrac{1}{n}\Sigma(x_i - \overline{x})^4$

In the case of frequency distribution or grouped frequency distribution, the k-th central moment or k-th moment is defined as

$$\mu_k = \frac{1}{N}\Sigma f_i(x_i - \overline{x})^k$$

where N = Σf_i = total frequency and $\overline{x}$ = A.M.

If $\qquad$ k = 1, $\quad \mu_1 = \dfrac{1}{N}\Sigma f_i(x_i - \overline{x}) = 0$

$\qquad\qquad$ k = 2, $\quad \mu_2 = \dfrac{1}{N}\Sigma f_i(x_i - \overline{x})^2 =$ Variance

$$k = 3, \quad \mu_3 = \frac{1}{N}\Sigma f_i\left(x_i - \overline{x}\right)^3$$

$$k = 4, \quad \mu_4 = \frac{1}{N}\Sigma\left(x_i - \overline{x}\right)^4$$

These moments are useful in measuring 'coefficient of skewness' and 'coefficient of kurtosis' which are given in the following sections.

5.2 Skewness

Skewness is defined as the asymmetry of curve. If a curve is bell shaped then it is considered as symmetric curve. If the curve bends or tilts towards right or left then it is said to be asymmetric curve.

Symmetric curve

A symmetric curve is one where the shape of the curve on either side of the mean is identical. In a frequency distribution the frequencies on either side of the mean should be equal. In this curve the measures of central tendency such as mean, median and mode will be equal and the ordinate drawn from the peak of the curve to the mean on the x-axis would bifurcate the area under curve into two equal halves. In this case the skewness of the curve is zero.

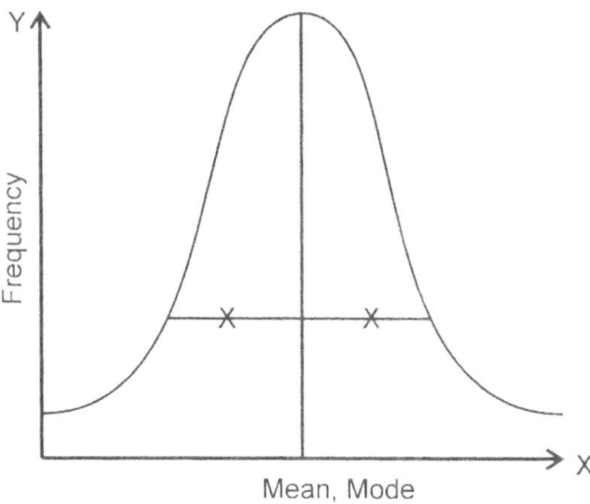

Fig. 5.1 Symmetric Curve.

Asymmetric curve

A curve which is not symmetric is called 'symmetric' or 'skewed' curve. If peak of the curve bends towards right of the mean and has a long tail on left is called 'negatively skewed curve'. This curve is shown in Fig. 5.2.

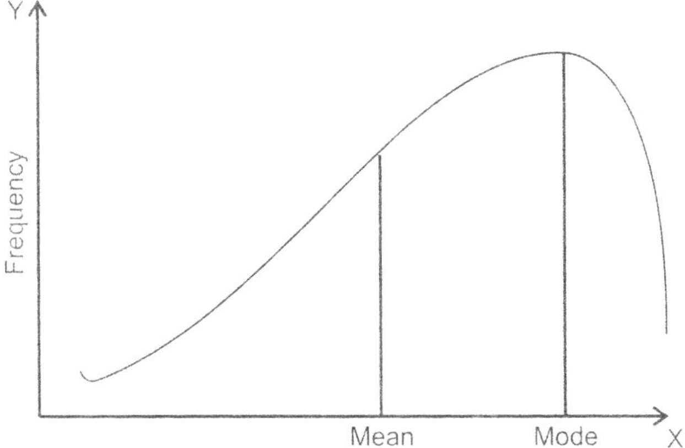

Fig. 5.2 Negative skewness.

If the curve bends towards left of the mean and has a long tail on right side of the mean then it is said to be 'positively skewed curve'. The curve is depicted in Fig. 5.3.

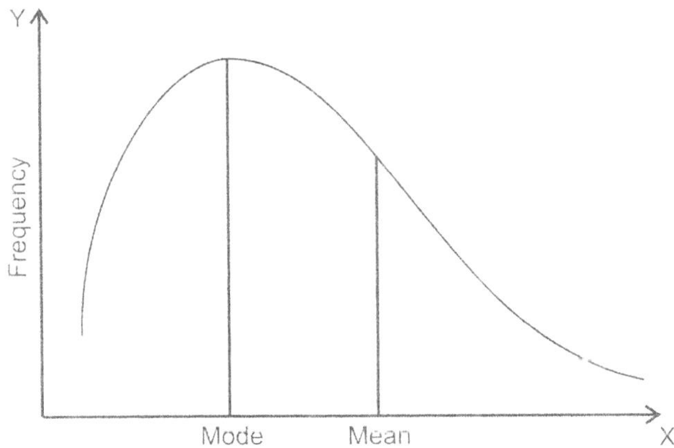

Fig. 5.3 Positive skewness.

The different measures of skewness are given here.

5.2.1 Pearson's coefficient of skewness

$$SK_{(p)} = \frac{\text{Mean} - \text{Mode}}{\text{S.D.}}$$

where 'Mode' is one of the measures of central tendency and is defined as the value having the highest frequency.

S.D. is standard deviation. This measure is independent of units.

If Mean > Mode, then the skewness is positive

If Mean < Mode, then the skewness is negative

If Mean = Mode, then the skewness is zero.

5.2.2   Moment coefficient of skewness

$$\beta_1 = \frac{\mu_3}{\mu_2^{3/2}} = \frac{\mu_3^2}{\mu_2^3}$$

where μ_3 = 3rd central moment

μ_2 = 2nd central moment or variance.

Since μ_2 is always positive, the positive or negative skewness is indicated by the value of 'μ_3'. This measure is also independent of units.

5.3   Kurtosis

The shape of the vertex of the curve is known as kurtosis. There are three types of kurtosis. The coefficient of kurtosis is denoted by 'β_2'.

5.3.1   Platykurtic

If the peak or vertex of the curve is flat compared to normal vertex and the tails are long then it is called platykurtic. Here $\beta_2 < 3$.

5.3.2   Mesokurtic

The peak of the curve is normal and tails on both sides of mean are also normal then it is called Meso kurtic. In this curve Mean = Median = Mode. Here $\beta_2 = 3$.

5.3.3   Leptokurtic

In this curve the peak or vertex of the curve is sharp or narrow and tails on both sides of mean are small. Here $\beta_2 > 3$.

These three curves are depicted in Fig. 5.4.

The measure of kurtosis is given by coefficient of kurtosis and is given by the formula as

$$\beta_1 = \frac{\mu_4}{\mu_2^2},$$

where μ_4 = 4-th central moment

μ_2 = 2nd central moment.

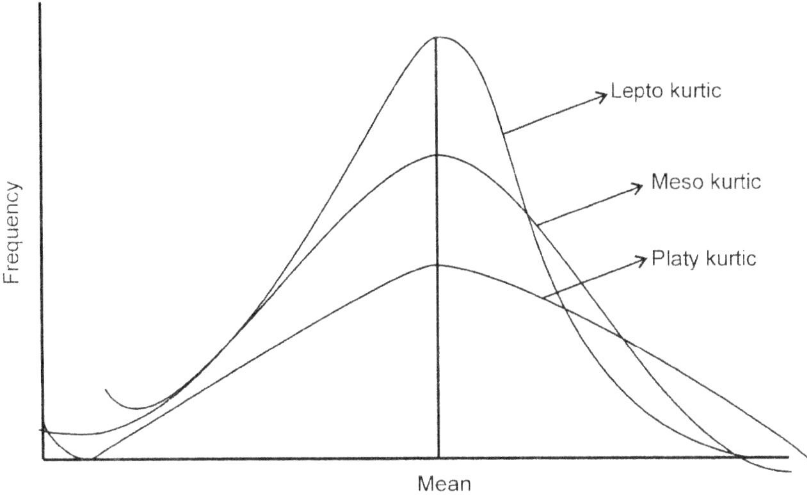

Fig. 5.4 Kurtosis.

This measure also is independent of units. This measure is always positive as both μ_2 and μ_4 are always positive.

Example

The following are the data on vitamin A content (percentage) in 10 samples of leafy vegetable (Amaranthus).

Compute Pearson's coefficient of skewness, Moment coefficient of skewness and coefficient of kurtosis.

Table 5.1

S.No.	Vitamin-A (x_i)	$(x_i - \bar{x})$	$(x_i - \bar{x})^2$	$(x_i - \bar{x})^3$	$(x_i - \bar{x})^4$
1	5	-2	4	-8	16
2	8	1	1	1	1
3	4	-3	9	-27	81
4	15	8	64	512	4096
5	8	1	1	1	1
6	6	-1	1	-1	1
7	10	3	9	27	81
8	3	-4	16	-64	256
9	2	-5	25	-125	625
10	9	2	4	8	16
Total	70		134	324	5174

Mean $= \dfrac{\Sigma x_i}{n} = \dfrac{70}{10} = 7$, Mode $= 8$ (8 is repeated twice where as other values are not repeated in the data).

Pearson's coefficient of skewness, $SK_{(p)} = \dfrac{\text{Mean} - \text{Mode}}{\text{S.D.}}$

Mean $= 7$, Mode $= 8$

$$S.D. = \sqrt{\frac{1}{n}\Sigma(x_i - \bar{x})^2} = \sqrt{\frac{134}{10}} = 3.66$$

$$SK(p) = \frac{(7-8)}{3.66} = \frac{-1}{3.66} = -0.27$$

The skewness is negative using this measure.

$$\mu_2 = 13.4$$

$$\mu_3 = \frac{1}{n}\Sigma(x_i - \bar{x})^3 = \frac{324}{10} = 32.4$$

$$\mu_4 = \frac{1}{n}\Sigma(x_i - \bar{x})^4 = \frac{5174}{10} = 517.4$$

Moment coefficient of skewness, $\beta_1^2 = \dfrac{\mu_3^2}{\mu_2^3}$

$$\beta_1^2 = \frac{(32.4)^2}{(13.4)^3} = \frac{1049.76}{2406.10} = 0.44$$

The skewness is positive using this measure. This measure is more accurate.

Coefficient of kurtosis, $\beta_2 = \dfrac{\mu_4}{\mu_2^2}$

$$\beta_2 = \frac{517.4}{(13.4)^2} = \frac{517.4}{179.56} = 2.88$$

Since $\beta_2 < 3$, the kurtosis is platy kurtic slightly as it is slightly lower than 3.

Exercises

1. Find the coefficient of skewness given the following results on weights (kgs) of patients admitted in cancer hospital,

   Mean = 64, Mode = 70, Varicance = 4

2. Compute Moment coefficient of skewness and coefficient of kurtosis for the following distribution of pigeon pea according to protein content.

Protein (%)	0-4	4-8	8-12	12-16	16-20
Samples	10	18	24	12	16

3. The following are the data on high B.P. for the patients admitted in heart disease specialty hospital. Obtain coefficient of skewness and kurtosis.

   130, 142, 160, 164, 170, 156, 154, 144, 142, 180,

   200, 142, 165, 210, 138, 136, 157, 220, 186, 134

4. Find the coefficients of skewness and kurtosis for the following distribution of serum cholesterol levels of patients in a hospital.

Serum cholesterol	50-60	60-70	70-80	80-90	90-100
Patients	6	10	24	22	18

5. The following is the distribution of leafy vegetable samples collected from different markets with respect to iron content (percent). Find moment coefficient of skewness and coefficient of kurtosis.

Iron content (%)	0-2	2.4	4-6	6-8	8-10
Samples	9	10	18	16	7

CHAPTER 6

Probability and Distributions

6.1 Introduction

We use the word 'probability' several times in our daily life. The doctor says that a particular patient has survival chance of 60 percent after operation. Sometimes the doctor says that a certain patient has 90 percent chance of having a particular disease. The parents say that we may have male child this time. We may have good harvest this year. These statements are based on chances of happening of an event. These statements are no longer subjective since the development of probability theory.

The concept of probability may be categorized into (i) classical or a priori probability and (ii) relative frequency or a posteriori probability.

6.1.1 A priori Probability

If an event can happen in 'a' ways and fails to happen in 'b' ways and all these cases are equally likely, then the probability of happening of an event is $\dfrac{a}{a+b}$ and probability of not happening an event is $\dfrac{b}{a+b}$. In other words, probability of happening of an event is defined as the ratio of number of 'favourable' cases to total number of equally likely cases.

If $$p = \frac{a}{a+b}, q = \frac{b}{a+b}$$
then $$p + q = 1$$

'p' always lies between 0 and 1. If p = 1 and q = 0 the event is certain to happen. If p = o, q = 1 the event certainly will not happen.

For example, if a card is drawn from a pack of cards at random, the probability of having a diamond card is $\dfrac{13}{52}$ since there are 13 diamond cards out of total

52 cards. Similarly a dice is thrown once the probability of turning up of '4' out of 6 numbers is $\dfrac{1}{6}$.

6.1.2 A posteriori Probability

The probability based on relative frequency of happening of an event is known as a posteriori probability.

For example, the probability of survival of patients is calculated after finding the number of cases of survival of patients out of total cases admitted. If 10 patients survive after operating on 15 patients then the probability of survival is $\dfrac{10}{15} = \dfrac{2}{3}$. In this case frequency of happening of an event is to be found after actual occurrence of an event.

6.2 Mutually Exclusive Events

Events are said to be mutually exclusive and exhaustive if the occurrence of any one of the events excludes the occurrence of other events at a particular occasion.

For example, an outpatient ward has persons suffering with eye, heart, ENT and gastro diseases. A person was called at random and if a person with heart disease comes to doctor then other persons of other diseases cannot come. These events are mutually exclusive. If a coin is tossed once if 'HEAD' turns up then 'TAIL' cannot come. Turning of 'HEAD' and 'TAIL' are mutually exclusive events. A dice is thrown once. Turning up any one out of 6 numbers excludes other numbers. These events are called mutually exclusive events.

6.2.1 Addition rule

Let $E_1, E_2,..., E_n$ be n mutually exclusive events. Then the probability of occurrence of any one of the events is the sum of the probability of the separate events.

$$P(E_1 \text{ or } E_2 \text{ or } ...\text{or } E_n) = P(E_1) + P(E_2) + ... + P(E_n)$$

Example 1

If there are 6 persons suffering from heart disease, 10 persons from ENT disease, 12 persons from eye disease and 2 from gastro disease in outpatient hall and a person is called at random from the group, what is the probability that the patient is either from eye or heart disease group.

$$P(\text{Eye}) = \dfrac{12}{30}, \ P(\text{Heart}) = \dfrac{6}{30}$$

$$P(\text{E or H}) = P(\text{E}) + P(\text{H})$$

$$= \dfrac{12}{30} + \dfrac{6}{30} = \dfrac{18}{30} = \dfrac{3}{5}$$

Example 2

What is the probability of drawing a card either of a diamond or club when it is drawn at random from a pack of cards.

A pack of cards contains 4 suits such as Heart, Spade, Diamond and Club and each suit contains 13 cards which makes 52 cards in all.

Probability of drawing a Diamond card = $\dfrac{13}{52}$

Probability of drawing a Club card = $\dfrac{13}{52}$

∴ probability of drawing either diamond or club card = $\dfrac{13}{52} + \dfrac{13}{52} = \dfrac{26}{52} = \dfrac{1}{2}$

6.3 Mutually Independent Events

Events are said to be mutually exclusive if the occurrence of any one of the events does not affect the occurrence of any other event.

A coin is tossed twice. The occurrence of 'Head' or 'Tail' on the second occasion does not depend upon the outcome of the first occasion. These two events are mutually independent.

Similarly one card is drawn from each of two packs of cards, two cards are drawn one after another from the same pack of cards by replacing the first card are mutually independent events.

6.3.1 Multiplication Rule

Let E_1, E_2,...,E_n be n mutually independent events then the probability of simultaneous occurrence of all the 'n' events is the product of all the probabilities of the individual events.

$$P(E_1, E_2, ... E_n) = P(E_1)\, P(E_2)\, ... \, P(E_n)$$

Example 1

What is the probability of having two male children in first two births of a couple?

Probability of having a male child in first birth = $\dfrac{1}{2}$

Probability of having male child in second birth = $\dfrac{1}{2}$

Probability of having male children in both births = $\dfrac{1}{2} \times \dfrac{1}{2} = \dfrac{1}{4}$

Example 2

Two dice are thrown simultaneously once. What is the probability of getting 6 on first die and 4 on the second die.

Probability of getting 6 on the first die $= \dfrac{1}{6}$

Probability of getting 4 on the second die $= \dfrac{1}{6}$

Probability of getting 6 on first die and 4 on second die $= \dfrac{1}{6} \times \dfrac{1}{6}$

$$= \dfrac{1}{36}$$

6.4   Not Mutually Exclusive Events

If E_1 and E_2 are not two mutually exclusive events then

$$P\,(E_1 \text{ or } E_2 \text{ or } E_1\,E_2) = P\,(E_1) + P\,(E_2) - P\,(E_1\,E_2)$$

or $\qquad\quad P\,(E_1 \cup E_2) = P\,(E_1) + P\,(E_2) - P\,(E_1\,E_2)$

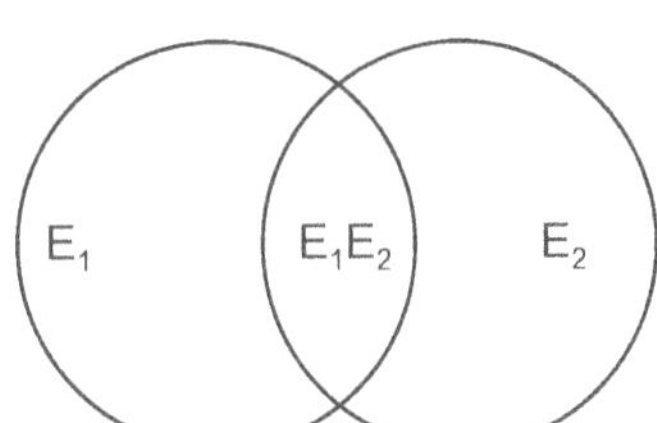

Example

A coin is tossed twice. What is the probability that they contain at least one 'Head'.

Probability of getting 'Head, in the first trial or $P(H_1) = \dfrac{1}{2}$

Probability of getting 'Head' in the second trial or $P(H_2) = \dfrac{1}{2}$

Probability of getting 'Heads' in the both trials or $P(H_1\,H_2) = \dfrac{1}{4}$

$\therefore$ the probability of obtaining at least one 'Head' in both the trials i.e.

$$P\,(H_1 \text{ or } H_2 \text{ or } H_1 H_2) = P\,(H_1) + P(H_2) - P(H_1 H_2)$$

$$= \dfrac{1}{2} + \dfrac{1}{2} - \dfrac{1}{4} = \dfrac{3}{4}$$

In the case of three events E_1, E_2 and E_3 which are not mutually exclusive events.

Then

$$P = (E_1 \text{ or } E_2 \text{ or } E_3 \text{ or } E_1E_2 \text{ or } E_1E_3 \text{ or } E_2E_3 \text{ or } E_1E_2E_3)$$

or $\quad P = (E_1 \cup E_2 \cup E_3) = P(E_1) + P(E_2) + P(E_3) - P(E_1E_2) - P(E_1E_3)$

$$- P(E_2E_3) + P(E_1E_2E_3)$$

Example

A coin is tossed thrice. What is the probability of obtaining at least one 'Head' out of three trials.

$$P(H_1) = \frac{1}{2}, \qquad P(H_2) = \frac{1}{2}, \qquad P(H_3) = \frac{1}{2}$$

$$P(H_1H_2) = \frac{1}{4}, \; P(H_1,H_3) = \frac{1}{4}, \; P(H_2H_3) = \frac{1}{4}, \; P(H_1H_2H_3) = \frac{1}{8}$$

$$P(H_1 \cup H_2 \cup H_3) = P(H_1) + P(H_2) + P(H_3) - P(H_1H_2) - P(H_1H_3)$$

$$- P(H_2H_3) + P(H_1H_2H_3)$$

$$= \frac{1}{2} + \frac{1}{2} + \frac{1}{2} - \frac{1}{4} - \frac{1}{4} - \frac{1}{4} + \frac{1}{8} = \frac{7}{8}$$

6.5   Conditional Probability

Dependent events: The events are said to be dependent if the occurrence of any one of them depends on the occurrence of any other event.

Let E_1 and E_2 are two dependent events then the probability of simultaneous occurrence of the two events is given by the relation.

$$P(E_1E_2) = P(E_1) . P(E_2/E_1)$$

$$P(E_1E_2) = P(E_2) . P(E_1/E_2),$$

where $P(E_2/E_1)$ is read as probability of E_2 given E_1 and $P(E_1/E_2)$ is read as probability of E_1 given E_2.

It may be noted that multiplication rule holds good if the events are dependent or independent.

Example

A basket contains 10 Mangoes, 15 Apples and 25 Oranges. Two fruits are drawn at random from the mix one after the other. What is the probability that there is one Mango and one Apple when the first fruit is not replaced ?

Case (i) Probability of drawing Mango fruit first = $\dfrac{10}{50}$

Probability of drawing Apple fruit second = $\dfrac{15}{49}$

Since the above two events are dependent,

the probability of drawing 1 Mango and 1 Apple fruit = $\dfrac{15}{50} \times \dfrac{10}{49}$

Case (ii) Probability of drawing Apple fruit first = $\dfrac{15}{50}$

Probability of drawing Mango fruit second = $\dfrac{10}{49}$

Since the above two events are dependent,

the probability of drawing 1 Mango and 1 Apple fruit = $\dfrac{15}{50} \times \dfrac{10}{49}$

Since case (i) and case (ii) are mutually exclusive the corresponding probabilities will be added.

Probability of drawing 1 Mango and 1 Apple fruit = $\dfrac{10}{50} \times \dfrac{15}{49} + \dfrac{15}{50} \times \dfrac{10}{49}$

$$= \dfrac{300}{50 \times 49}$$

6.5.1 Bayes Theorem

An event A can be described by a set of n exhaustive and mutually exclusive hypotheses B_1, B_2,..., B_n. Given

(i) a priori probabilities $P(B_1)$, $P(B_2)...P(B_n)$; $P(B_i) \neq 0$ for i = 1, 2,...,n corresponding to a total absence of a knowledge regarding the occurrence of A and

(ii) conditional probabilities $P(A/B_1)$, $P(A/B_2)...P(A/B_n)$

The a posteriori probabilities $P(B_i/A)$ are obtained as

$$P(B_i/A) = \dfrac{P(B_i)\,P(A/B_i)}{\sum\limits_{i=1}^{n} P(B_i)\,P(A/B_i)}$$

Example

A factory has 3 machines A, B and C. A produces 4000 injection needles, B produces 5000 and C produces 3000 per day. Machine A produces 2%, B produces 1% and C produces 3% defective needles. A needle is checked at random at the end of a day and is found to be defective. What is the probability that it is produced by machine B.

Let P(A), P(B) and P(C) be the probabilities of production of injection needles by machines A, B and C, respectively.

$$P(A) = \frac{4000}{4000 + 5000 + 3000} = \frac{1}{3}$$

$$P(B) = \frac{5000}{4000 + 5000 + 3000} = \frac{5}{12}$$

$$P(C) = \frac{3000}{4000 + 5000 + 3000} = \frac{3}{12} = \frac{1}{4}$$

Let P(D/A) P(DIB) and P(D/C) be the probabilities of producing defective needles from machines A, B and C, respectively.

$$P(D/A) = \frac{2}{100} = 0.02, \; P(D/B) = \frac{1}{100} = 0.01, \; P(D/C) = \frac{3}{100} = 0.03$$

$$P(B/D) = \frac{P(B).P(D/B)}{P(A).P(D/A) + P(B).P(D/B) + P(C).P(D/C)}$$

$$= \frac{\frac{5}{12} \times 0.01}{\frac{1}{3} \times 0.02 + \frac{5}{12} \times 0.01 + \frac{3}{12} \times 0.03} = \frac{0.05}{0.22} = 0.23$$

Exercises

1. Basket A contains 20 Mangoes, 15 Apples and 10 Oranges and another basket B contains 10 Mangoes, 20 Apples and 15 Oranges. A fruit is drawn at random from the basket A and transferred to B basket. If a fruit is drawn from B basket what is the probability that it is Apple?

2. There are two boxes, one of which contains 100 packets of antibiotic injections and 80 packets of vitamin B injections and the other box contains 120 packets of antibiotic injections and 100 packets of vitamin B injections. A packet of injection is drawn at random from one or other of the two boxes. Find the probability that it is vitamin B.

3. Three dairy farms A, B and C produce milk with 40, 25 and 35 percent, respectively in a city. A milk packet is found defective if it contains fat percentage 3 or less. Three farms A, B and C produce defective packets in the ratio 2 : 4 : 4. A milk packet is drawn at random from the mix and it is found defective. What is the probability that it is from B?

4. A box contains 40 Vitamin B and 60 Vitamin C packets. A packet is drawn at random and in its place a packet of other Vitamin is put in the box. Now one packet is drawn at random from the box. Find the probability that it is Vitamin B.

5. A coin is tossed 4 times. Find the probability that it contains at least one 'HEAD'.

6. A box contains 50 calcium, 40 Vitamin B and 130 antibiotic strips of tablets. A strip of tablets is drawn at random. Find the probability that it is either vitamin B or antibiotic.

7. What is the probability of not obtaining 'HEAD' by tossing a coin 3 times?

8. What is the probability of having one male child out of 4 births in a family assuming that the probability is equal for having male or female child ?

9. Three machines M_1, M_2, M_3 produce identical items of their respective output of which 5%, 4%, 3% of items are faulty. On a certain day M_1 produced 25% of the total output, M_2 produced 30% and M_3 the remainder. An item that is selected at random is found to be faulty. What are the chances that it was produced by the machine with the highest output.

10. In a bolt factory machines P, Q, R manufacture 25%, 35% and 40% of the total. Of their output 5%, 4% and 2% are defective bolts. A bolt is drawn at random from the product and is found to be defective. What are the probabilities that it was manufactured by machines P, Q and R.

6.6   Binomial Distribution

Bernoulli Trials : Repeated independent trials with two possible outcomes at each trial are known as Bernoulli trials. Binomial distribution is based upon Bernoulli trials.

For example, if a coin is tossed 5 times, each time the outcome may be 'head' or 'tail'. The outcome of each trial is independent of the other. If 'head' turns up is considered as 'success' and, 'tail' as failure then the probability of success or failure is same throughout the 5 trials. These trials are considered as Bernoulli trials.

The probability of success at each trial can be computed as follows.

The Probability '0' successes i.e. TTTTT is $\dfrac{1}{2}.\dfrac{1}{2}.\dfrac{1}{2}.\dfrac{1}{2}.\dfrac{1}{2} = \left(\dfrac{1}{2}\right)^5$

Since probability of success or failure is $\dfrac{1}{2}$.

The probability '1' success out of 5 trials i.e. HTTTT, THTTT, TTHTT, TTTHT, TTTTH is

$$\dfrac{1}{2}.\dfrac{1}{2}.\dfrac{1}{2}.\dfrac{1}{2}.\dfrac{1}{2} + \dfrac{1}{2}.\dfrac{1}{2}.\dfrac{1}{2}.\dfrac{1}{2}.\dfrac{1}{2} + \dfrac{1}{2}.\dfrac{1}{2}.\dfrac{1}{2}.\dfrac{1}{2}.\dfrac{1}{2} + \dfrac{1}{2}.\dfrac{1}{2}.\dfrac{1}{2}.\dfrac{1}{2}.\dfrac{1}{2} + \dfrac{1}{2}.\dfrac{1}{2}.\dfrac{1}{2}.\dfrac{1}{2}.\dfrac{1}{2}$$

$= 5 \left(\dfrac{1}{2}\right)^5$ which can be written $5C_1 \left(\dfrac{1}{2}\right)\left(\dfrac{1}{2}\right)^4$ where $5C_1 = \dfrac{5!}{1!(5-1)!} = 5$

The probability of '2' successes out of 5 trials i.e.

HHTTT, HTHTT, HTTHT, HTTTH, THTTH, TTHTH, TTTHH, TTHHT, THHTT,

$HHTTT = 10 \left(\dfrac{1}{2}\right)^5$ which can be written as $5C_2 \left(\dfrac{1}{2}\right)^2\left(\dfrac{1}{2}\right)^3$

The probability of '3' successes out of 5 trials i.e.,

HHHTT, HHTTH, HTTHH, THTHH, HTHHT, THHTH, THTHH, TTHHH,

$THHHT, HTHTH = 5C_3 \left(\dfrac{1}{2}\right)^3\left(\dfrac{1}{2}\right)^2 = 10\left(\dfrac{1}{2}\right)^3\left(\dfrac{1}{2}\right)^2$

The probability of 4 successes out of 5 trials i.e.,

$HHHHT, HHHTH, HHTHH, HTHHH, THHHH = 5C_4 \left(\dfrac{1}{2}\right)^4\left(\dfrac{1}{2}\right) = 5\left(\dfrac{1}{2}\right)^4\left(\dfrac{1}{2}\right)$

The probability of 5 successes out of 5 trials i.e., HHHHH is $\left(\dfrac{1}{2}\right)^5$

These probabilities with respect to successes are arranged in Table 6.1.

Table 6.1

Success	Probability
0	$\left(\dfrac{1}{2}\right)^5$
1	$5C_1 \left(\dfrac{1}{2}\right)\left(\dfrac{1}{2}\right)^{5-1}$
2	$5C_2 \left(\dfrac{1}{2}\right)^2\left(\dfrac{1}{2}\right)^{5-2}$
3	$5C_3 \left(\dfrac{1}{2}\right)^3\left(\dfrac{1}{2}\right)^{5-3}$
4	$5C_4 \left(\dfrac{1}{2}\right)^4\left(\dfrac{1}{2}\right)^{5-4}$
5	$\left(\dfrac{1}{2}\right)^5$

In general, if probability of success is denoted by 'p' and failure by 'q' then

$p + q = 1$. If a coin is tossed 'n' times the probability of 'r' successes out of 'n' trials is given as

$$P_r = nc_r \, p_r \, q^{n-r}$$

where $\qquad nc_r = \begin{pmatrix} n \\ r \end{pmatrix} = \dfrac{n!}{r!(n-r)!}$

The successive probabilities can be obtained for $r = 0, 1, 2, \ldots n$ in the above expression and they are arranged in the Table 6.2.

Table 6.2

Success	Probability	Frequency
0	q^n	$N.\, q^n$
1	$\begin{pmatrix} n \\ 1 \end{pmatrix} p\, q^{n-1}$	$N \begin{pmatrix} n \\ 1 \end{pmatrix} p\, q^{n-1}$
2	$\begin{pmatrix} n \\ 2 \end{pmatrix} p^2\, q^{n-2}$	$N \begin{pmatrix} n \\ 2 \end{pmatrix} p^2\, q^{n-2}$
$\vdots$		$\vdots$
r	$\begin{pmatrix} n \\ r \end{pmatrix} p^2\, q^{n-r}$	$N \begin{pmatrix} n \\ r \end{pmatrix} p^r\, q^{n-r}$
$\vdots$	$\vdots$	$\vdots$
n	p^n	Np^n
Total	1	N

The probabilities in Table 6.2 are equivalent to successive terms of a well-known expansion called Binomial expansion, which is given by

$$(q + p)^n = q^n + \begin{pmatrix} n \\ 1 \end{pmatrix} pq^{n-1} + \begin{pmatrix} n \\ 2 \end{pmatrix} p^2 q^{n-2} + \ldots + \begin{pmatrix} n \\ r \end{pmatrix} p^r\, q^{n-r} + \ldots + p^n \qquad \ldots(6.1)$$

It can be verified that the terms in expansion in eq. (6.1) are equivalent to successive probabilities in Table 6.2. The total of the terms in equation (6.1) is equal to '1' as $(q+p)^n = 1^n = 1$. Therefore the total of the probability column in Table 6.2 is 1.

Hence, the distribution of probabilities with respect to successes in Table 6.2 is known as Binomial distribution.

If 'N' coins are tossed simultaneously 'n' times the frequencies of probabilities can be obtained by multiplying 'N' with each of the probabilities and these are given in column (3) of Table 6.2 under 'Frequency'.

The frequency distribution is represented by diagram in Fig. 6.1. Since this distribution is discrete distribution the diagram is called line diagram.

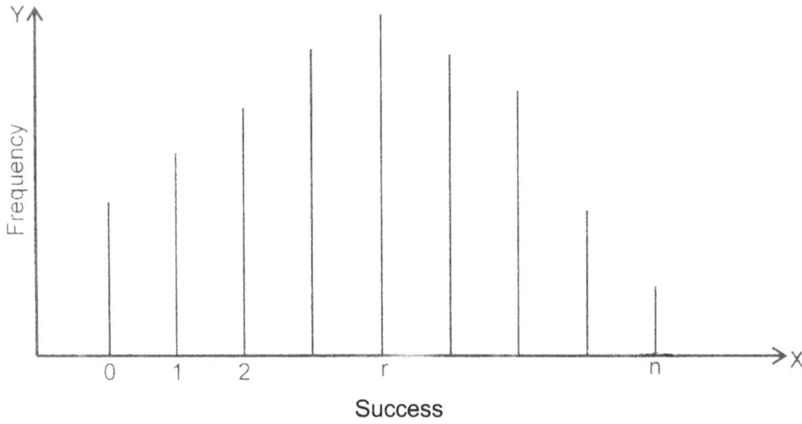

Fig. 6.1

6.6.1 Properties of Binomial Distribution

Mean = np, μ_2 = npq, S.D, $\sigma = \sqrt{npq}$

μ_3 = npq (q − p), $\mu_4 = 3n^2p^2q^2$ + npq (1 − 6pq)

Coefficient of skewness, $\beta_1 = \dfrac{(q-p)}{\sqrt{npq}}$

coefficient of kurtosis, $\beta_2 = 3 + \dfrac{(1-6\,pq)}{npq}$

'n' and 'p' are called parameters of the Binomial distribution.

As r takes values from 0 to n, the value of p_r increases monotonically and reaches maximum when r = s, where 's' lies between (n + 1)p − 1 and (n + 1)p. However, when r = s where s = (n + 1)p, then $p_r = p_r − 1$ and later on decreases monotonically.

Example

If a coin is tossed 3 times and turning up of 'head' is considered as success, find the probability of having exactly 2 successes.

Two 'heads' may turn up in 3 trials as HHT, HTH, THH. The probability of getting head is $\dfrac{1}{2}$ and probability of getting tail is $\dfrac{1}{2}$ then the probabilities for the above combinations can be written as (Table 6.3).

Table 6.3

Combination	Probability	Probability
HHT	$\dfrac{1}{2}\cdot\dfrac{1}{2}\cdot\dfrac{1}{2}$	$=\left(\dfrac{1}{2}\right)^{2}\dfrac{1}{2}$
HTH	$\dfrac{1}{2}\cdot\dfrac{1}{2}\cdot\dfrac{1}{2}$	$=\left(\dfrac{1}{2}\right)^{2}\dfrac{1}{2}$
THH	$\dfrac{1}{2}\cdot\dfrac{1}{2}\cdot\dfrac{1}{2}$	$=\left(\dfrac{1}{2}\right)^{2}\dfrac{1}{2}$

The above combinations in Table 6.3 are equally likely and mutually exclusive events. Therefore, the probability of 2 successes out of 3 trials will be obtained by adding these 3 probabilities.

$$P3 = \left(\frac{1}{2}\right)^{2}\left(\frac{1}{2}\right)+\left(\frac{1}{2}\right)^{2}\left(\frac{1}{2}\right)+\left(\frac{1}{2}\right)^{2}\left(\frac{1}{2}\right)$$

$$= 3\left(\frac{1}{2}\right)^{2}\left(\frac{1}{2}\right)=\binom{3}{1}\left(\frac{1}{2}\right)^{2}\left(\frac{1}{2}\right)$$

Example

Find the probability of getting at least 3 heads by tossing a coin 4 times.

The combinations of 3 heads out of 4 trials are HHHT, HHTH, HTHH and THHH.

The probability of getting 3 heads out of 4 trials is obtained by adding the probabilities of these 4 combinations i.e.

$$= \binom{4}{3}\left(\frac{1}{2}\right)=\left(\frac{1}{2}\right)^{3}\left(\frac{1}{2}\right)+\left(\frac{1}{2}\right)^{3}\left(\frac{1}{2}\right)+\left(\frac{1}{2}\right)^{3}\left(\frac{1}{2}\right)+\left(\frac{1}{2}\right)^{3}\left(\frac{1}{2}\right)$$

Since in question the probability of getting at least 3 heads is asked therefore we have to consider probability of getting 4 heads also.

The combination of getting 4 heads is HHHH.

The probability of getting 4 heads is $\left(\dfrac{1}{2}\right)^{4}$.

$\therefore$ the probability of getting at least 3 heads out of 4 trials

$$= \binom{4}{3}\left(\frac{1}{2}\right)^3\left(\frac{1}{2}\right) + \left(\frac{1}{2}\right)^4 \qquad \text{where} \quad \binom{4}{3} = 4 \ C_3 = \frac{4!}{3!(4-3)!}$$

$$= \frac{1\times2\times3\times4}{1\times2\times3\times1} = 4$$

$$= 4\times\frac{1}{16} + \frac{1}{16} = \frac{5}{16}$$

6.6.2 Fitting of the Binomial Distribution

From the sample data 'p' is estimated. The probabilities for different successes can be obtained by knowing the values of 'n' and p. Expected frequencies can be obtained by multiplying the probabilities with 'N' the total frequency. Further the difference between observed and expected frequencies can be tested for its significance with the help of chi-square test. If chi-square test is found not significant at a given level of significance, the given distribution follows Binomial Distribution. Otherwise it does not follow Binomial Distribution.

The above procedure of fitting can be illustrated with the following example.

Example

The following is the distribution of persons who got relief from headache by consuming tablets of a chemical composition supplied by pharmaceutical company in a hospital.

No. of tablets	0	1	2	3	4	5
Persons	2	6	14	9	5	4

Fit a Binomial distribution to the above data.

Table 6.4

No. of tablets (x_i)	Persons (f_i)	$f_i x_i$	Probability	Expected frequency
0	2	0	.02825	1.13
1	6	6	.14700	5.88
2	14	28	.30600	12.24
3	9	27	.31850	12.74
4	5	20	.16575	6.63
5	4	20	.03450	1.38
	40	101	1.00000	40.00

$$\text{Mean} = np = \frac{\Sigma f_i x_i}{\Sigma f_i} = \frac{101}{40} = 2.525, \ n = 5$$

$$p = \frac{2.525}{5} = 0.505 \simeq 0.51 \text{ (rounded off to second decimal place)}$$

$$q = 1 - p = 1 - 0.51 = 0.49$$

The chi-square test will be used to test whether there is significant difference between observed frequencies in column (2) and expected frequencies in column (5). If the difference is not significant at a specified level of significance then the above distribution follows Binomial distribution. The chi-square test is described in a later chapter of this book.

6.7   Poisson Distribution

If 'n' increases and 'p' decreases and np remains fixed the Binomial distribution tends to Poisson distribution. This distribution was developed by S.D. Poisson in 1837.

If$\qquad$$np = m = \text{mean}$

$$p_r = \frac{m^r}{r!} e^{-m}$$

where p_r is the probability of 'r' successes and 'e' is the exponential function.

If$\qquad$$r = 0, \qquad p_0 = \frac{m^0}{0!} e^{-m} = e^{-m}$

$$r = 1, \qquad p_1 = \frac{m}{1!} e^{-m} = me^{-m}$$

$$r = 2, \qquad p_2 = \frac{m^2}{2!} e^{-m} = \frac{m^2}{2} e^{-m}$$

$$r = 3, \qquad p_3 = \frac{m^2}{3!} e^{-m} = \frac{m^3}{6} e^{-m}$$

and so on

6.7.1 Properties

Mean $= m$, $\mu_2 = m$, $\mu_3 = m$, $\mu_4 = 3m^2 + m$

$$\text{Coefficient of skewness, } \beta_1 = \frac{1}{\sqrt{m}},$$

$$\text{coefficient of kurtosis, } \beta_2 = 3 + \left(\frac{1}{m} \right)$$

It may be noted that the first three moments are equal for this distribution. 'm' is the parameter of this distribution.

This distribution is found useful when the probability of success is small. For example, number of deaths of persons due to rare disease like AIDS in a month, number of car accidents in a day, number of defective medical kits produced by pharmaceutical company in a day, number of printing mistakes in a page of a book, bacteria count on a petri plate where the plate is divided into small squares, number of weed seeds in seed packet etc., follow Poisson distribution.

6.7.2 Fitting of Poisson Distribution

We would like to know whether sample distribution follows poisson distribution or not. First the parameter of the distribution 'm' is estimated. Using the value of m the probabilities of each success can be computed. Further expected frequencies can be calculated by multiplying probabilities with 'N' the total frequency.

The above procedure is illustrated with the following example.

Example

The following (Table 6.5) is the distribution of hospitals in a city with respect to number of persons who reported to have positive symptoms of AIDS on a particular day.

Table 6.5

Effected persons (x_i)	hospitals (f_i)	$f_i x_i$	Probability	Expected frequency
0	6	0	0.1225	6.1250
1	10	10	0.25725	12.8625
2	18	36	0.27011	13.5055
3	9	27	0.18908	9.4900
4	5	20	0.09927	4.9635
5	2	10	0.04169	2.0845
Total	50	103	0.9799	49.031

$$\text{Mean} = np = \frac{103}{50} = 2.06 \approx 2.1 \text{ (Rounded off to first decimal place)}.$$

If $m = 2.1$ $e^{-2.1}$ $= 0.1225$

If $r = 0,$ $P_0 = e^{-m} = e^{-2.1}$ $= 0.1225$

            $r = 1,$ $P_1 = m.e^{-m}$ $= 0.25725$

            $r = 2,$ $P_2 = \dfrac{m^2}{2!} e^{-m}$ $= 0.27011$

            $r = 3,$ $P_3 = \dfrac{m^3}{3!} e^{-m}$ $= 0.18908$

            $r = 4,$ $P_4 = \dfrac{m^4}{4!} e^{-m}$ $= 0.09927$

            $r = 5,$ $P_5 = \dfrac{m^5}{5!} e^{-m}$ $= 0.04169$

The exponential values for different values of m i.e. e^{-m} values can be obtained directly from scientific calculators or through logarithmic tables.

The computed values of e^{-m} for different values of m from 1.0 to *5.3* are presented in the Table 6.6.

Table 6.6

m	e^{-m}	m	e^{-m}	m	e^{-m}	m	e^{-m}
1.0	0.3679	2.1	0.1225	3.2	0.0408	4.3	0.0136
1.1	0.3329	2.2	0.1108	3.3	0.0369	4.4	0.0123
1.2	0.3012	2.3	0.1003	3.4	0.0334	4.5	0.0111
1.3	0.2725	2.4	0.0907	3.5	0.0302	4.6	0.0101
1.4	0.2466	2.5	0.0821	3.6	0.0273	4.7	0.0091
1.5	0.2231	2.6	0.0743	3.7	0.0247	4.8	0.0083
1.6	0.2019	2.7	0.0672	3.8	0.0224	4.9	0.0074
1.7	0.1827	2.8	0.0608	3.9	0.0202	5.0	0.0067
1.8	0.1653	2.9	0.0550	4.0	0.0183	5.1	0.0061
1.9	0.1496	3.0	0.0498	4.1	0.0166	5.2	0.0055
2.0	0.1353	3.1	0.0450	4.2	0.0150	5.3	0.0050

Poisson distribution is also a discrete distribution like Binomial distribution. The diagram depicting the frequency distribution is a line diagram and is presented in Fig. 6.2.

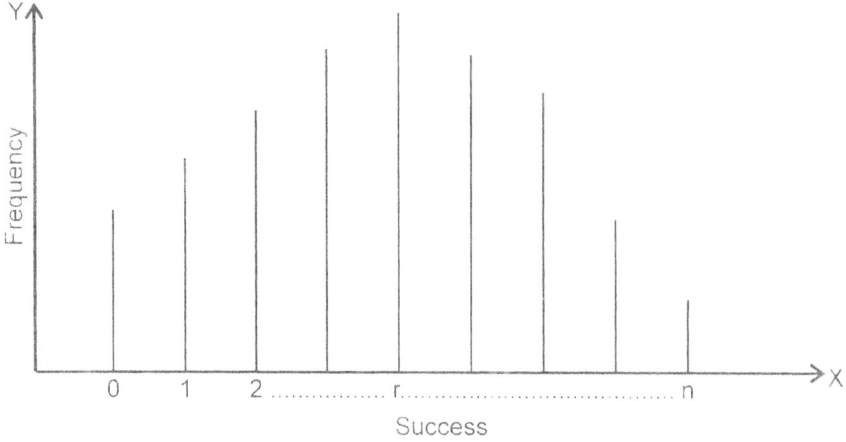

Fig. 6.2

6.8   Normal Distribution

In Binomial distribution the number of trials, n is large and number of successes, r is also large and probability of success, p is fixed then Binomial distribution tends to Normal distribution. This distribution was given by A. Demoivre in 1718, later independently by Laplace in 1812 and Gauss (1777-1855). This distribution is also known as Gaussian distribution.

The density function of Normal distribution for the variable, x is f(x)

where
$$f(x) = \frac{1}{\sigma\sqrt{2\pi}}e^{\frac{-(x-\mu)^2}{2\sigma^2}}$$

Here μ is mean and σ is standard deviation, are the parameters of the normal distribution. The curve for f(x) is called normal probability curve or normal curve of error. The curve is depicted in Fig. 6.3.

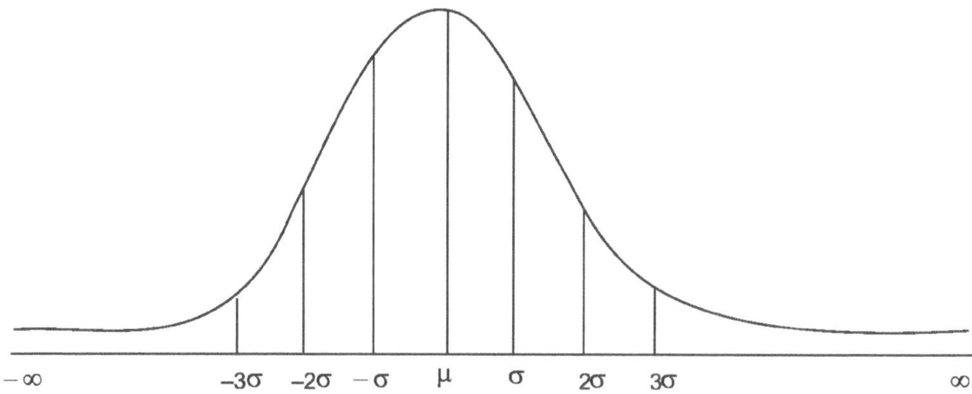

Fig. 6.3 Normal curve.

The area under the normal curve from -3σ to 3σ in Fig. 6.3 is 99.7 percent of the total area. The area under the normal curve from -2σ to 2σ in Fig. 6.3 is 95.5 percent of the total area. The area under the normal curve from $-\sigma$ to σ in Fig. 6.3 is 68.3 percent of the total area.

Standard Normal Distribution

If x is the normal variate then $Z = \dfrac{x-\mu}{\sigma}$ is called standard normal deviate or standard normal variate which follows normal distribution with mean zero and standard deviation unity.

The density function of z is given by,

$$f(z) = \frac{1}{\sqrt{2\pi}} e^{-\frac{1}{2}z^2}$$

The standard normal curve is depicted in Fig. 6.4

The area under the curve is 1 sq. unit. The maximum ordinate is at mean and is equal to $\dfrac{1}{\sqrt{2\pi}}$.

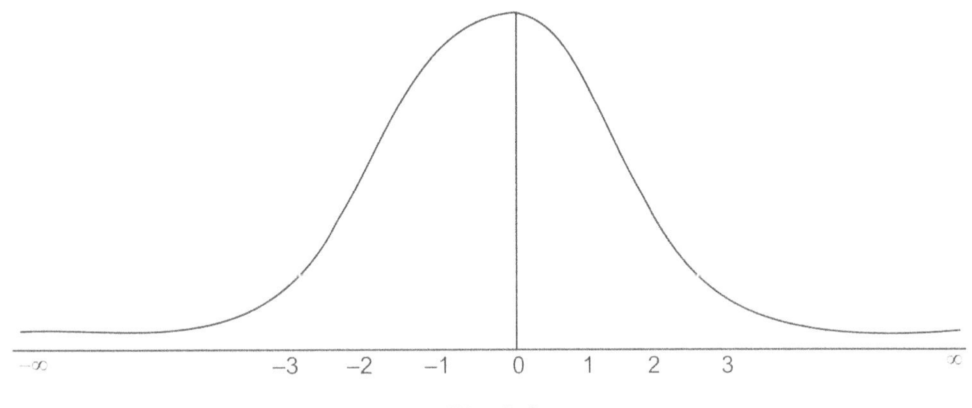

Fig. 6.4

6.8.1 Frequency Function

If N is the total frequency then the frequency function of normal distribution for variable, x is given by

$$f_r(x) = \frac{N}{\sigma\sqrt{2\pi}} e^{\frac{-(x-\mu)^2}{2\sigma^2}}$$

The frequency function is useful in finding out the expected frequencies in fitting of normal distribution.

6.8.2 Properties

(i)   The curve is bell shaped and tails of symmetrically on both sides of the mean.

(ii)   The mean, median and mode will have same value or they are equal.

(iii)   The area under the curve is divided into two equal halves by the ordinate at mean.

(iv)   The curve extends from $-\infty$ to $+\infty$.

(v)   The value or length of the ordinate at mean is equal to $\dfrac{N}{\sigma\sqrt{2\pi}}$.

(vi)   The second moment about mean $\mu_2 = \sigma^2$.

(vii)   All odd moments are equal to zero, i.e., $u_1 = u_3 = u_5 = \ldots\ldots = 0$.

(viii)   The fourth central moment, $\mu_4 = 3\sigma^4$.

(ix)   The coefficient of skewness, $\beta_1 = 0$.

(x)   The coefficient of kurtosis, $\beta_2 = 3$.

6.8.3 Distribution Function

The distribution function of the variable x is F(x) which is given by,

$$F(x) = \int_{-\infty}^{x} \frac{1}{\sigma\sqrt{2\pi}} e^{-\frac{(x-\mu)^2}{2\sigma^2}}$$

where the symbol '$\int$' indicates the integration.

F(x) gives the area under normal curve from $-\infty$ to x.

If $z = \dfrac{x-\mu}{\sigma}$, the distribution function of standard normal distribution is F(z) and is given by,

$$f(z) = \int_{-\infty}^{z} \frac{1}{\sqrt{2\pi}} e^{-\frac{1}{2}z^2}$$

For different values of z, the values of F(z) are provided in the table called Normal Probability Integral table. The values of F(z) are given in proportions and the corresponding frequencies are obtained by multiplying F(z) values with N, the total frequency.

Example : The random blood sugar of 200 patients admitted in corporate hospital is assumed to follow normal distribution with mean as 150 and standard deviation as 10.

Find the number of patients whose blood sugar is (i) between 160 and 180, (ii) below 125 and (iii) 173 and above.

Here $\mu = 150$, $\sigma = 10$

Let $x_1 = 160$ then $z_1 = \dfrac{x_1 - \mu}{\sigma} = \dfrac{160 - 150}{10} = 1.0$

$x_2 = 180$ then $z_2 = \dfrac{x_2 - \mu}{\sigma} = \dfrac{180 - 150}{10} = 3.0$

The area between 1.0 and 3.0 can be obtained by entering into probability Integral table.

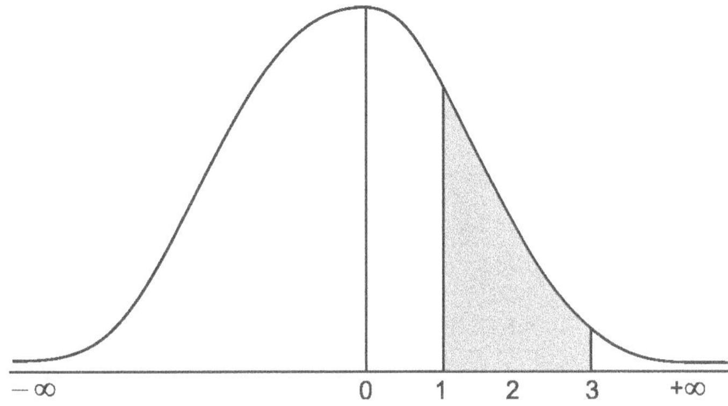

Fig. 6.5

z	Area to the left of z
1.0	$1.0 - 0.15866 = 0.841340$
3.0	$1.0 - 0.001349 = 0.998651$

The area between 3.0 and 1.0 is $(0.998651 - 0.841340) = 0.157311$

(i) The number of patients whose random blood sugar ranges from 160 to 180 is

$0.157311 \times 200 = 31.46 \simeq 32$ (approximately).

(ii) Let $x = 125$ then $z = \dfrac{125 - 150}{10} = -2.5$

The area to the left of z is obtained from the Normal Probability Integral table as:

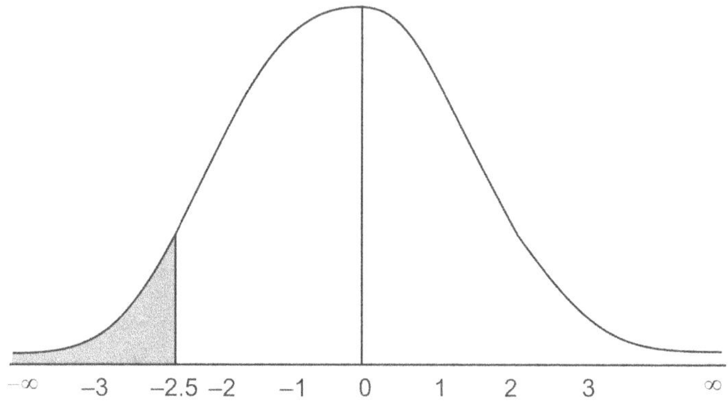

Fig. 6.6

z	Area to the left of z
–2.5	0.0062097

The number of patients whose random blood sugar is below 125 is

$$0.0062097 \times 200 = 1.24 \simeq 1 \text{ (approximately)}.$$

(iii)   Let x = 173 then $z = \dfrac{173 - 150}{10} = 2.3$

The area to the right of z is obtained by entering into the Normal Probability Integral table.

z	Area to the right of x
2.3	0.010724

$$0.010724 \times 200 = 2.14 \simeq 2 \text{ (approximately)}.$$

6.8.4   Fitting of Normal Distribution

In order to know whether the given grouped frequency distribution follows normal distribution or not, following procedure is adopted by computing mean and standard deviation. The method is illustrated with an example.

Example: The following is the grouped frequency distribution of ages of patients already admitted in Government college teaching hospital recorded on a particular day (Table 6.7).

Table 6.7

Age	Patients (f_i)	Mid-value (x_i)	$f_i x_i$	$f_i\, x_i^2$	Limits x	$z = \dfrac{x - \mu}{\sigma}$	Area to the left of Z	Area between the limits	Expected frequencies
0-10	8	5	40	200	$-\infty$	$-\infty$	0.000000	0.040930	8.2
10-20	24	15	360	5400	10	-1.74	0.040930	0.07609	15.2
20-30	20	25	500	12500	20	-1.19	0.117020	0.144070	28.8
30-40	36	35	1260	44100	30	-0.64	0.261090	0.203050	40.6
40-50	42	45	1890	85050	40	-0.09	0.464140	0.213100	42.6
50-60	38	55	2090	114950	50	0.46	0.677240	0.164100	32.8
60-70	20	65	1300	84500	60	1.00	0.841340	0.098089	19.6
70 and above	12	75	900	67500	70	1.55	0.939429	0.060571	12.1
	200		8340	414200	∞	∞	1.00000.		199.9

$$\text{Mean} = \frac{\Sigma f_i x_i}{\Sigma f_i} = \frac{8340}{200} = 41.7$$

$$\text{S.D.} = \sqrt{\frac{1}{200}\left[414200 - \frac{(8340)^2}{200}\right]} = 18.22$$

It may be noted that total of observed frequencies in column (2) and total of expected or theoretical frequencies in column (10) are almost equal. The differences between them can be tested with the help of chi-square test. If chi-square test is found not significant then the given distribution follows normal distribution and vice-versa.

Exercises

Binomial and Poisson Distributions

1. In a city 0.2 percent of population were effected by a rare disease. Find the probability that 5 persons are effected in a locality consisting of 10,000 population.

2. In a mango orchard consisting of 400 trees, 2 percent of them were effected by fruit drop disease. Find the number of trees effected by the disease, standard deviation, coefficient of skewness and coefficient of kurtosis assuming that fruit drop disease follows binomial distribution.

3. The following were the results obtained by conducting an experiment of chromosome interchanges induced by X-ray irradiation of the experiment.

Cells with K interchanges	0	1	2	3
Observed number of cells	653	266	49	15

Fit a Poisson distribution to the above data.

4. The following are the observed number of squares on a petri plate with K dark spots (counts of Bacteria) in first experiment.

Fit a Poisson distribution to it.

K counts of bacteria	0	1	2	3	4	5
Observed number of squares	4	12	20	24	18	2

5. Each strip of 10 tablets each were tested for relief in 100 families who were suffering from cold and cough. The following is the distribution of families who were relieved from cold and cough with respect to the number of tablets consumed.

No. of tables consumed	1	2	3	4	5	6	7	8
No. of families	4	10	14	18	20	16	10	8

Fit a Binomial distribution to the above data.

6. The number of accidents in a year to taxi drivers in a city follows Poisson distribution with mean equal to 4. Out of 500 taxi drivers, find approximately the number of drivers with:

(i) no accidents in a year   (ii) more than 4 in a year.

7. The number of people affected by AIDS disease in a year in a locality follows Poisson distribution with mean equal to 10. Out of 10000 people in a locality, find approximately the number of people with:

(i) No incidence in a year,   (ii) more than 4 in a year.

Normal Distribution

1. The following is the data on blood sugar level in 50 patients in a hospital :
    120, 130, 160, 180, 140, 190, 136, 110, 108,
    136, 132, 130, 138, 142, 130, 164, 160, 144,
    130, 112, 116, 164, 170, 172, 118, 114, 171,
    156, 150, 138, 151, 132, 117, 140, 146, 144,
    180, 174, 171, 170, 116, 126, 122, 125, 128,
    119, 130, 127, 128 and 143.

    Verify the above data on blood sugar level follows normal distribution using all the properties of normal distribution.

2. The ages of patients in a Government teaching hospitals assumed to follow normal distribution with mean age as 45 years and standard deviation as 16 years. In a hospital consisting of 250 patients find the number of patients:

   (i) having age between 35 to 45,

   (ii) above 60 years,

   (iii) below 40 years.

3. The following is the distribution of days with respect to number of Gelusil Mps tablet strips sold by a medical shop in a city.

No. of strips sold	0-4	4-8	8-12	12-16	16-20	20-24
No. of days	6	10	24	32	18	10

   Fit a normal distribution to the above data.

4. Fit a normal distribution to the following distribution of weights of patients in a hospital on a particular day:

Weight (kg)	0-10	10-20	20-30	30-40	40-50	50-60	60-70	70 & above
Patients	8	12	24	30	34	40	22	20

5. The antibiotic production of 200 pharmaceutical companies follows normal distribution with mean number of boxes produced per day is 80 with a standard deviation of 10 boxes. Find the number of companies producing:

   (i)   between 70 and 90 boxes,

   (ii) above 90 boxes, and

   (iii) below 70 boxes.

6. In a sampling a large number of parts manufactured by a machine, the mean number of defective in a sample of 20 is 2. Out of 1000 such samples, how many would be expected to contain at least 3 defective parts.

7. The mean and standard deviation of the marks obtained by 1000 students in an examination are respectively 34.4 and 16.5. Assuming the normality of distribution, find the approximate number of students expected to obtain marks between 30 and 60.

8. In a bombing action there is 50% chance that any bomb will strike the target. Two direct hits are needed to destroy the target completely. How many bombs are required to be dropped to give a 90% chance or better completely destroying the target.

9. The mean height of 500 students is 151 cm and the standard deviation is 15 cm. Assuming that heights are normally distributed, find how many students heights lie between 120 and 155 cm.

CHAPTER 7

Correlation and Regression

7.1 Correlation

If variable x changes in sympathy with other variable y, then it is said that x and y variables are related or correlated. In other words it can be said that there exists correlation between the two variables x and y. For example, if weight increases in individuals as height increases then it can be said that 'height' and 'weight' variables are correlated. If both variables change in same direction then it is known as positive correlation and if they change in opposite direction then it is called negative correlation. This can be depicted in Fig. 7.1 and 7.2, respectively.

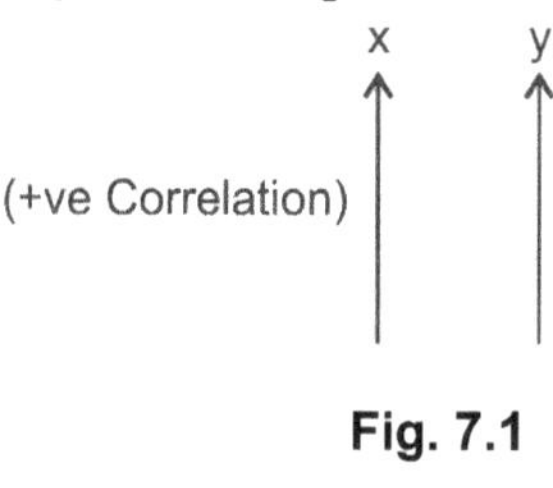

Fig. 7.1

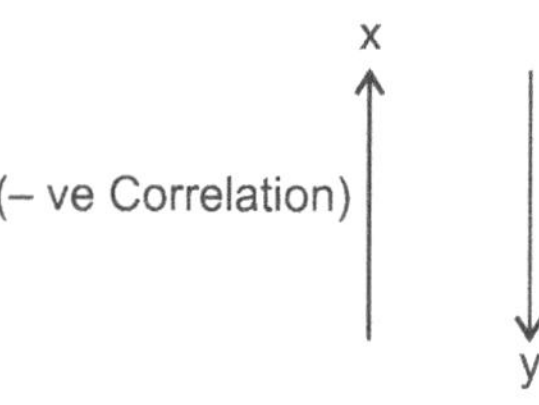

Fig. 7.2

In order to know whether the two variables are correlated or not this can be observed with the help of graph. The sample data of related variables can be plotted in a graph sheet as shown in Fig. 7.3.

The diagram shown in Fig. 7.3 is called scatter diagram as the bivariate points are scattered. If the scattered points indicate a straight line, a line can be drawn in between

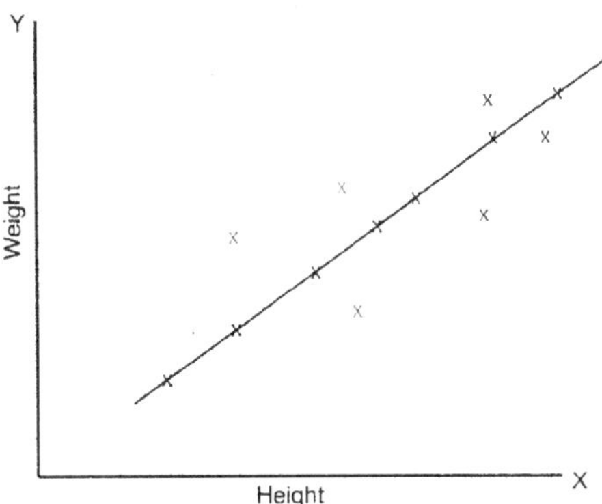

Fig. 7.3 Scatter diagram.

the points then it is known as 'linear correlation'. If the points indicate a curve instead of a straight line then it is called 'non-linear correlation'.

If the scatter diagram indicates square or circle then it is can be concluded that there is no correlation between the two variables as shown in Fig. 7.4 and Fig. 7.5, respectively.

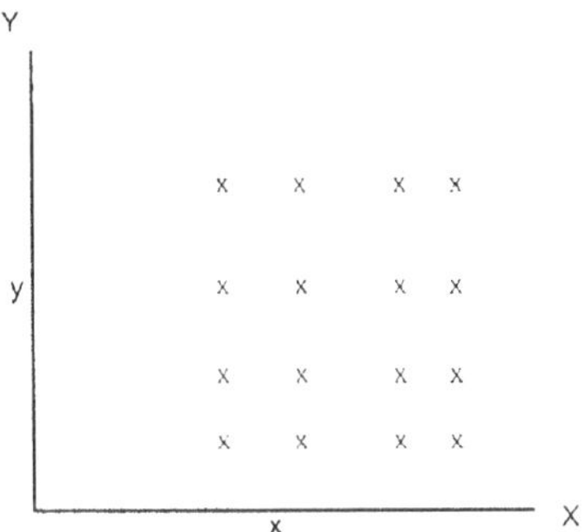

Fig. 7.4 No correlaton.

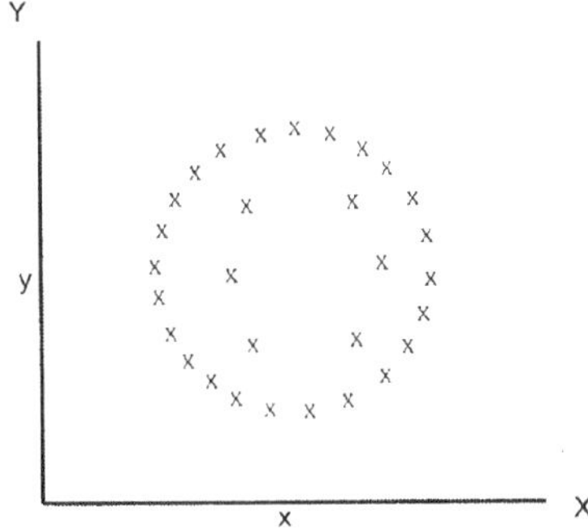

Fig. 7.5 No correlaton.

The correlation can be positive or negative. If body weight increases when height increases then it is a positive correlation. If the production of medicine increases in a pharmaceutical company and the corresponding price decreases over a period of time then it is an example of negative correlation.

The amount of correlation between the related variables or the extent of associationship between them is called coefficient of correlation or correlation coefficient. This is denoted by 'r' which is called as the sample linear correlation coefficient and is given by,

$$r = \frac{\text{covariance}(xy)}{\sqrt{\text{variance}(x)\,\text{variance}(y)}}$$

$$= \frac{\sum_{i=1}^{n}(x_i - \bar{x})(y_i - \bar{y})}{\sqrt{\sum_{i=1}^{n}(x_i - \bar{x})^2 \sum_{i=1}^{n}(y_i - \bar{y})^2}}$$

$$= \frac{\sum_{i=1}^{n} x_i y_i - \dfrac{\left(\sum_{i=1}^{n} x_i\right)\left(\sum_{i=1}^{n} y_i\right)}{n}}{\sqrt{\left[\sum_{i=1}^{n} x_i^2 - \dfrac{(\Sigma x_i)^2}{n}\right]\left[\sum_{i=1}^{n} y_i^2 - \dfrac{\left(\sum_{i=1}^{n} y_i\right)^2}{n}\right]}} \,,$$

where 'Σ' indicates summation over n pairs of observations of x and y variables, r always lies between -1 and 1. If r = 1 then it is called perfect positive correlation between the two variables, if r = -1 then it is perfect negative correlation and if r = 0 there exists no correlation between two variables. The perfect positive or perfect negative correlations are depicted in Figs. 7.6 and 7.7, respectively.

In the above Figs. 7.6 and 7.7 all points will lie on the line.

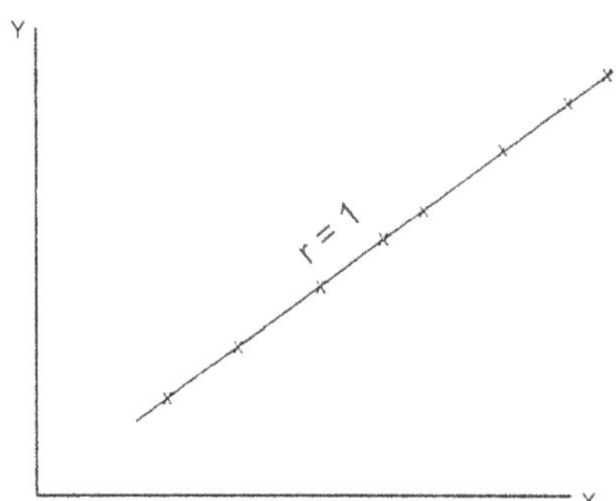

Fig. 7.6 Perfect positive correlation.

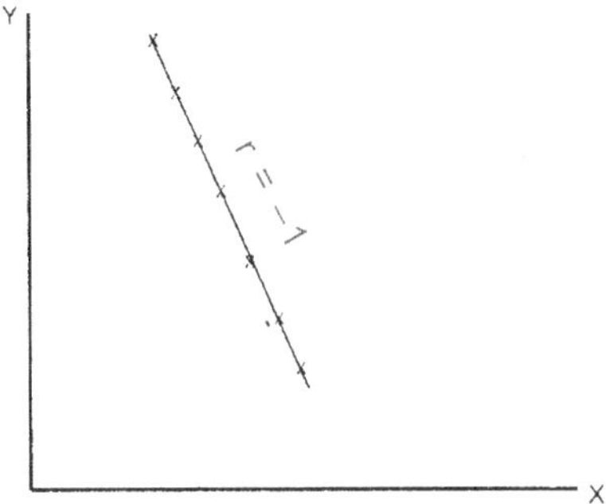

Fig. 7.7 Perfect negative correlation.

7.1.1 Test of significance

The correlation coefficient can be tested for its significance with the help of student's t-test. Sometime the correlation coefficient value may be high but it may not be found significant due to small number of observations.

Null Hypothesis, H_0: p = 0,

where p is called the population correlation coefficient.

Alternative Hypothesis, $H_1 : \rho \neq 0$

$$t = \frac{|r|}{\sqrt{\dfrac{1-r^2}{(n-2)}}}$$

Conclusion

If t (calculated) value > t (tabulated) value with (n – 2) degrees of freedom at chosen level of significance, the null hypothesis is rejected and alternative hypothesis, H_1 is accepted. That is there is significant correlation between the two variables. Otherwise, null hypothesis is accepted.

It may be noted that if correlation coefficient is computed even though two variables are not related then it is called spurious correlation.

Example 1

The following is the data on protein content (percent) in diet and gain in weight (100 gm) of 8 pre-school going children in tribal area. The gain in weights were recorded after 3 months of administration of diet.

Protein	2.0	3.0	4.0	5.0	5.5	6.0	7.0	7.5
Weights	8	10	14	18	22	25	28	35

Compute the correlation coefficient and test its significance at probability level 0.05.

Table 7.1

S.No.	x_i	y_i	$(x_i-\bar{x})$	$(y_i-\bar{y})$	$(x_i-\bar{x})(y_i-\bar{y})$	$\Sigma(x_i-\bar{x})^2$	$(y_i-\bar{y})^2$	$x_i\,y_1$	x^2	y^2
1	2.0	8	− 3	− 12	36.0	9	144	16.0	4	64
2	3.0	10	− 2	− 10	20.0	4	100	30.0	9	100
3	4.0	14	− 1	− 6	6.0	1	36	56.0	16	196
4	5.0	18	0	− 2	0	0	4	90.0	25	324
5	5.5	22	0.5	2	1.0	0.25	4	121.0	30.25	484
6	6.0	25	1.0	5	5.0	1.00	25	150.0	36.00	625
7	7.0	28	2.0	8	16.0	4.00	64	196.0	49.00	84
8	7.5	35	2.5	15	37.5	6.25	225	262.5	56.25	1225
Total	40.0	160			121.5	25.50	602	921.5	225.20	3802
	5.0	20								

$$\bar{x} = \frac{40}{8} = 5, \quad \bar{y} = \frac{160}{8} = 20$$

$$r = \frac{\Sigma(x_i-\bar{x})(y_i-\bar{y})}{\sqrt{\Sigma(x_i-\bar{x})^2\,\Sigma(y_i-\bar{y})^2}}$$

$$= \frac{121.5}{\sqrt{25.5\times602}} = \frac{121.5}{123.90} = 0.98$$

Alternatively,

$$r = \frac{\Sigma x_i y_i - \dfrac{(\Sigma x_i)(\Sigma y_i)}{n}}{\sqrt{\left[\Sigma x_i^2 - \dfrac{(\Sigma x_i)^2}{n}\right]\left[\Sigma y_i^2 - \dfrac{(\Sigma y_i)^2}{n}\right]}}$$

$$= \frac{921.5 - \dfrac{(40)(160)}{8}}{\sqrt{\left[225.5 - \dfrac{(40)^2}{8}\right]\left[3802 - \dfrac{(160)^2}{8}\right]}}$$

$$= \frac{121.5}{\sqrt{25.5\times602}} = \frac{121.5}{123.90} = 0.98$$

The correlation coefficient between protein content in diet and gain in weight of tribal children was found to be 0.98. Though it is very high correlation which is nearer to 1 but it needs to be tested for its significance as it was obtained from the results of only 8 children.

Test of Significance

Null hypothesis H_o $\rho = 0$

Alternative hypothesis H_1 $\rho \neq 0$

$$t = \frac{|r|}{\sqrt{\dfrac{1-r^2}{(n-2)}}}$$

$$t = \frac{0.98}{\sqrt{\dfrac{1-(0.98)^2}{(8-2)}}} = \frac{0.98}{0.98} = 12.25$$

Conclusion

Here t (calculated) value i.e., 12.25 > t (tabulated) value i.e., 2.447 with (8 – 2) degrees of freedom at 5 percent level of significance or probability level 0.05. Therefore H_0 is rejected and H_1 is accepted. Hence it can be concluded that there is significant correlation between protein content in diet and gain in weight of children.

Example 2

The following is the data on the dose of medicine administered to patients and the days to recover from illness. Compute the correlation between the two variables and test its significance at probability level 0.01.

Dose (mg)	100	150	200	250	300	500
Days to recover	18	15	10	8	6	3

Table 7.2

S.No.	Dose x_i	Days y_i	$(x_i - \bar{x})$	$(y_i - \bar{y})$	$(x_i - \bar{x})$ $(y_i - \bar{y})$	$\Sigma(x_i - \bar{x})^2$	$(y_i - \bar{y})^2$	$x_i y_i$	y_i^2	x_i^2
1	100	18	– 150	8	– 1200	2,2500	64	10000	324	10000
2	150	15	– 100	5	– 500	10000	25	2250	225	22500
3	200	10	– 50	0	0	2500	0	2000	100	40000
4	250	8	0	– 2	0	0	4	2000	64	62500
5	300	6	50	– 4	– 200	2500	16	1800	36	90000
6	500	3	250	– 7	– 1750	62500	49	1500	9	250000
	1500	60			–3650	100000	158	11350	758	475000

$$\bar{x} = \frac{1500}{6} = 250, \quad \bar{y} = \frac{60}{6} = 10$$

$$r = \frac{\Sigma(x_i - \bar{x})(y_i - \bar{y})}{\sqrt{\Sigma(x_i - \bar{x})^2 \, \Sigma(y_i - \bar{y})^2}}$$

$$= \frac{-3650}{\sqrt{100000 \times 158}} = \frac{-3650}{3974.92} = -0.92$$

Alternatively,

$$r = \frac{\Sigma x_i y_i = \dfrac{(\Sigma x_i)(\Sigma y_i)}{n}}{\sqrt{\left[\Sigma x_1^2 - \dfrac{(\Sigma x_i)^2}{n}\right]\left[\Sigma y_i - \dfrac{(\Sigma y_i)^2}{n}\right]}}$$

$$= \frac{11350 - \dfrac{(1550)(60)}{6}}{\sqrt{\left[475000 - \dfrac{(1500)^2}{6}\right]\left[758 - \dfrac{(60)^2}{6}\right]}}$$

$$= \frac{-3650}{\sqrt{100000 \times 158}} = -0.92$$

It can be seen that both methods will give same result of r and the one which is convenient can be chosen by the individual.

Test of Significance

Null hypothesis $\qquad$ $H_o \;\; \rho = 0$

Alternative hypothesis $\quad$ $H_1 \;\; \rho \neq 0$

$$t = \frac{|r|}{\sqrt{\dfrac{1-r^2}{(n-2)}}}$$

$$t = \frac{|-0.92|}{\sqrt{\dfrac{1-(0.92)^2}{(6-2)}}} = \frac{0.92}{0.20} = 4.6$$

Conclusion

Here t (calculated) value i.e., 4.6 < t (tabulated) value i.e. 4.604 with (6 – 2) degrees of freedom at probability level 0.01. Therefore there is no significant correlation between the two variables.

Example 3

The following is the data on head and body weights of 10 insects (*drosophila melanagoster*).

Head weight (mg)	18	20	25	28	19	27	30	34	36	33
Body weight (mg)	52	54	60	62	59	63	65	70	78	77

Compute the correlation coefficient between 'head' and 'body' weights of insects and test its significance.

Table 7.3

S.No.	Head Weight (x_i)	Body Weight (y_i)	$x_i y_i$	x_i^2	y_i^2	$(x_i - \bar{x})$	$(y_i - \bar{y})$	$(x_i - \bar{x})(y_i - \bar{y})$	$(x_i - \bar{x})^2$	$(y_i - \bar{y})^2$
1	18	52	936	324	2704	− 9	− 12	108	81	144
2	20	54	1080	400	2916	− 7	− 10	70	49	100
3	25	60	1500	625	3600	− 2	− 4	8	4	16
4	28	62	1736	784	3844	1	− 2	− 2	1	4
5	19	59	1121	361	3481	− 8	− 5	40	64	25
6	27	63	1701	729	3969	0	− 1	0	0	1
7	30	65	1950	900	4225	3	1	3	9	1
8	34	70	2380	1156	4900	7	6	42	49	36
9	36	78	2808	1296	6084	9	14	126	81	196
10	33	77	2541	1089	5929	6	13	78	36	169
	270	640	17753	7664	41652			473	374	692
Mean	27	64								

$$\bar{x} = \frac{270}{10} = 27, \quad \bar{y} = \frac{640}{10} = 64$$

$$r = \frac{\Sigma(x_i - \bar{x})(y_i - \bar{y})}{\sqrt{\Sigma(x_i - \bar{x})^2 \Sigma(y_i - \bar{y})^2}}$$

$$= \frac{473}{\sqrt{374 \times 692}} = \frac{473}{508.73} = 0.93$$

Alternatively,

$$r = \dfrac{\Sigma x_i y_i - \dfrac{(\Sigma x_i)(\Sigma y_i)}{n}}{\sqrt{\left[\Sigma x_i^2 - \dfrac{(\Sigma x_i)^2}{n}\right]\left[\Sigma y_i^2 = \dfrac{(\Sigma y_i)^2}{n}\right]}}$$

$$= \dfrac{17753 - \dfrac{(270)(640)}{10}}{\sqrt{\left[7664 - \dfrac{(270)^2}{10}\left[41652 - \dfrac{(640)^2}{10}\right]\right]}}$$

$$= \dfrac{473}{\sqrt{374 \times 692}} = \dfrac{473}{508.73} = 0.93$$

Test of Significance

Null hypothesis $\qquad$ H_o $\rho = 0$

Alternative hypothesis $\quad$ H_1 $\rho \neq 0$

$$t = \dfrac{|r|}{\sqrt{\dfrac{1-r^2}{(n-2)}}}$$

$$= \dfrac{0.93}{\sqrt{\dfrac{1-(0.93)^2}{(10-2)}}} = \dfrac{0.93}{0.13} = 7.15$$

Conclusion

Here t (calculated) value i.e., 7.15 > t (tabulated) value i.e. 3.355 with (10 − 2) degrees of freedom at probability level 0.01. Therefore the null hypothesis H_0 is rejected. Hence it can be concluded that there is significant correlation between head and body weights.

7.2 Regression

Galton while studying the heights of grand-fathers, fathers and sons, found that sons, heights were more closely associated or related to grandfather's heights than father's heights. This type of backward relationship he termed as 'regression'. Here son's height is considered as dependent variable and grandfather's height is independent variable. The points plotted on a graph sheet with son's height on Y-axis and grandfathers height on X-axis and if the scatter diagram indicates straight line then it can be said that there exists linear regression between son's heights and grandfather's heights. This relationship can be depicted in Fig. 7.8.

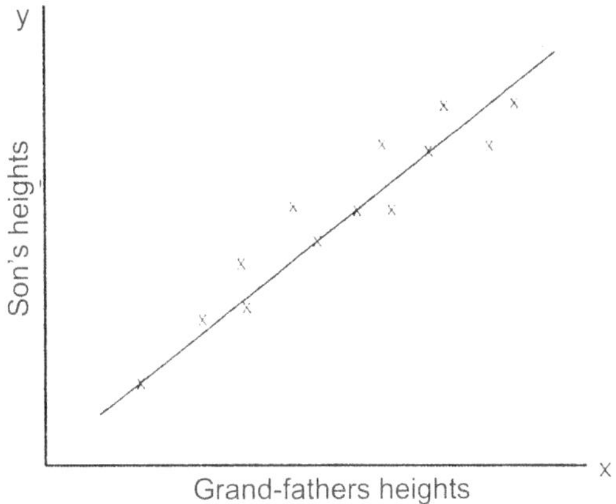

Fig. 7.8 Linear Regression.

If the relation between dependent and independent variables shows a curve on scatter diagram then it is called curvilinear regression. This can be observed in Fig. 7.9.

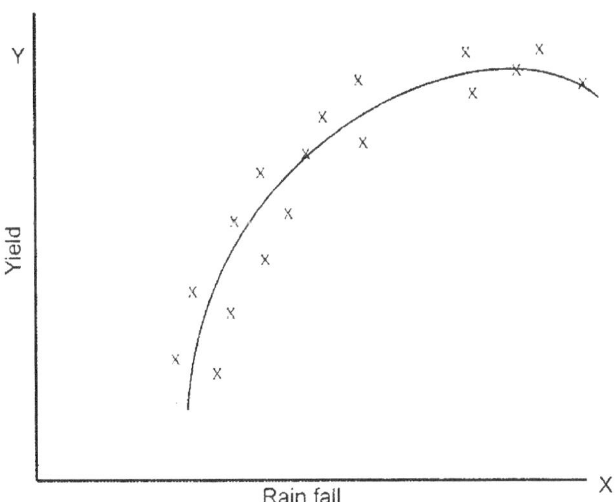

Fig. 7.9 Curvilinear regression.

From Fig. 7.9 it can be observed that the yield of crop is increasing as the rainfall is increasing up to certain point and then yield is decreasing even though rainfall is increasing.

The equation of a straight line in Fig. 7.8 for linear regression is given by,

$$y = a + bx$$

where y is dependent variable (effect), x is independent variable (cause), a = intercept or constant and b = regression coefficient of y on x (slope)

$$b = \frac{covariance(xy)}{variance(x)}$$

$$b = \frac{\Sigma(x_i - \bar{x})(y_i - \bar{y})}{\Sigma(x_i - \bar{x})^2}$$

$$= \frac{\Sigma x_i y_i - \dfrac{(\Sigma x_i)(\Sigma y_i)}{n}}{\Sigma x_i^2 - \dfrac{(\Sigma x_i)^2}{n}}$$

where n = number of paired observations

$$a = \bar{y} - b\bar{x}$$

where $\qquad \bar{y} = \dfrac{\Sigma y_i}{n}$ = mean of y

$$\bar{x} = \frac{\Sigma x_i}{n} = \text{mean of x}$$

The value of b measures the change in dependent variable for a unit change in independent variable. For example, if x is the dose of medicine to be administered to patient and y is the number of days to recover from illness then b measures the number of days reduced for recovering from illness if dose is increased by say 100 mg at a time.

Sometimes if both variables x and y are dependent on each other and the rate of change is to be calculated. If one is dependent and the other is independent then two regression equations will be fitted.

If x is dependent variable and y is independent variable, then the regression equation of x on y is given by,

$$x = a' + b'y$$

where
$$b' = \frac{\text{covariance}(xy)}{\text{variance}(y)}$$

$$b' = \frac{\Sigma(x_i - \overline{x})(y_i - \overline{y})}{\Sigma(y_i - \overline{y})^2}$$

$$= \frac{\Sigma x_i y_i - \dfrac{(\Sigma x_i)(\Sigma y_i)}{n}}{\Sigma y_i^2 - \dfrac{(\Sigma y_i)^2}{n}}$$

and
$$a' = \overline{x} - b'\,\overline{y}$$

where
$$\overline{x} = \frac{\Sigma x_i}{n} = \text{mean of } x$$

$$\overline{y} = \frac{\Sigma y_i}{n} = \text{mean of } y$$

b' is called the regression coefficient of x on y and a' is called the intercept or constant. The two regression lines y on x and x on y are shown in Fig. 7.10. The point of intersection of two regression lines is $(\overline{x}, \overline{y})$.

$$r = \sqrt{b.b'}$$

The geometric mean of two regression coefficients is the correlation coefficient between the two variables.

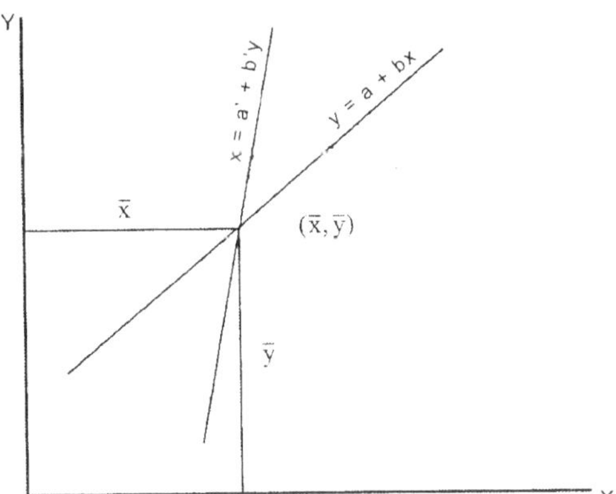

Fig. 7.10 Regression lines.

If two regression lines intersect at right angles then r = 0 and is depicted in Fig. 7.11.

If two regression lines coincide on positive side then r = 1 and is shown in Fig. 7.12.

If two regression lines coincide on negative side then r = – 1 and is depicted in Fig. 7.13.

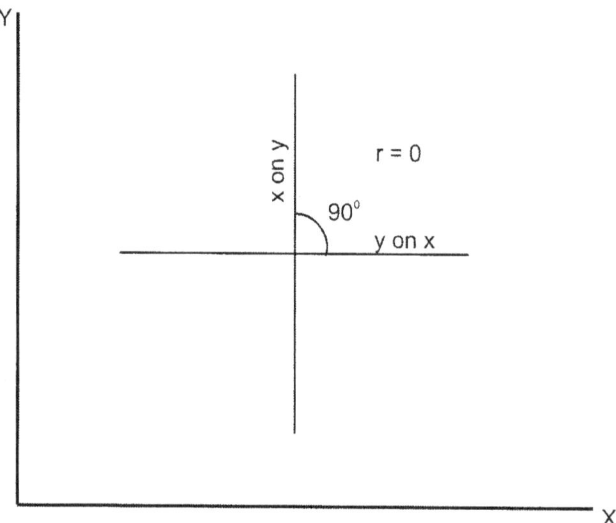

Fig. 7.11 Two regression lines.

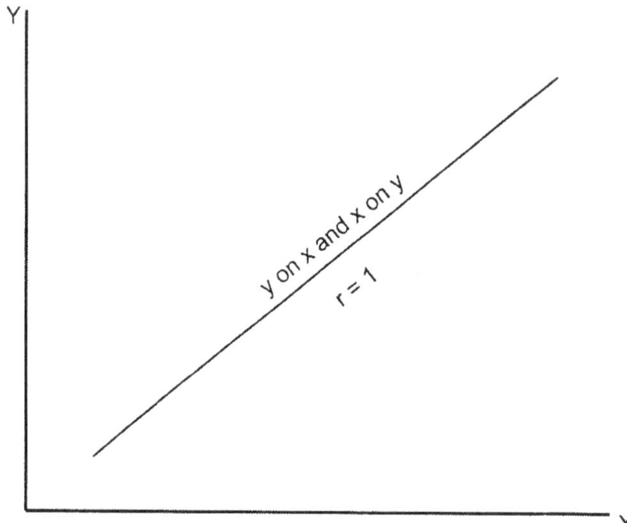

Fig. 7.12 Regression lines on Positive side.

Test of significance of b

Null hypothesis, $H_0 : \beta = 0$

Alternative hypothesis, $H_1 : \beta \neq 0$

where 'β' is known as the population regression coefficient of y on x

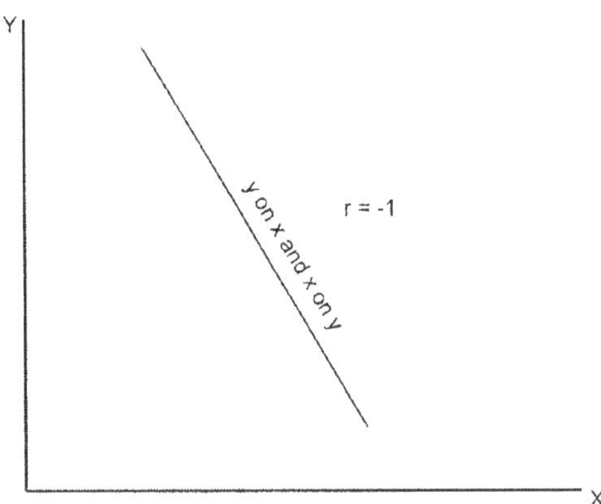

Fig. 7.13 Regression lines on negative side.

$$t = \frac{|b|}{SE \text{ of } b}$$

$$= \frac{|b|}{\sqrt{\dfrac{\Sigma(y_i - \bar{y})^2 - b^2\,\Sigma(x_i - \bar{x})^2}{(n-2)\Sigma(x_i - \bar{x})^2}}}$$

where n is the number of paired observations in the sample.

Conclusion

If t (calculated) value > t (tabulated) value with (n – 2) degrees of freedom at chosen level of significance, the null hypothesis is rejected. Otherwise it is accepted.

If null hypothesis is rejected then it can be concluded that there is significant regression of y on x.

7.2.1   Test of significance of b'

Null hypothesis, $H_0 : \beta' = 0$

Alternative hypothesis, $H_1 : \beta' \neq 0$

where β' is the regression coefficient of x on y,

$$t = \frac{|b'|}{SE \text{ of } b'}$$

$$= \frac{b'}{\sqrt{\dfrac{\Sigma(x_i - \bar{x})^2 - b'^2 \Sigma(y_i - \bar{y})^2}{(n-2)\Sigma(y_i - \bar{y})^2}}}$$

Conclusion : Same as in the case of b.

7.3   Regression vs Correlation

In correlation, dependent and independent variables need not be identified whereas it is necessary in the case of regression. Correlation coefficient is independent of units whereas regression coefficient is measured in units of dependent variable. Correlation coefficient always lie between -1 and 1 whereas regression coefficient can take any value between $-\infty$ and $+\infty$.

From regression coefficient the dependent variable value can be predicted given the value of independent variable but that is not possible in the case of correlation.

r^2 is known as coefficient of determination and $\sqrt{1-r^2}$ is called coefficient of alienation. The sign of correlation coefficient and both regression coefficients is same as all the three have same covariance value.

Example

The following are the data on 'chest' and 'arm' circumference of 8 tribal children in the age group between *5* to 10 years.

Circumference	1	2	3	4	5	6	7	8
Arm (cm)	30	28	22	23	27	20	18	16
Chest (cm)	10	9	4	6	7	4	5	3

Compute the correlation coefficient and also fit both the regression equations and the point of intersection of two regression lines. Also test the significance of correlation coefficient and regression coefficients.

Table 7.4

S.No.	Chest (x_i)	Arm (y_i)	$x_i y_i$	x_i^2	y_i^2	$(x_i - \bar{x})$	$(y_i - \bar{y})$	$(x_i - \bar{x})(y_i - \bar{y})$	$(x_i - \bar{x})^2$	$(y_i - \bar{y})^2$
1	30	10	300	900	100	7	4	28	49	16
2	28	9	252	784	81	5	3	15	25	9
3	22	4	88	484	16	-1	-2	2	1	4
4	23	6	138	529	36	0	0	0	0	0
5	27	7	189	729	49	4	1	4	16	1
6	20	4	80	400	16	-3	-2	6	9	4
7	18	5	90	324	25	-5	-1	5	25	1
8	16	3	48	256	9	-7	-3	21	49	9
Total	184	48	1185	4406	332			81	174	44
Mean	23	6								

$$x = \frac{\Sigma x_i}{n} = \frac{184}{8} = 23, \quad \overline{y} = \frac{\Sigma y_i}{n} = \frac{48}{8} = 6$$

$$r = \frac{\Sigma(x_i - \overline{x})(y_i - \overline{y})}{\sqrt{\Sigma(x_i - \overline{x})^2\,\Sigma(y_i - \overline{y})^2}}$$

$$= \frac{81}{\sqrt{174 \times 44}} = \frac{81}{87.5} = 0.93$$

Alternatively,

$$r = \frac{\Sigma x_i y_i - \dfrac{(\Sigma x_i)(\Sigma y_i)}{n}}{\sqrt{\left[\Sigma x_i^2 - \dfrac{(\Sigma x_i)^2}{n}\right]\left[\Sigma y_i^2 - \dfrac{(\Sigma y_i)^2}{n}\right]}}$$

$$= \frac{81}{\sqrt{[174 \times 44]}} = \frac{81}{87.50} = 0.93$$

Test of significance

Null hypothesis, $\qquad$ $H_0 : \rho = 0$

Alternative hypothesis, $\;$ $H_1 : \rho \neq 0$

$$t = \frac{|r|}{\sqrt{\dfrac{1-r^2}{(n-2)}}}$$

$$= \frac{0.93}{\sqrt{\dfrac{(1-(0.93)^2)}{(0.82)}}} = \frac{0.93}{0.15} = 6.2$$

Here t (calculated) value i.e., 6.2 > t (tabulated) value i.e., 3.707 with (8 – 2) degrees of freedom at 1 percent level of significance. Therefore there is significant correlation between 'chest' and 'arm' circumference.

Regression equation of y on x :

$$b = \frac{\Sigma(x_i - \overline{x})(y_i - \overline{y})}{\Sigma(x_i - \overline{x})^2}$$

$$= \frac{81}{174} = 0.47$$

The regression coefficient b = 0.47 indicates that if there is one cm increase in arm circumference then there will be an increase of 0.47 cm in chest circumference.

$$a = \bar{y} - b\bar{x}$$

$$= 6 - 0.47 \times 23 = -4.81$$

The fitted regression equation of y on x is

$$y = -4.81 + 0.47\, x$$

The regression equation of x on y :

$$b' = \frac{\Sigma(x_i - \bar{x})(y_i - \bar{y})}{\Sigma(y_i - \bar{y})^2}$$

$$= \frac{81}{44} = 1.84$$

The regression coefficient b' = 1.84 indicates that if there is 1 cm increase in arm circumference there will be an increase of 1.84 cm in chest circumference.

$$a' = \bar{x} - b'\bar{y}$$

$$= 23 - 1.84 \times 6 = 11.96$$

The fitted regression equation of x on y is

$$x = 11.96 + 1.84\, y$$

$$r = \sqrt{bb'}$$

$$= \sqrt{0.47 \times 1.84} = 0.93$$

The point of intersection of two regression lines,

$$y = -4.81 + 0.47\, x$$

$$x = 11.96 + 1.84\, y$$

$$y = -4.81 + 0.47\,(11.96 + 1.84\, y)$$

$$= .81 + 0.86\, y$$

$$y - 0.86y = 0.81$$

$$0.14\, y = 0.81$$

$$y = \frac{0.81}{0.14} = 5.79$$

The value obtained here 5.79 is due to rounding off figures up to second decimal place and is close to the actual value $\bar{y} = 6$.

Substitute y = 5.79 in the regression equation

$$x = 11.96 + 1.84\, y,$$

$$x = 11.96 + 1.84\,(5.79)$$

$$= 22.61$$

Therefore $\bar{x} = 22.61$

Here also $\bar{x}$ value obtained as 22.61 due to rounding off figures up to second decimal place which is close to actual value $\bar{x} = 23$.

Test of significance of b :

Null hypothesis, $H_0 : \beta = 0$

Alternative hypothesis, $H_1 : \beta \neq 0$

$$t = \frac{b}{SE \text{ of } b}$$

$$= \frac{0.47}{\sqrt{\dfrac{44 - (0.47)^2 \times 174}{(8-2) \times 174}}}$$

$$= \frac{0.47}{\sqrt{\dfrac{5.5634}{6 \times 174}}} = \frac{0.47}{0.07} = 6.71$$

Conclusion

Here t (calculated) value i.e., 6.71 > t (tabulated) value i.e., 3.707 with (8–2) degrees of freedom at 1 per cent level of significance. Therefore null hypothesis is rejected. Hence it can be concluded that there is significant regression of 'arm circumference' on 'chest circumference'.

Test of significance of b′ :

Null hypothesis, $H_0 : \beta' = 0$

Alternative hypothesis, $H_1 : \beta' \neq 0$

$$t = \frac{1.84}{\sqrt{\dfrac{174 - (1.84)^2 \times 44}{(8-2) \times 44}}}$$

$$= \frac{1.84}{\sqrt{\dfrac{25.03}{264}}} = \frac{1.84}{0.31} = 5.94$$

Conclusion

Here t (calculated) value i.e., 5.94 > t (tabulated) value i.e., 3.707 with (8–2) degrees of freedom at 1 per cent level of significance. Hence it can be concluded that there is significant regression of 'chest circumference' on 'arm circumference.'

Example 2

The following is the data on patients with respect to their age (x) and number of days of convalescence (y) in fever hospital.

Age	64	56	50	48	46	35	38	31
Days	18	12	10	9	6	5	8	4

Fit the regression equation of number of days of convalescence and age of patients and test the regression coefficient at probability level 0.05 and estimate the days of convalescence when the age is 60.

Table 7.5

S.No.	Age (x_i)	Days (y_i)	$x_i y_i$	x_i^2	$(x_i - \bar{x})$	$(y_i - \bar{y})$	$(x_i - \bar{x})(y_i - \bar{y})$	$(x_i - \bar{x})^2$	$(y_i - \bar{y})^2$
1	64	18	1152	4096	18	9	162	324	81
2	56	12	672	3136	10	3	30	100	9
3	50	10	500	2500	4	1	4	16	1
4	48	9	432	2304	2	0	0	4	0
5	46	6	276	2116	0	− 3	0	0	9
6	35	5	175	1225	− 11	− 4	44	121	16
7	38	8	304	1444	− 8	− 1	8	64	1
8	31	4	124	961	− 15	− 5	75	225	25
Total	368	72	3635	17782			323	854	142
Mean	46	9							

$$\bar{x} = \frac{\Sigma x_i}{n} = \frac{368}{8} = 46, \quad \bar{y} = \frac{\Sigma y_i}{n} = \frac{72}{8} = 9$$

$$b = \frac{\Sigma(x_i - \bar{x})(y_i - \bar{y})}{\Sigma(x_i - \bar{x})^2}$$

$$= \frac{323}{854} = 0.38$$

$$a = \bar{y} - b\bar{x}$$

$$= 9 - 0.38 \times 46 = -8.48$$

The fitted regression equation is

$$y = -8.48 + 0.38\, x$$

From the value of regression coefficient $b = 0.38$, it can be inferred that if the age increases by one year there will be an increase of 0.38 days for convalescence.

If age 60, the estimate of number of days of convalescence is given as

$$y = -8.48 + 0.38 \times 60$$

$$= 14.32$$

The number of days required for convalescence is 14.32 when the age of patient is 60 years.

Test of significance of b

Null hypothesis, $\qquad H_0 : \beta = 0$

Alternative hypothesis, $\quad H_1 : \beta \neq 0$

$$t = \frac{0.38}{\sqrt{\dfrac{142 - (0.38)^2 \times 854}{(8-2) \times 854}}}$$

$$= \frac{0.38}{\sqrt{\dfrac{18.6824}{6 \times 854}}} = \frac{0.38}{0.06} = 6.33$$

Conclusion

Here t (calculated) value i.e., 6.33 > t (tabulated) value i.e., 2.447 with (8 –2) degrees of freedom at 5 per cent level of significance. Therefore the null hypothesis is rejected. Hence it can be concluded that there is significant regression of number of days of convalescence on age of patients.

Exercises

1. Find the correlation coefficient between x and y for the given values.

x	1	2	3	4	5	6	7	8	9	10
y	10	12	16	28	25	35	41	49	40	50

2. Two random variables have the regression lines with equations $3x + 2y = 26$ and $6x + y = 31$. Find the mean values and the correlation between x and y.

3. Find the correlation coefficient between x and y for the given data.

x	78	89	97	69	59	79	68	57
y	125	137	156	112	107	138	123	108

4. The regression equations of two variables x and y are $x = 0.7y + 5.2$, $y = 0.3x + 2.8$. Find the means of the variables and the correlation between them.

5. The following are the percentage of survival of coconut seedlings and depth of plantation (cm) in 10 gardens.

Depth (cm)	35	54	62	68	74	81	90	112	124	100
Survival (%)	41	48	52	54	60	65	70	74	80	76

Fit the regression equation of survival percentage of seedlings on depth of planting and estimate the survival percentage when the depth of plantation is 110 cm.

6. Fit the regression equation of yield on average number of tillers of 10 paddy samples and also find the correlation coefficient between them and test its significance.

Yield (10 gm)	13	8	9	14	16	20	24	22	18	24
Average number of tillers	4.4	3.5	4.0	5.6	6.0	8.2	9.0	8.6	7.2	8.1

7. The following are the marks obtained by 10 students in mid-term and final examinations.

Marks	1	2	3	4	5	6	7	8	9	10
Mid-term	60	56	82	74	89	70	68	94	90	67
Final	70	64	78	72	80	76	56	86	84	74

Find the correlation coefficient between mid-term and final examination marks and also fit the regression equation of final examination marks on mid-term examination and test the significance of correlation and regression coefficients.

8. The following are the data on 'heights' and weights of 10 male children admitted in hospital.

Height (cm)	143	140	139	132	125	138	136	128	139	142
Weight (kg)	40	42	38	37	32	34	39	30	41	43

Fit both the regression equations of weight on height and height on weight and find the point of intersection of these lines. Also compute the correlation coefficient and test the significance of correlation coefficient and both regression coefficients.

9. The following are the data on average yield (100 gm) and average ear length (cm) of 10 samples of hills selected at random from paddy field.

Average yield	8	7	5	10	6	4	12	14	15	9
Average ear length	7	5	4	12	4	5	10	13	14	6

Fit the regression equations of 'yield' on 'ear length' and test the regression coefficient for its significance. Also, compute the correlation coefficient and test its significance.

10. Find the correlation coefficient between supply and price of onions in 10 markets and test its significance.

Supply (quintals)	18	22	26	20	12	14	16	19	23	25
Price (Rs/kg)	12	10	8	11	13	15	14	12	9	8

CHAPTER 8

Tests of Hypotheses

8.1 Introduction

The estimate based on sample will not be equal to population value due to inherent variation in the population. The samples drawn will have different estimates compared to the true value. It has to be verified that whether the difference between the sample estimate and population value is due to sampling fluctuation or real difference. If the difference is due to sampling fluctuation only then it can safely be concluded that sample belongs to the population with respect to character under question. Otherwise the sample does not belong to population with respect to the character under study. This will be decided with the help of tests of hypotheses. If the sample is one then the tests are called one sample test, and if there are two samples then they are called two sample tests.

8.1.1 Null Hypothesis

It is the statement about parameter or parameters which is likely to be rejected after testing. This is also called as hypothesis of no difference.

For example if we want to compare the performance of private management hospital and Government-run hospital, the null hypothesis can be stated as both hospitals are equally good with respect to their performance in treating patients.

8.1.2 Degree of Freedom

It is defined as the difference between total number of observations and total number of constraints.

For example if 5 numbers are to be selected with a condition that the total number should be 50 then 4 numbers can be chosen at will or with freedom and 5th number has to be chosen such that the total of five numbers should be 50. The fifth number to be chosen has no 'freedom'.

The degrees of freedom (d.f.) is $5 - 1 = 4$.

More mathematically degrees of freedom can be defined as the total number of linearly independent contrasts that can be formed from given number of observations. If 'n' is the total number of observations and k linearly independent contrasts that can be formed from 'n' observations then degrees of freedom (d.f.) is (n – k).

There are two types of errors committed in decision-making by applying tests of hypotheses. There are Type I and Type II errors.

Type I error : Rejecting the hypothesis when it ought to be accepted.

Type II error : Accepting the hypothesis it ought to be rejected.

8.1.3 Level of Significance

The maximum probability at which we will be risking type I error is known as level of significance.

In practice 5 percent or 1 percent are taken as levels of significance in tests of hypotheses, thereby specifying that our decision may go wrong 5 out of 100 or 1 out of 100 cases respectively. The decision will have 95 percent confidence at 5 percent level of significance and 99 percent confidence at 1 percent level of significance. This is depicted in Fig. 8.1.

The region of rejection is also known as critical region.

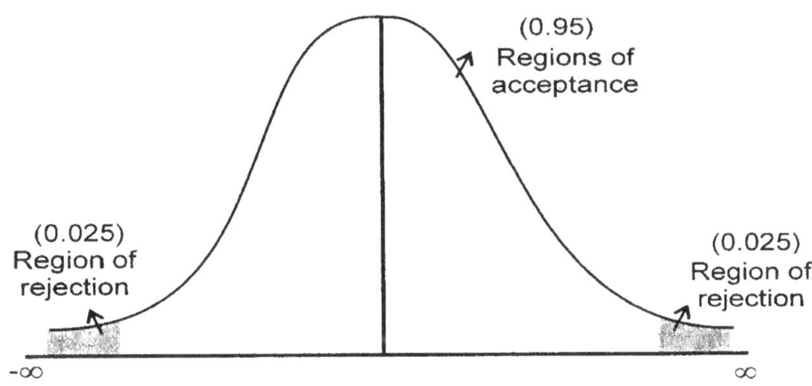

Fig. 8.1 Normal curve.

8.2 Standard Normal Deviate tests

If x follows normal distribution with mean, μ and S.D., σ then $\bar{x}$ also follows normal distribution with mean, μ and S.D., $\dfrac{\sigma}{\sqrt{n}}$, where n is the sample size. This can be written as

$$x \sim N(\mu,\ \sigma) = \bar{x} \sim N\left(\mu, \frac{\sigma}{\sqrt{n}}\right)$$

where symbol '~' indicates follows.

Then
$$\frac{\bar{x}-\mu}{\dfrac{\sigma}{\sqrt{n}}} \sim N(0,\,1)$$

The expression on the left hand side is called standard normal deviate which follows normal distribution mean as zero and standard deviation unity. The test of hypothesis based on standard normal deviate is called standard normal deviate test or S.N.D test in short form.

Confidence limits

The confidence limits or 'fiducial' limits for the population mean, μ are given as,

$$\bar{x} \pm 1.96\,\frac{\sigma}{\sqrt{n}}$$

where $\bar{x}+1.96\,\dfrac{\sigma}{\sqrt{n}}$ is the upper limit and $\bar{x}-1.96\,\dfrac{\sigma}{\sqrt{n}}$ is the lower limit. In other words, the population mean lies between these two limits. The figure 1.96 is the tabulated value of Z at 5 per cent level of significance.

Usually the population S.D. is not known and hence it is estimated by sample. If size of sample is large say > 30, then confidence limits are given by,

$$\bar{x} \pm 1.96\,\frac{s}{\sqrt{n}}$$

where
$$s = \sqrt{\frac{1}{n}\Sigma\left(x_i - \bar{x}\right)^2}$$

If the sample size is small say $\leq$ 30, then the confidence limits are given by,

$$\bar{x} \pm t_{(n-1)}\,\frac{s}{\sqrt{n}}$$

where $t_{(n-1)}$ is the tabulated value of t-distribution with (n–1) degrees of freedom at required level of significance and

$$s = \sqrt{\frac{1}{n-1}\Sigma\left(x_i - \bar{x}\right)^2}$$

8.2.1   Two-Sample S.N.D test

This test is used when common population S.D. is not known and sizes of samples are large i.e. n_1, n_2 > 30 where n_1 and n_2 are the sizes of 1st and 2nd samples respectively.

Assumptions : (i) Populations are normal

(ii) Samples are drawn independently and at random.

Conditions   : (i) Common population S.D, σ is not known

(ii) Sizes of samples are large i.e. n_1, $n_2 > 30$.

Null hypothesis, $H_0 :$ $\mu_1 = \mu_2$

Alternative hypothesis, $H_1 :$ $\mu_1 \neq \mu_2$

where μ_1, μ_2 are means of 1st and 2nd populations respectively.

$$Z = \frac{|\bar{X}_1 - \bar{X}_2|}{\sqrt{\dfrac{S_1^2}{n_1} + \dfrac{S_2^2}{n_2}}}$$

where $S_1^2 = \dfrac{1}{n_1}\Sigma(x_{1i} - \bar{x}_1)^2, S_2^2 = \dfrac{1}{n_2}\Sigma(x_{2i} - \bar{x}_2)^2$ are the variances for the 1st and 2nd samples respectively, n_1, n_2 are the sizes of 1st and 2nd samples respectively and $\bar{x}_1$ and $\bar{x}_2$ are the means of 1st and 2nd samples respectively.

Conclusion

If z (calculated) value > z (tabulated) value at required level of significance, the null hypothesis, H_0 is rejected. Otherwise H_0 is accepted.

If H_0 is rejected it can be concluded that there is significant difference between the two samples with respect to characteristic under consideration.

Example

A random sample of 40 mothers gave birth to children with an average weight of 2.8 kg, at the time of birth in hospital A in an year with S.D. of 0.6 kg and another random sample of 60 mothers gave birth to children with an average weight of 3.2 kg at the time of birth in hospital B in the same year with S.D. of 0.8 kg. Test whether there is any significant difference between the weights of the two groups of mothers at 5 percent level of significance.

Null hypothesis, $H_0 : \mu_1 = \mu_2$

$$Z = \frac{|2.8 - 3.2|}{\sqrt{\dfrac{(0.6)^2}{40} + \dfrac{(0.8)^2}{60}}}$$

$$Z = \frac{0.4}{0.14} = 2.86$$

Conclusion

Here z (calculated) value i.e., 2.86 > z (tabulated) value i.e. 1.96 at 5 percent level of significance. Therefore H_0 is rejected. Hence it can be concluded that there is significant difference between two groups of mothers with respect to birth weight of their children.

8.3   Two-Sample t - test

If the common population S.D. σ is not known and sizes of samples are small say n_1, $n_2 \leq 30$ then the test of hypothesis will be two - sample t- test instead of Z-test. The t-test is based on t-distribution which was developed by W.S. Gosset.

The curve of this distribution is symmetric about the mean, unimodal and extends from $-\infty$ to $+\infty$. In this curve the tabulated values will change as the sample size or degrees of freedom changes.

Assumptions :   (i) Populations are normal

(ii) Samples are drawn independently and at random.

Conditions   :   (i) Common population S.D., σ is not known

(ii) Sizes of samples are small say n_1, $n_2 \leq 30$.

Null hypothesis, $H_0 :$ $\mu_1 = \mu_2$

Alternative hypothesis, $H_1 :$ $\mu_1 \neq \mu_2$

where μ_1, μ_2 are means of 1st and 2nd populations respectively.

$$t = \frac{|\bar{x}_1 - \bar{x}_2|}{\sqrt{s_c^2 \left(\dfrac{1}{n_1} + \dfrac{1}{n_2} \right)}}$$

where
$$s_c^2 = \frac{(n_1 - 1)s_1^2 + (n_2 - 1)s_2^2}{n_1 + n_1 - 2}$$

$$= \frac{\Sigma(x_{1i} - \bar{x}_1)^2 + \Sigma(x_{2i} - \bar{x}_2)^2}{n_1 + n_1 - 2}$$

where
$$s_1^2 = \frac{1}{n_1 - 1}\Sigma(x_{1i} - \bar{x}_1)^2, s_2^2 = \frac{1}{n_2 - 1}\Sigma(x_{2i} - \bar{x}_2)^2$$

is called the combined estimate of variance. $\bar{x}_1$, $\bar{x}_2$ are the means of 1st and 2nd samples respectively and n_1, n_2 are the sizes of 1st and 2nd samples respectively.

Conclusion

If t (calculated) value > t (tabulated) value with $(n_1 + n_2 - 2)$ degrees of freedom at the required level of significance, the null hypothesis, H_0 is rejected. Otherwise it is accepted.

If H_0 is rejected, it can be concluded that there is significant difference between the two samples with respect to character under consideration.

Example

Two brands of foods were administered to two groups of children of age between 1 to 3 years and their gain in weight (100 gm) were recorded after 6 months of administration.

Food	1	2	3	4	5	6	7	8
A	6	8	10	7	12	9	5	7
B	10	14	8	6	15	7		

Test whether there is any significant difference between brands of food A and B at probability level 0.01.

Null hypothesis, H_0 : $\mu_1 = \mu_2$

Table 8.1

S.No.	Age (x_{1i})	Days (x_{2i})	$(x_{1i} - \bar{x}_1)$	$(x_{1i} - \bar{x}_1)^2$	$(x_{2i} - \bar{x}_2)$	$(x_{2i} - \bar{x}_2)^2$	x_1^2	x_2^2
1	6	10	−2	4	0	0	36	100
2	8	14	0	0	4	16	64	196
3	10	8	2	4	−2	4	100	64
4	7	6	−1	1	−4	16	49	36
5	12	15	4	16	5	25	144	225
6	9	7	1	1	−3	9	81	49
7	5		−3	9			25	
8	7		−1	1			49	
Total	64	60		36		70	548	670
Mean	8	10						

Mean, $x_1 = \dfrac{\Sigma x_1}{n_1} = \dfrac{64}{8} = 8, \ \bar{x}_2 = \dfrac{\Sigma x_2}{n_2} = \dfrac{60}{6} = 10$

$$s_c^2 = \dfrac{36 + 70}{8 + 6 - 2} = \dfrac{106}{12} = 8.83$$

Alternatively

$$s_c^2 = \frac{\left[548 - \frac{(64)^2}{8}\right] + \left[670 - \frac{(60)^2}{6}\right]}{8 + 6 - 2}$$

$$= \frac{36 + 70}{8 + 6 - 2} = \frac{106}{12} = 8.83$$

$$t = \frac{|8 - 10|}{\sqrt{8.83\left(\frac{1}{8} + \frac{1}{6}\right)}} = \frac{2}{1.60} = 1.25$$

Conclusion

t (calculated) value i.e., 1.25 < t (tabulated) value i.e. 3.055 with (8 + 6 − 2) d.f. at 1 per cent level of significance. Therefore H_0 is accepted. Hence it can be concluded that there is no significant difference between two brands of food with respect to gain in weight.

8.3.1   Paired t - Test

This test is used as a special case of two sample t - test. This test is also called as a dependent t-test. When two samples are dependent on each other and are of equal size and small then this test is used in preference to two sample t-test.

Same patients may be used for comparison of two drugs, rats from the same litter may be considered for comparison of two diets, branches of same tree or plant for comparison of nitrogen uptake, neighbouring plots of the experimental field etc., are some of the situations where paired t - test can be used. This test is more sensitive since all experimental conditions are same except the treatments are under comparison.

Assumptions :   (i) Populations are normal

(ii) Samples are drawn independently and at random

Conditions   :   (i) Samples are small, related and of equal size

(ii) Common population S.D. is not known.

Null hypothesis, $H_0 : \quad \mu_1 = \mu_2$

Alternative hypothesis, $H_1 : \quad \mu_1 \neq \mu_2$

$$t = \frac{|\bar{d} - 0|}{\sqrt{\frac{s_d^2}{n}}}$$

where $d_i = (x_{1i} - x_{2i})$, $\overline{d} = \dfrac{\Sigma d_i}{n}$

n = size of the paired sample

$$s_d^2 = \frac{1}{n-1}\Sigma(d_i - \overline{d})^2$$

$$= \frac{1}{n-1}\left[\Sigma d_i^2 - \frac{(\Sigma d_i)^2}{n}\right]$$

Conclusion

If t (calculated) value > t (tabulated) value with (n–1) degree of freedom at the chosen level of significance then the null hypothesis, H_0 is rejected. Otherwise, it is accepted.

Example

The following is the data of number of minutes taken to recover to normal after consuming antacid tablet for acidity complaint in 10 patients, one tablet from each of two different pharmaceutical companies to each of the patients.

Drug	1	2	3	4	5	6	7	8	9	10
A	20	15	18	17	30	25	14	20	26	15
B	14	10	12	11	21	20	9	12	22	16

Test whether there is any significant difference between two drugs at 1 percent level of significance.

Table 8.2

S.No.	Drug A x_{1i}	Drug B x_{2i}	d_i $(x_{1i} - x_{2i})$	d_i^2
1	20	14	6	36
2	15	10	5	25
3	18	12	6	36
4	17	11	6	36
5	30	21	9	81
6	25	20	5	25
7	14	9	5	25
8	20	12	8	64
9	26	22	4	16
10	15	16	−1	1
Total			53	345

$$\overline{d} = \frac{53}{10} = 5.3, \; n = 10$$

$$s_d^2 = \frac{1}{(10-1)}\left[345 - \frac{(53)^2}{10}\right]$$

$$= \frac{64.1}{9} = 7.12$$

Null hypothesis, $H_0: \quad \mu_1 = \mu_2$

$$t = \frac{|5.3|}{\sqrt{\dfrac{7.12}{10}}} = \frac{5.3}{\sqrt{0.712}}$$

$$t = \frac{5.3}{0.84} = 6.31$$

Conclusion

Here t (calculated) value i.e. 6.31 > t (tabulated) value i.e. 3.25 with (10 − 1) d.f. at 1 percent level of significance. Therefore H_0 is rejected. Hence it can be concluded that there is significant difference between two drugs with respect to their effectiveness.

8.4   S.N.D Test for Proportions

Sometimes there is need to test the proportion of individuals in two samples instead of averages. The proportion in the sample follows Binomial distribution. The standard error for the difference of two proportions is taken based on Binomial distribution. For example proportion of individuals effected with a particular disease in two samples can be tested by using the test given in this section.

8.4.1   Two-sample test

Here the proportion in the population is assumed to be not known.

If p_1 and p_2 are the proportions having an attribute in the two samples of sizes n_1 and n_2 respectively then P, its proportion having the same attribute in the populations is estimated by p taking weighted averages of p_1 and p_2

$$p = \frac{n_1 p_1 + n_2 p_2}{n_1 + n_2}$$

Assumptions :   (i) Populations are normal

(ii) Samples are drawn independently and at random

Conditions :   (i) P the proportion in the population is not known.

(ii) sizes of samples may be small or large.

Null hypothesis, $H_0 : P_1 = P_2 = P$

Alternative hypothesis, $H_1 : P_1 \neq P_2$

where P_1 and P_2 are proportions in the 1st and 2nd populations

$$z = \frac{|p_1 - p_2|}{\sqrt{pq\left(\dfrac{1}{n_1} + \dfrac{1}{n_2}\right)}}$$

where $q = 1 - p$

Conclusion

If z (calculated) value > z (tabulated) value at chosen level of significance, the H_0 is rejected. Otherwise it is accepted. If H_0 is rejected then it can be concluded that there is significant difference between the proportions in the two samples having an attribute.

Example

In a survey conducted in a city 4 percent of people were affected with heart ailment in one locality consisting of 10,000 people and in another locality of the same city consisting of 12,000 people 2 percent of the people were effected with the same disease. Test whether the first locality is significantly more affected than second locality at 5 percent level of significance.

Null hypothesis, $H_0 : P_1 = P_2 = P$

Alternative hypothesis, $H_1 : P_1 \neq P_2$

$$p = \frac{n_1 p_2 + n_2 p_2}{n_1 + n_2}$$

$$= \frac{10{,}000 \times \dfrac{4}{100} + 12{,}000 \times \dfrac{2}{100}}{10{,}000 + 12{,}000}$$

$$= \frac{400 + 240}{22{,}000} = 0.03$$

$q = 1 - p = 1 - 0.03 = 0.97$

$$Z = \frac{|0.04 - 0.02|}{\sqrt{0.03 \times 097\left(\dfrac{1}{10{,}000} + \dfrac{1}{12{,}000}\right)}}$$

$$= \frac{0.02}{\sqrt{0.03 \times 0.97\,(0.0001 + 0.000083)}}$$

$$= \frac{0.02}{0.0023} = 8.7$$

Conclusion

Here Z (calculated) value i.e. 8.7 > Z (tabulated) value i.e. 1.833 at 5 percent level of significance for one tailed test. Therefore H_0 is rejected. Hence it can be concluded that the first locality is significantly more affected than second locality.

Exercises

1. The average number of seeds set per pod in red gram were determined for top and bottom branches in 10 red gram plants are presented here.

Branch	1	2	3	4	5	6	7	8	9	10
Top	4.5	3.2	4.0	3.2	4.4	3.6	4.6	5.0	6.0	5.2
Bottom	6.0	5.8	7.5	5.0	6.8	5.8	6.4	7.0	5.4	7.8

Test the significant difference between two branches of red gram plants with respect to average number of seeds set per pod.

2. The daily production (100 boxes) of vitamin tablets of two pharmaceutical companies was recorded as follows.

Company	1	2	3	4	5	6	7	8	9	10
A	6	8	10	12	5	13	9	4	13	20
B	12	14	6	13	15	18	19	15		

Test whether there is any significant difference between two companies with respect to daily production.

3. Two stimuli were administered to two groups of patients and the changes in blood pressure were recorded as

Stimuli										
A	0	2	3	5	8	7	1	−2	−1	4
B	2	− 4	5	3	7	8	5	9		

Test the significant difference between two stimuli with respect to changes in blood pressure at the probability level 0.01.

4. In a pharmacy college the average marks scored by 2004 batch students in 1st year consisting of 80 students was 68 with a standard deviation of 12 marks. The average marks scored by 2005 batch in 1st year consisting of 120 students was 72 with a standard deviation of 8 marks. Test whether there is any significant difference between the two batches with respect to their performance with probability level 0.05.

5. In a particular village consisting of 1000 people 2 percent were affected with malaria. In another village of the same mandal consisting of 800 people 4 percent were affected with malaria. Test whether there is any significant difference between the two villages with respect to incidence of malaria.

6. Two methods of preparation of same leaf vegetable gave the iron content (mg) when 10 pairs of samples were studied.

Method	1	2	3	4	5	6	7	8	9	10
I	0.22	0.14	0.04	0.12	0.14	0.08	0.09	0.15	0.20	0.05
II	0.18	0.20	0.06	0.25	0.20	0.10	0.14	0.10	0.24	0.14

Test whether there is any significant difference between the two methods with respect to iron content at 5 percent level.

7. Fruit dropping for a particular variety of mango was found to be 6 percent/tree in a garden of 220 trees in a village. In another garden consisting of 180 trees the fruit dropping was recorded as 4 percent in the same village. Test whether there is any significant difference between the two gardens at probability level 0.01.

8. The daily production (tons) of two pesticide factories of the same corporation for different days were recorded as follows.

Factory

A	14	18	20	19	21	13	17	22	20	16
B	18	22	24	20	19	25	18	16		

Test whether Factory B is significantly producing more than Factory A at 5 percent level of significance.

CHAPTER 9

Chi-Square Test

9.1 Introduction

In the tests such as Z and t dealt with in previous chapter are called parametric tests, since these tests are used for data of measurement level of at least interval scale level. Further these tests are used with the assumption that population of observations or variate values follows normal distribution. It is not always possible to have data at least at the level of interval scale and also the population of these variate values follow normal distribution in biological and agricultural research. In such situations non-parametric tests including Chi-square test can be used. Chi-square test can be used for enumeration data given in contingency tables. Chi-square test can be used in :

   (i)   Goodness of fit of distributions

   (ii)   Test of independence of attributes

   (iii)   Genetic problems such as segregation and linkage

   (iv)   Test of homogeneity

  Chi-square test is based on Chi-square distribution which was developed by Karl Pearson in 1900. This test is therefore used as parametric as well as non-parametric test.

9.2 Chi-Square Distribution

Let x_1, x_2, ... x_n be n independent normal variates and each is distributed normally with mean zero and standard deviation unity, then $x_1^2 + x_2^2 ... + x_n^2 = \Sigma x_i^2$ is distributed as Chi-square χ^2 with n degrees of freedom (d.f.) where n is large. The Chi-square curve for d.f. n = 1, 2 , ... 6 are given in Fig. 9.1.

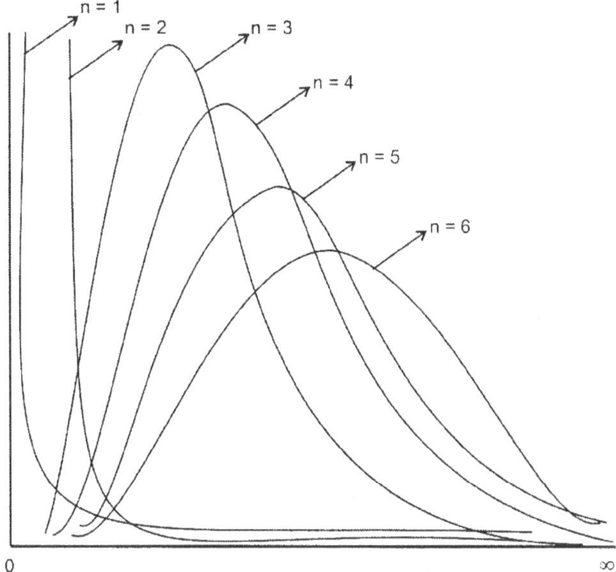

Fig. 9.1 Chi-square curves.

9.2.1 Properties

1. For n > 2, the Chi-square curve has mode at (n – 2). For n = 2, the distribution is L - shaped with maximum ordinate at zero, while for 0 < n < 2 the distribution is L - shaped and has infinite ordinate at the origin.

2. Chi-square distribution is having the additive property. If $\chi_1^2, \chi_2^2 \ldots \chi_k^2$ are k independent vaiates with n_1, n_2 ..... n_k d.f. respectively then $\chi_1^2 + \chi_2^2 + \ldots + \chi_k^2$ is a χ^2 variate with $n_1 + n_2 + \ldots + n_k$ d.f.

3. The central moments $\mu_2 = 2n$, $\mu_3 = 8n$ and $\mu_4 = 48n + 12n^2$.

4. The coefficient of skewness $\beta_2 = \left(\dfrac{8}{n}\right)^{\frac{1}{2}}$ and

   coefficient of kurtosis, $\beta_2 = \dfrac{12}{n} + 3$

As n tends to infinity, the Chi-square distribution tends to normal distribution.

9.2.2 Chi-Square Test for Goodness of Fit

Chi-square test is used to test whether the given distribution follows certain theoretical distribution or not. For example, if the given frequency distribution follows Binomial, Poisson or Normal distribution or not, Chi-square test is used.

The Chi-square test formula for goodness of fit is :

Null hypothesis, H_0 : The given distribution follows theoritical distribution

Alternative hypothesis, H_1 : The given distribution does not follow theoritical distribution.

$$x^2 = \sum_{i=1}^{k} \frac{(O_i - E_i)^2}{E_i}$$

where O_i = observed frequency of i-th item

E_i = expected frequency of i-th item and i = 1, 2 ... , k items.

Here 'item' is used for class interval for grouped frequency distribution and category for enumeration data.

Conclusion

If x^2 (calculated) value > x^2 (tabulated) value with (k – 1) d.f. at chosen level of significance the null hypothesis is rejected, otherwise it is accepted.

If the null hypothesis is accepted then it can be concluded that the given distribution follows theoritical distribution.

Example

The example in Table 6.4 of chapter 6 is taken as illustration for Chi-square test of goodness of fit.

Table 9.1

No.of tablets	Persons (O_i)	Expected frequency (E_i)	$(O_i - E_i)$	$(O_i - E_i)^2$	$\dfrac{(O_i - E_i)^2}{E_i}$
0	2	1.13	0.87	0.7569	0.670
1	6	5.88	0.12	0.0144	0.002
2	14	12.24	1.76	3.0976	0.253
3	9	12.74	–3.74	13.9876	1.098
4	5	6.63	–1.63	2.6569	0.401
5	4	1.38	2.62	6.8644	4.974
	40	40.00			7.398

H_0 : The frequency distribution in the Table 9.1 follows binomial distribution.

Conclusion

Here x^2 (calculated) value i.e 7.398 < x^2 (tabulated) value i.e. 9.488 with (5-1) d.f. at 5 percent level of significance. Therefore H_0 is accepted. Hence it can be concluded that the distribution in Table 9.1 follows binomial distribution.

It may be noted that the same procedure is adopted for testing the goodness of fit for Poisson and Normal distributions also.

9.3   Chi-Square test of Independence

Chi-square test is used for test of independence of two attributes or qualitative characters based on enumeration data. For example if shape and colour are associated or not to be tested based on enumeration data of flowers then chi-square test can be used.

9.3.1   Two × Two Contingency table

When the individuals or objects are classified according to two attributes and each attribute is further subdivided into two categories then it is called 2 x 2 contingency table. In this table there are two rows and two columns and in all 4 cells. The cells are filled up with enumeration (counting) data called frequencies.

Example

Suppose the flowers in a garden are classified according to colour and shape as shown in Table 9.2.

Table 9.2

Colour	Shape		Total
	Flat	**Wrinkled**	
Red	a	b	R_1
White	c	d	R_2
Total	C_1	C_2	N

Here a, b, c and d are the frequencies of flowers in different categories. R_1, R_2 are the row totals and C_1, C_2 are column totals and N is the grand total.

Null hypothesis, H_0 : The two attributes 'Colour' and 'Shape' are independent.

Alternative hypothesis, H_1 : The two attributes are not independent.

$$\chi^2 = \sum_i \sum_j \frac{\left(O_{ij} - E_{ij}\right)^2}{E_{ij}}$$

where O_{ij} = observed frequency of $(i, j)^{th}$ cell

           E_{ij} = expected frequency of $(ij)^{th}$ cell

           i = 1, 2 and j = 1, 2

Since observed frequencies are known, the expected frequencies are obtained as

$$E(o_{11}) = \frac{R_1 \times C_1}{N}$$

$$E(o_{12}) = \frac{R_1 \times C_2}{N}$$

$$E(o_{21}) = \frac{R_2 \times C_1}{N}$$

$$E(o_{22}) = \frac{R_2 \times C_2}{N}$$

Here $o_{11} = a$, $o_{12} = b$, $o_{21} = c$, $o_{11} = d$ in Table 9.2.

Usin the above calculated expected frequencies the X^2 (calculated) value is obtained.

X^2 (calculated) value can also be obtained in 2×2 contingency table without computing expected frequencies of different cells by using the direct formula as

$$X^2 = \frac{(ad - bc)^2 N}{R_1 R_2 C_1 C_2}$$

Conclusion

If x^2 (calculated) value > x^2 (tabulated) value with $(2 - 1)(2 - 1)$ d.f. at chosen level of significance, H_0 is rejected. Otherwise, H_0 is accepted.

If H_0 is rejected then it can be concluded that there is significant association between the two attributes say colour and shape.

Example

Rose flowers are classified according to colour and shape plucked from a garden. The data are presented in the 2 x 2 contingency table.

Table 9.3 Shape

Colour	Shape		Total
	Flat	Wrinkled	
Red	24	26	50
White	36	44	80
	60	70	130

Test whether there is any significant association or relationship between 'colour' and 'shape' of rose flowers.

$$E(o_{11}) = \frac{50 \times 60}{130} = 23.1 \text{ (Rounded off to 1}^{st}\text{ decimal place)}$$

$$E(o_{12}) = \frac{50 \times 70}{130} = 26.9$$

$$E(o_{21}) = \frac{80 \times 60}{130} = 36.9$$

$$E(o_{22}) = \frac{80 \times 70}{130} = 43.1$$

$$X^2 = \frac{(24 - 23.1)^2}{23.1} + \frac{(26 - 26.9)^2}{26.9} + \frac{(36 - 36.9)^2}{36.9} + \frac{(44 - 43.1)^2}{43.1}$$

$$= 0.04 + 0.03 \; 0.02 + 0.02$$

$$= 0.11$$

Conclusion

Here X^2 (calculated) value i.e. $0.11 < X^2$ (tabulated) value i.e. 3.841 with $(2 - 1)(2 - 1)$ d.f. at 5 percent level of significance. Therefore H_0 is accepted. Hence it can be concluded that the attributes 'colour' and 'shape' are independent.

It may be noted that the number of expected frequencies in contingency table can be computed based on the degrees of freedom. If d.f. is (1) then only one expected frequency need to be calculated and other expected frequencies are obtained by subtraction from corresponding marginal totals. For example, E_{11} is known, then $E_{12} = R_1 - E_{11}$, $E_{21} = C_1 - E_{11}$ and $E_{22} = C_2 - E_{12}$. Using direct formula, x^2 (calculated) value for the example in Table 9.3 is given as

$$x^2 = \frac{(24 \times 44 - 26 \times 36)^2 \times 130}{50 \times 80 \times 60 \times 70}$$

$$x^2 = \frac{14400 \times 13x^2}{50 \times 80 \times 60 \times 70} = \frac{187200}{1680000}$$

$$= 0.11$$

Conclusion

same as given above.

9.3.2 Yate's Correction for Continuity

In 2×2 contingency table the expected frequencies are small say less than 5 then the Chi-square test cannot be used. In that case the direct formula of Chi-square test is modified and is given as,

$$X^2 = \frac{\left[\,|ad - bc| - \frac{N}{2}\,\right]^2 N}{R_1 R_2 C_1 C_2}$$

9.3.3   m x n Contingency table

The formula of Chi-square test can be used for m x n contingency table where m is the number of rows and n is the number of columns. However the direct formula cannot be used in this case. In conclusion the degrees of freedom for consulting tabulated value of Chi-square is (m − 1) (n − 1).

Example

The following is the data classified according to vaccination and recovery of children in a hospital from a particular disease.

Table 9.4

	Recovered	Not-recovered	Total
Vaccinated	18	2	20
Non-Vaccinated	4	10	14
Total	22	12	34

Test whether there is any significance association of vaccination and recovery from disease of children.

From Table 9.4 it can be observed that the expected frequency of $(2, 2)^{th}$ cell is $\dfrac{12 \times 14}{34}$ = 4.9 which is less than 5. Therefore the Yates correction for continuity may be used for this example.

Null hypothesis, H_0 : Vaccination has no effect on the disease for recovery.

Alternative hypothesis, H_1 : Vaccination has an effect on the disease for recovery.

$$\chi^2 = \frac{\left[|18 \times 10 - 2 \times 4| - \dfrac{34}{2}\right]^2 34}{20 \times 14 \times 22 \times 12} = \frac{816850}{73920} = 11.05$$

Conclusion

Here χ^2 (calculated) value i.e. 11.05 > χ^2 (tabulated) i.e. 6.635 with (2-1 (2-1) d.f. at 1 percent level of significance. Therefore H_0 is rejected. Hence it can be concluded that vaccination does effect in controlling the disease.

9.4   Chi-Square test for Genetic Problems

Genetic theory states that different genes segregate independently and in a specific phenotypic ratios depending upon the cross. A dominant gene segregates from its recessive allels in the ratio 3 : 1 in F_2 generation and in the ratio 1: 1 in back cross. If two genes are responsible for a particular character then there are four types of pheotypic combinations in F_2 generation and back cross. These are (3 : 1) × (3 : 1) = 9 : 3 : 3 : 1 and (1: 1) × (1: 1) = 1 : 1 : 1 : 1 in F_2 generations and back cross respectively.

Example

A cross between two varieties of sorghum one giving high yield and the other high amount of fodder was made. The number of plants observed in F_2 generation are 82, 162 and 88. Test whether this sample data is in agreement with Mendelian ratio 1 : 2 : I or not.

Null hypothesis, H_0 :   The sample data follows I : 2 : 1 ratio.

Alternative hypothesis, H_1 :   The sample data does not follow Mendelian ratio 1:2: 1.

Table 9.5

Observed Freq. O_i	Expected Freq. E_i	$(O_i - E_i)$	$\dfrac{(O_i - E_i)^2}{E_i}$
82	$332 \times \dfrac{1}{4} = 83$	-1	0.0120
162	$332 \times \dfrac{2}{4} = 166$	-4	0.0964
88	$332 \times \dfrac{1}{4} = 83$	5	0.3012
332	332		0.4096

Conclusion

Here x^2 (calculated) value i.e. $0.4096 < x^2$ (tabulated) value i.e. 5.991 with (3-1) d.f. at 5 per cent level of significance. Therefore H_0 is accepted. Hence it can be concluded that the sample data in F_2 generation is in agreement with Mendelian ratio 1 : 2 : 1.

9.5   Chi-Square test for Homogeneity

Chi-square test can be used also to test whether the occurrence of events follow uniformly or not. For example the admission of patients in Government hospital in all days of week is uniform or not can be tested with the help of Chi-square test.

Example

The number of patients admitted in Government hospital on 7 days of a week in May month of year is presented in Table 9.6.

Table 9.6

	SUN	MON	TUE	WED	THUR	FRI	SAT
Patients	24	20	16	18	22	19	21

Test whether the admission of patients on all 7 days is uniform or not at 5 percent level of significance.

Null hypothesis, H_0 : The admission of patients is uniform for all 7 days of a week.

Alternative hypothesis, H_1 : The admission of patients is not uniform.

Table 9.7

	SUN	MON	TUE	WED	THUR	FRI	SAT	TOTAL
O_i	24	20	16	18	22	19	21	140
E_i	20	20	20	20	20	20	20	140
$(O_i - E_i)$	4	0	-4	-2	2	-1	1	
$\dfrac{(O_i - E_i)^2}{E_i}$	0.8	0	0.8	0.2	0.2	0.05	0.05	2.1

Where the expected frequency $E_i = 140 \times \dfrac{1}{7} = 20$

Conclusion

Here x^2 (calculated) value i.e. $2.1 < x^2$ (tabulated) value i.e. 12.592 with (7-1) d.f at 5 percent level of significance. Therefore H_0 is accepted. Hence it can be concluded that the admission of patients in the hospital is uniform throughout the week.

9.6   Non-Parametric tests

When the scale of measurement is nominal or ordinal the parametric tests cannot be applied for such data since parametric tests require data based on interval scale at least and also certain assumptions like normality of population distribution. In such situations non-parametric tests can be applied for data based on nominal or ordinal scale without any rigorous assumptions.

9.6.1   Wilcoxon test

This test is used when two samples are related and data of scores are available for both the samples, when the size of paired sample is more than 25.

Null hypothesis H_0 : There is no significant difference between 'Morning' and 'Evening' Doctors with respect to their performance.

Alternative hypothesis, H_1 : There is significant difference between 'Morning' and 'Evening' Doctors.

$$Z = \frac{\left| S - \dfrac{n(n+1)}{4} \right|}{\sqrt{\dfrac{n(n+1)(2n+1)}{24}}}$$

where S = total of all the positive or negative ranks whichever is smaller and n is the number of pairs of observations.

Conclusions

If Z calculated value > Z (tabulated) value then H_0 is rejected. Otherwise H_0 is accepted. If H_0 is rejected then it can be concluded that there is significant difference between the scores of two samples.

Example

Thirty patients were randomly selected and interviewed with respect to treatment and behaviour of 'Morning' and 'Evening' duty Doctors in a hospital. The scores given by the patients were recorded and presented in Table 9.8.

Test whether there is any significant difference between the two shifts Doctors with respect to their performance in the opinion of patients.

Table 9.8

S.No	Morning	Evening	S.No.	Morning	Evening
1	80	76	16	74	76
2	70	78	17	69	68
3	64	60	18	79	81
4	90	80	19	86	80
5	76	82	20	94	92
6	80	70	21	65	60
7	94	90	22	74	71
8	68	70	23	95	89
9	79	75	24	92	85
10	86	80	25	69	71
11	94	92	26	78	79
12	84	81	27	89	87
13	76	82	28	94	90
14	70	68	29	86	81
15	84	85	30	91	87

Table 9.9

S.No. (1)	Difference (2)	Rank (3)	S (4)	S.No. (5)	Difference (6)	Rank (7)	S (8)
1	4	16.5		16	−2	−7.5	7.5
2	−8	−28.0	28.0	17	1	2	
3	4	16.5		18	−2	−7.5	7.5
4	10	29.5		19	6	24.0	
5	−6	−24.0	24.0	20	2	7.5	
6	10	29.5		21	5	20.5	
7	4	16.5		22	3	12.5	
8	−2	−7.5	7.5	23	6	24.0	
9	4	16.5		24	7	27.0	
10	6	24.0		25	−2	−7.5	7.5
11	2	7.5		26	−1	−2	2.0
12	3	12.5		27	2	7.5	
13	−6	−24.0	24.0	28	4	16.5	
14	2	7.5		29	5	20.5	
15	−1	−2	2.0	30	4	16.5	
			85.5				24.5

$$S = 85.5 + 24.5 = 110.0$$

In Table 9.9 ranks in columns (3) and (7) were given based on the differences in columns (2) and (6) without considering negative signs. If the differences are equal for first three ranks then the average of ranks 1, 2 and 3 i.e. 2 is given to first three differences. The differences are equal for next 5 values then subsequent ranks average is to be given for the 5 values. For example the average of ranks 4, 5, 6, 7 and 8 i.e. 6 is to be given to next five equal differences, and so on. Then the negative sign is given to the ranks of negative differences. If negative ranks are small in number comparative to positive ranks then S is the total of negative ranks.

$$Z = \frac{\left|110 - \dfrac{30(30+1)}{4}\right|}{\sqrt{\dfrac{30(31)(61)}{24}}}$$

$$= \frac{|110 - 232.5|}{\sqrt{2563.75}} = \frac{87.5}{50.63} = 1.73$$

Conclusion

Here Z (calculated) value i.e., 1.73 < Z (tabulated) value i.e., 1.96 is at 5 per cent level of significance. Therefore H_0 is accepted. Hence it can be concluded that there is no significant difference between 'Morning' and 'Evening' duty Doctors with respect to their performance in the opinion of patients.

9.6.2 Mann - Whitney test

This test is used to test the significant difference between two independent samples when the data are measured on ordinal scale. If scores are given based on the opinion of judges for two independent groups with respect to character under consideration then this test is applied. This is a powerful non-parametric test for two independent samples just as two-sample t-test in parametric case.

Let n_1, n_2 be sizes of small and large groups respectively out of the two groups to be tested for their difference. Common ranking is done for all the $(n_1 + n_2)$ scores such that lowest score would be given 1 and next higher score would be given 2, and so on.

The scores of both the groups would be arranged in ascending order of magnitude starting from highest negative value, if any. The ranks would be awarded to these scores giving 1 to the highest negative value, and so on. Then these ranks would be placed in their respective groups. W can be calculated as follows.

$$W = n_1 n_2 + \frac{n_1(n_1 + 1)}{2} - T_1$$

or

$$W_1 = n_1 n_2 + \frac{n_2(n_2 + 1)}{2} - T_2$$

where T_1, T_2 are the sum of the ranks in the groups of sizes n_1, n_2 respectively.

If $n_2 > 20$ irrespective of size of n_1 the following test is used.

Null hypothesis, H_0 : There is no significant difference between two groups with respect to character under consideration.

Alternative hypothesis, H_1 : There is significant difference between two groups.

$$Z = \frac{\left| W - \frac{n_1 n_2}{2} \right|}{\sqrt{\frac{n_1 n_2 (n_1 + n_2 + 1)}{12}}}$$

Conclusion

If Z (calculated) value > z (tabulated) value at chosen level of significance then H_0 is rejected. Otherwise, it is accepted.

If H_0 is rejected then it can be concluded that there is significant difference between the two groups.

Example

The following are the scores obtained by two Medical Colleges final year students in medical camps conducted in villages.

Medical college

A	65	80	72	68	84	65	56	78	
	(7.5)	(20)	(16)	(11.5)	(24)	(9.5)	(2)	(19)	
B	68	54	75	84	81	71	70	84	
	(11.5)	(1)	(18)	(24)	(21)	(14.5)	(13)	(24)	
	59	65	71	86	90	82	59	64	61
	(3.5)	(9.5)	(14.5)	(26)	(28)	(22)	(3.5)	(7.5)	(5)
	89	91	95	73	62				
	(27)	(29)	(30)	(17)	(6)				

Common ranking is done for all the scores in two groups giving rank 1 to lowest score. These ranks are written underneath the scores.

$$T_1 = 109.5, \quad n_1 = 8, \quad n_2 = 22, \quad T_2 = 355.5$$

$$W = n_1 n_2 + \frac{n_1(n_1 + 1)}{2} - T_1$$

$$= 8 \times 22 + \frac{8(8 + 1)}{2} - 109.5$$

$$= 102.5$$

$$Z = \frac{\left| 102.5 - \dfrac{8 \times 22}{2} \right|}{\sqrt{\dfrac{8 \times 22(8 + 22 + 1)}{12}}} = \frac{14.5}{21.32}$$

$$Z = 0.68$$

Conclusion

Here Z (calculated) value i.e. 0.68 < Z (tabulated) value i.e. 1.96 at 5 per cent level of significance. Therefore H_0 is accepted. Hence it can be concluded that there is no significant difference between two groups of students from two colleges for their performance in conducting medical camps.

Exercises

1. To prevent eye disease in children an experimental diet was recommended. In a survey of children in school the following results were obtained.

	Prevented	Not prevented
Experimental diet	24	6
Control diet	10	30

Test whether experimental diet has any effect in controlling the eye disease in children.

2. Tobacco leaves were classified according to shape and quality in grading at a tobacco company and the results are presented as follows.

	Shape		
Quality	Large	Medium	Narrow
Good	26	18	6
Satisfactory	20	24	12
Poor	8	18	30

Test whether there is any significant association between 'shape' and 'quality' of tobacco leaves.

3. The following are the 'observed' and 'expected' frequencies in normal distribution.

Observed	8	14	20	36	17	10	5
Expected	6	17	22	34	16	12	3

Test whether expected frequencies are in close agreement with observed frequencies at I per cent level of significance.

4. Patients are expected to be admitted in corporate hospital with heart ailment and other complaints in the ratio 2:1. In a survey conducted in one corporate hospital the number of patients admitted as heart patients was 38 and other patients 16. Test whether the observed patients are in agreement with expected ratio at 5 per cent level of significance.

5. The following are the number of seeds germinated in each pot when 10 seeds of barley were sown in glasshouse experiment consisting of 10 pots.

Plot										
	1	2	3	4	5	6	7	8	9	10
Germinated	6	4	8	7	3	10	2	5	9	0

Test whether seeds germinated uniformly in all the pots at 1 per cent level of significance.

6. The number of scores awarded to 'private' and Government hospitals in a city by Indian Council of Medical Research (ICMR) are given as follows.

Government	84	70	64	58	60	46	50	68
Private	54	65	84	80	72	78	64	60
	86	90	57	51	68	74	76	85
	81	69	64	76	73	71	62	

Test whether there is any significant difference between Government and private hospitals with respect to the scores obtained at 5 per cent level of significance.

7. In an experiment conducted on Tomatoes, Red and Round were crossed with Pink and Elongated and the progeny in F_2 generation were observed. Red and round tomatoes were 42, red and elongated 80, pink and round 66 and pink and elongated 32. Test whether the progeny in F_2 generation is in agreement with ratio 9 : 3 : 3 : 1 according to Mendel.

8. In an experiment on chillies the following results were obtained.

Shape	Pungent	Not-Pungent
Long	26	34
Short	34	16

Test whether there is significant association between 'shape' and 'pungentness' at 1 percent level of significance.

CHAPTER 10

Analysis of Variance

10.1 Introduction

When more than two treatments are under study t-test has to be applied for every pair of treatments for testing the null hypothesis. If 4 treatments (objects of comparison) are to be compared then t-test has to be used $4c_2 = 6$ times for testing the equality of treatment means. Sir R.A Fisher developed technique called Analysis of Variance (ANOVA) which can be used for testing more than two treatments at a time using F-test. In this method the total variation in the experimental data is analysed into different sources of variation. The variation due to different sources is compared with experimental error variation with F-test. If F-test shows significant then the source is causing significant variation compared to experimental error variation. For example in a pond there will be a variation or movement of water underneath due to movement of fishes, snakes, frogs etc. If we throw a stone in the pond there will be a violent movement of water creating ripples caused by violent movement of fishes, snakes, frogs etc., in water. Analysis of variance will help us to detect whether there is a significant disturbance of water due to violent movement of fishes, snakes, frogs etc., compared to movement of water without outside interference such as act of throwing a stone in the pond.

This technique is extensively used in agricultural, biological, medical, research etc. The model used in Analysis of Variance technique is given as

$$y_{ijk} = \mu + \alpha_i + \beta_i + e_{ijk}$$

where y_{ijk} is the response value of k-th experimental unit of the jth level of factor B and i-th level of factor A for i = 1, 2,……., p, j = 1, 2 ...., q and k = 1, 2 ...., r and μ is the general mean, α_i is the effect of i-th level of factor A and β_i is the effect of j-th level of factor B. e_{ijk} is the experimental error effect or residual effect on (I, j, k)th unit. μ, α_i, β_i, are unknown constants (parameters) and these are estimated with the help of 'least squares method'.

Assumptions underlying in the Analysis of Variance model:

(i) The effects of factors A and B, experimental effect and general mean are additive. The implication of this assumption is that the levels of factors A and B can be compared without interference from outside factors.

(ii) The residual effect e_{ijk} are independent from observation to observation and are assumed to follow normal distribution with zero mean and common variance σ^2.

The following are some of the concepts used in Analysis of Variance technique.

10.1.1   Randomization

Ramdom allocation of treatments to experimental units is called randomization. The allotment of treatments to experimental units can be done with the help of random numbers tables. Randomization ensures the validity of statistical tests like F-test, t-test etc. F-test and t-test require the assumption of normality of population. Randomization provides the assumption of independence of experimental errors and assumption of normality of experimental errors. Therefore randomization of treatments is essential for analyzing the data using Analysis of Variance technique.

10.1.2   Replication

Repetition of treatment to experimental units is known as Replication. Replication of treatment reduces experimental error and also provides experimental or residual variance which is essential for carrying out F-test.

10.1.3   Local Control

Grouping of homogeneous experimental units is called 'Local Control'. The 'Local control' also helps in reduction of experimental error variance. In medical research if same patient is used for comparing two or more drugs then local control concept is used. In agricultural field experiment neighbouring plots will be grouped into blocks based on soil fertility gradient and hence local control concept is used.

10.2   One-Way Analysis of Variance

If one factor is used in testing levels of that factor, then it is known as one-way analysis of variance. For example when different doses of same drug is tested on patients then it is called as one-way classification of Analysis of Variance.

The Analysis of Variance model is

$$y_{ij} = \mu + \alpha_i + e_{ij}$$

where y_{ij} is the response value of j-th patient having i-th dose of drug, μ is general mean, α_1 is the effect of i-th dose of drug and e_{ij} is the experimental or residual effect on (i, j)-th patient for i = 1, 2, … p and j = 1, 2, … r_i and $\Sigma ri = n$.

The procedure of method of Analysis of Variance is given as follows.

Table 10.1 Drug Dose

	1	2	.....	i	.....	p	
	Y_{11}	Y_{21}		Y_{i1}		Y_{p1}	
	Y_{21}	Y_{22}		Y_{i2}		Y_{p2}	
	.	.		.		.	
	.	.		.		.	
	.	.		.		.	
	Y_{1r1}	Y_{2r2}		Y_{iri}		Y_{prp}	
Total	$Y_1.$	$Y_2.$		$Y_i.$		$Y_p.$	$Y..$

Correction Factor (C.F.) $= \dfrac{Y^2..}{n}$

where y.. is the grand total and $n = \Sigma r_i$ is the total number of observations.

Drug sum of Squares

$$(\text{D.S.S}) = \frac{y_{1.}^2}{r_1} + \frac{y_{2.}^2}{r_2} + ... + \frac{y_{p.}^2}{r_p} - \text{C.F.}$$

where $Y_i.$ is the total of i-th dose of Drug.

Total sum of squares (T.S.S.) $= \left[y_{11}^2 + y_{12}^2 + ...y_{rrp}^2 \right] - \text{C.F}$

Where y_{ij} is the response value of the j-th patient having i-th dose of Drug.

Error sum of squares (E.S.S) $= (\text{T.S.S} - \text{D.S.S})$

The sums of squares are presented in the Table 10.2 for carrying out F-test.

$$H_0 = y_1. = y_2. = ...y_p.; \quad H_1.y_1 \neq y_2. \neq ... \neq y_p.$$

where $y_i.$ is the mean of i-th dose of drug.

Table 10.2 (ANOVA)

Source	d.f	S.S	M.S	F_{cal}	F_{tab} (d.f.)
Drug doses	p – 1	D.S.S	D.M.S	$\dfrac{\text{D.M.S}}{\text{E.M.S}}$	(p – 1), (n – p)
Error	n – p	E.S.S	E.M.S		
Total	n – 1	T.S.S			

where $\quad \text{D.M.S} = \dfrac{\text{D.S.S}}{(P-1)}, \quad \text{E.M.S} = \dfrac{\text{E.S.S}}{(n-P)}$

Conclusion

If F(calculated) value > F (tabulated) value with $(p - 1)$, $(n - p)$ d.f. at chosen level of significance, the null hypothesis, H_0 is rejected and H_1 is accepted.

If H_0 is rejected then it can be concluded that there is significant difference between doses of drug. The pair wise comparison of doses of drug can be done with the help of student t-test when the number of patients considered for each dose of drug is not equal.

If the number of patients is equal for each dose of drug then the dose means are arranged in ascending order of magnitude and the difference between each pair of means is tested with the critical difference (C.D.) or least significant difference (L.S.D) value which is given as

$$C.D = t_{(n-p)} \times \sqrt{\frac{2\,(E.M.S)}{r}}$$

where $r_1 = r_2 = \ldots = r_p = r$ and $t_{(n-p)}$ is the tabulated value with $(n-p)$ d.f. at required level of significance. E.M.S value is obtained from Table 10.2. If the difference between two doses means is greater than C.D. value then they are significantly different from each other. Otherwise there is no significant difference between them.

When the number of patients is not equal to the doses of drug the usual t-test would be conducted for testing the significant difference between each pair of doses by taking standard error between them as $\sqrt{E.M.S\left(\dfrac{1}{r_i} + \dfrac{1}{r_j}\right)}$, where r_i and r_j are the number of patients used for testing i-th and j-th doses of drug.

The standard error of doses means is $\sqrt{\dfrac{E.M.S}{r}}$

where $r = r_1 = r_2 .= \ldots = r_p$ and

$C.V. = \sqrt{\dfrac{E.M.S}{\dfrac{Y..}{n}}} \times 100$ is the coefficient of variation in the experiment.

Example

The following (Table 10.3) is the data of number of days required to come to normal body temperatures by administering different doses 50 mg, 100 mg, 250 mg and 500 mg of crocin. These tablets are administered to different patients. Test the significant difference between the doses at 5 percent level using Analysis of variance technique.

Table 10.3

Patient	50 mg	100 mg	250 mg	500 mg	
1	6	4	3	2	
2	8	5	4	3	
3	10	7	6	5	
4	12	8	7	6	
Total	36	24	20	16	96

H_0 : All doses means are equal

H_1 : All doses means are not equal.

Correction Factor (C.F.) = $\dfrac{Y_{..}^{2}}{n} = \dfrac{(96)^2}{16} = 576$

where $n = r_1 + r_2 + r_3 + r_4 = 4 + 4 + 4 + 4 = 16$

Dose sum of squares (D.S.S) = $\dfrac{Y_{1.}^{2}}{r_1} + \dfrac{Y_{2.}^{2}}{r_2} + \dfrac{Y_{3.}^{2}}{r_3} + \dfrac{Y_{4.}^{2}}{r_4} - CF$

$$= \dfrac{(36)^2}{4} + \dfrac{(24)^2}{4} + \dfrac{(20)^2}{4} + \dfrac{(16)^2}{4} - 576$$

$$= 632 - 576 = 56$$

Total sum of squares (T.S.S) = $y_{11}^{2} + y_{12}^{2} + ... y_{prp}^{2} - C.F.$

$$= [(6)^2 + (8)^2 + ... + (6)^2] - 576$$

$$= 682 - 576 = 106$$

Error sum of squares (E.S.S) = T.S.S – D.S.S = 106 – 56 = 50.

The sums of square are furnished in Analysis of Variance (ANOVA) (Table 10.4)

Table 10.4 ANOVA

Source	d.f.	S.S.	M.S.	F_{cal}	F_{tab} (d.f.)
Drug	4 – 1 = 3	56.0	18.67	4.48	3.49 (3, 12)
Error	16 – 4 = 12	50.0	4.17		
Total	16 – 1 = 15	106.0			

Conclusion

Here F (calculated) value i.e., 4.48 > F(tabulated) value i.e., 3.49 with (3, 12) d.f. at 5 percent level of significance. Therefore H_0 is rejected and H_1 is accepted. Hence it can be concluded that there is significant difference between doses of drug.

In order to know which dose is superior and which dose is inferior the doses means are arranged in ascending order of magnitude as in Table 10.5.

Table 10.5

50 mg	250 mg	100 mg	500 mg
b	ab	a	a
9	6	5	4

The L.S.D or C.D. value is given as

$$C.D. = t_{12} \times \sqrt{\frac{2 \times 4.17}{4}}$$

$$= 2.179 \times \sqrt{\frac{2 \times 4.17}{4}} = 3.14$$

The difference between each pair of doses means is compared with C.D. value. If the difference of means is greater than C.D. value then different superscripts are placed above the means. Otherwise same superscript is used as shown in Table 10.5.

From Table 10.5 it can be observed that 50 mg tablet is significantly inferior to other tablets having potency 100 mg, 250 mg and 500 mg in reducing the number of days to come to normal temperature of patient and the doses 100 mg, 250 mg and 500 mg tablets are not significantly different from each other in reducing the temperatures.

Example

Table 10.6 shows the life time in hours of samples from three different types of television tubes manufactured by a company. Using the long method, test at 0.05 significance level whether there is a difference in the three types.

Sample 1 : 407   411   409

Sample 2 : 404   406   408   405   402

Sample 3: 410   408   406   408

Method 1 :

The data are arranged in Table 10.6.

Table 10.6 Sample

	1	2	3	
	407	404	410	
	411	406	408	
	409	408	406	
		405	408	
		402		
Total	1227 (3)	2025 (5)	1632 (4)	4884

$$\text{C.F.} = \frac{(4884)^2}{12} = 1987788$$

Total sum of squares (T.S.S) $= (407)^2 + (411)^2 + ... + (408)^2 - \text{C.F.}$

$$= 1987860 - 1987788 = 72$$

Error sum of squares (E.S.S) $= (\text{T.S.S} - \text{S.S.S})$

$$= 72 - 36 = 36$$

The above sums of squares are furnished in the ANOVA Table 10.7.

Table 10.7

Source	d.f.	S.S.	M.S.	F_{cal}	F_{tab} (d.f.)
Samples	2	36	18	4.5	$4.26_{(2, 9)}$
Error	9	36	4		
Total	11	72			

Conclusion

Here F (calculated) value i.e., 4.5 > F (tabulated) value i.e., 4.26. Therefore H_0 is rejected and H_1 is accepted. Hence it can be concluded that there is a significant difference between three types of television tubes.

Method 2 :

The analysis for the above example can be done by simplifying the data by subtracting 400 from each of the observation as the values are around 400 and the conclusions will remain same.

Table 10.8 Sample

	1	**2**	**3**	
	7 (49)	4 (16)	10 (100)	
	11 (121)	6 (36)	8 (64)	
	9 (81)	8 (64)	6 (36)	
		5 (25)	8 (64)	
		2 (4)		
Total	27 (251) (3)	25 (145) (5)	32 (264) (4)	84

$$C.F. = \frac{(84)^2}{12} = 588$$

$$T.S.S = (7)^2 + (11)^2 + ... + (8)^2 - C.F. =$$

$$= (251 + 145 + 264) - 588 = 72$$

$$S.S.S = \frac{(27)^2}{3} + \frac{(25)^2}{5} + \frac{(32)^2}{4} - C.F.$$

$$= (243 + 125 + 256) - 588 = 36$$

$$E.S.S : 72 - 36 = 36$$

The above sums of squares are arranged in ANOVA Table 10.8 for carrying out F-test.

Table 10.9

Source	d.f.	S.S.	M.S.	F_{cal}	2
Samples	2	36	18	4.5	$4.26_{(2, 9)}$
Error	9	36	4		
Total	11	72			

Conclusion

same as in Method 1.

10.3   Two-Way Analysis of Variance

When two factors are used in testing levels within these factors then it is known as two-way analysis. For example when two drugs are tested at different levels of doses with respect to their efficacy on patients then two-way analysis of variance is a useful tool.

The Analysis of Variance model is

$$Y_{ij} = \mu + \alpha_i + \beta_i + e_{ij}$$

where Y_{ij} is the response value of j-th level of factor B and i-th level of factor A for i = l, 2,...p, j = 1, 2,..q, μ is overall mean, α_i is the effect of i-th level of factor A, β_i the effect of j-th level of factor B and e_{ij} is the experimental error effect of (i, j)th observation.

The procedure of analysis is given as follows.

The Y_{ij} values are presented in Table 10.10.

Table 10.10

A	1	2	...	j	...	q	Total
1	Y_{11}	Y_{12}	...	Y_{1j}		Y_{1q}	$Y_{1.}$
2	Y_{21}	Y_{22}	...	Y_{2j}	...	Y_{2q}	$Y_{2.}$
⋮	⋮	⋮	⋮	⋮	⋮	⋮	⋮
i	Y_{i1}	Y_{i2}	...	Y_{ij}	...	Y_{iq}	$Y_{i.}$
⋮	⋮	⋮	⋮	⋮	⋮	⋮	⋮
⋮	⋮	⋮	⋮	⋮	⋮	⋮	⋮
p	Y_{p1}	Y_{p2}	...	Y_{pj}	...	Y_{pq}	$Y_{p.}$
Total	$Y_{.1}$	$Y_{.2}$	...	$Y_{.j}$	...	$Y_{.q}$	$Y_{..}$

$$\text{Correction Factor (C.F.)} = \frac{Y_{..}^2}{pq}$$

where $Y_{..}$ is the grand total

$$\text{Total sum of squares (T.S.S)} = \left(Y_{11}^2 + Y_{12}^2 + ... Y_{ij}^2 + ... + Y_{pq}^2\right) - \text{C.F.}$$

$$\text{Factor A S.S.} = \left(\frac{Y_{1.}^2}{q} + \frac{Y_{2.}^2}{q} + ... + \frac{Y_{p.}^2}{q}\right) - \text{C.F,}$$

where $y_{1.}$, $y_{2.}$, etc are the totals of 1st and 2nd etc levels of factor A.

$$\text{Factor B S.S} = \left(\frac{Y_{.1}^2}{p} + \frac{Y_{.2}^2}{p} + ... + \frac{Y_{.q}^2}{p}\right) - \text{C.F.}$$

where $Y_{.1}$, $y_{.2}$, etc. are the totals of 1st and 2nd etc. levels of factor B.

$$\text{Error S.S.} = \text{T.S.S} - (\text{A.S.S} + \text{B.S.S})$$

The sums of squares obtained above are presented in Table 10.11 for carrying out the F-test.

(i) $H_0 : \alpha_1 = \alpha_2 = \ldots \alpha_p,$ $\qquad$ $H_1 : \alpha_1 \neq \alpha_2 \neq \ldots \neq \alpha_p$

(ii) $H_0 : \beta_1 = \beta_2 = \ldots = B_q,$ $\qquad$ $H_1 : \beta_1 \neq \beta_2 \neq \ldots \neq \beta_q$

Table 10.11

Source	d.f.	S.S.	M.S.	F_{cal}	F_{tab} (d.f.)
A	p − 1	A.S.S	A.M.S	$\dfrac{A.M.S}{E.M.S}$	(p − 1), (p − 1) (q − 1)
B	q − 1	B.S.S	B.M.S	$\dfrac{B.M.S}{E.M.S}$	(q − 1), (p − 1) (q − 1)
Error	(p − 1) (q − 1)	E.S.S	E.M.S		
Total	pq − 1	T.S.S			

where A.M.S = A.S.S/(p − l), $\qquad$ B.M.S = B.S.S/(q −1) $\qquad$ and

E.M.S = E.S.S/(p − 1) (q − 1)

Conclusion

If F (calculated) value > F (tabulated) value with (p − 1), (p − 1)(q − 1) d.f. for factor A and (q − 1), (p − 1) (q − 1) d.f for factor B at chosen level of significance, the H_0 is rejected. Otherwise the H_0 is accepted.

If H_0 is rejected then it can be concluded that there is significant difference between the levels of each factor. If H_0 is accepted then it can be concluded that there is no significant difference between the levels of each factor.

If H_0 is rejected, then the levels means of each factor are arranged in ascending order of magnitude separately and the difference between each pair of means will be compared with corresponding critical difference (C.D.) value, which are given as follows.

$$C.D \ (A) = t_{(p-1)(q-1)} \times \sqrt{\frac{2(EMS)}{q}}$$

$$C.D \ (B) = t_{(p-1)(q-1)} \times \sqrt{\frac{2(EMS)}{p}}$$

where $t_{(p-1)(q-1)}$ is the tabulated value of student's t-distribution with (p − 1) (q − 1) d.f. at the required level of significance.

If the difference between pair of means for each factor is greater than C.D. value then different superscripts are placed above the mean values. Otherwise same superscript will be used.

Example

Two drugs simultaneously were administered to patients to control body temperature. The number of days required to come to normal temperature were recorded and presented in Table 10.12. Test the significant difference between doses of two drugs A and B using two-way analysis of variance technique at 5 percent level of significance.

Table 10.12 Drug B

Drug A	50 mg	100 mg	250 mg	Total
50 mg	10	8	7	25
100 mg	9	6	5	20
250 mg	8	4	3	15
500 mg	7	3	2	12
Total	34	21	17	72

1. H_0 : In drug A all doses are equal in their effectiveness

2. H_0 : In drug B all doses are equal in their effectiveness

Correction Factor (C.F.) $= \dfrac{Y_{..}^2}{pq} = \dfrac{(72)^2}{4 \times 3} = 432$

where Y.. = grand total, p = 4, q = 3

Total S.S. (T.S.S) $= \left(Y_{11}^2 + Y_{12}^2 + ... + Y_{pq}^2\right) - C.F.$

$$= [(10)^2 + (8)^2 + ... + (2)^2 - 432 = 506 - 432 = 74$$

Drug A S.S $= \left[\dfrac{y_{1.}^2}{q} + \dfrac{y_{2.}^2}{q} + ... + \dfrac{y_{p.}^2}{q}\right] - C.F.$

$$= \dfrac{1}{3}\,[(25)^2 + (20)^2 + (15)^2 + (12)^2] - 432$$

$$= 464.67 - 432 = 32.67$$

Drug B S.S $= \dfrac{1}{4}\,[(34)^2 + (21)^2 + (17)^2] - 432$

$$= 471.5 - 432 = 39.5$$

Error S.S = T.S.S − (A.S.S + B.S.S)

$$= 74 − (32.67 + 39.5) = 1.83$$

The above sums of squares are furnished in Table 10.13 for carrying out the F-test.

Table 10.13

Source	d.f.	S.S.	M.S.	F_{cal}	F_{tab} (d.f.)
A	4 − 1 = 3	32.67	10.89	35.13	4.76 (3, 6)
B	3 − 1 = 2	39.50	19.75	63.71	5.14 (2, 6)
Error	3 × 2 = 6	1.83	0.31		
Total	**4 × 3 − 1 =11**				

Conclusion

Here F (calculated) value i.e., 35.13 > F (tabulated) value i.e., 4.76 with (3,6) d.f. at *5* percent level of significance. Hence H_0 is rejected. Therefore it can be concluded that there is significant difference between doses of drug A.

Here F(calculated) value i.e. 63.71 > F(tabulated) value i.e., 5.14 with (2,6) d.f. at *5* percent level of significance. Therefore H_0 is rejected. Hence it can be concluded that there is significant difference between doses of drug B.

In order to find out which is the most effective dose for drugs A and B the doses means are calculated and arranged in ascending order of magnitude and the differences between each pair of means are compared with corresponding critical difference values.

$$\text{C.D(A)} = t_{(p-1)(q-1)} \times \sqrt{\frac{2(EMS)}{q}}$$

$$= 2.447 \times \sqrt{\frac{2 \times 0.31}{3}} = 1.10$$

The doses means of drug A are arranged in ascending order of magnitude as in Table 10.14.

Table 10.14

50 mg	100 mg	250 mg	500 mg
c	b	a	a
8.33	6.67	5.00	4.00

From Table 10.14, it can be observed that doses 250 mg and 500 mg are not significantly different from each other and are most effective and dose 50 mg is the least effective.

The doses means of drug B are arranged in ascending order of magnitude as in Table 10.15.

Table 10.15

50 mg	100 mg	250 mg
c	b	a
8.5	5.25	4.25

$$C.D\ (B) = t_{(p-1)(q-1)} \times \sqrt{\frac{2(E.M.S)}{p}}$$

$$= 2.447 \times \sqrt{\frac{2 \times 0.31}{4}} = 0.95$$

It can be observed that from Table 10.15 dose 250 mg is the most effective followed by 100 mg and 50 mg doses.

Exercises

1. The following are the data on number of seeds germinated in pot culture experiment conducted in glass-house at different temperatures. Ten seeds were sown in each pot and kept at different temperatures.

20 °C	25 °C	30 °C	35 °C
6	8	10	7
5	9	9	3
3	7	5	2
2	6	6	4
4	5	4	1
	4		2

   Test the significant difference between temperatures using Analysis of variance technique at 5 percent level of significance.

2. Table shows the yields in tonnes per hectare of a certain variety of vegetable crop sown in a particular type of soil treated with chemicals A, B or C. Find (a) the mean yields for the different treatments (b) the grand mean for all treatments (c) the total variation (d) the variation between treatments and (e) the variation within treatments.

A	48	49	50	49
B	47	49	48	48
C	19	51	50	50

3. The following are the data of number of buds that appeared on rose plants which were maintained in different pots kept at different levels of temperatures and different levels of relative humidity by giving uniform basal dose of fertilizer and irrigation schedules.

Temperatures

R.H.	20 °C	25 °C	30 °C	35 °C
40	4	6	8	5
60	6	8	10	6
70	7	10	12	8
75	5	6	7	4

Test the significant difference between temperatures and also between levels of relative humidity with respect to appearance of rose buds using two-way analysis of variance technique at 1 percent level of significance.

4. The following are the data on gain in weight (100 gm) of weight of preschool going children after 3 months when they were administered the diets with different levels of protein content and different levels of carbohydrates.

Carbohydrate (%)	**Protein** (%)		
	5	10	15
20	4	6	10
30	7	10	12
40	8	14	16
50	12	18	20

Test the significant difference between levels of Carbohydrates and also between levels of protein content in diet at 1 percent level of significance using two-way analysis technique.

5. The following are the results obtained by conducting experiment in pots kept under glass-house. In this experiment different soils and different levels of irrigation were used for barley crop and the yields (100 gms) were recorded as follows.

	Number of Irrigations		
Soil	4	6	8
Sandy	10	14	9
Loamy	16	20	12
Clay	18	14	13

Test the significant difference between different soils and different levels of irrigation at 5 percent level of significance using two-way analysis of variance technique.

6. The following are the results of an experiment conducted on grapes with different number of prunings. The yields (100 gm) of bunches of seedless variety on different wines are given as follows.

Prunings

2	**4**	**6**	**8**
6	10	14	7
8	9	16	6
11	13	9	10
14	6	11	5
5	8	10	12
	15		11

Test the significant difference between the prunings with respect to yields of grapes at 5 percent level using one-way analysis of variance technique.

CHAPTER 11

Experimental Designs

11.1 Introduction

When more than two treatments are to be tested in an experiment in the agricultural field then a separate layout is used. This layout is generally called design. Different layouts are employed in different field situations and therefore different designs are used. In all the designs, analysis of variance technique is used as developed by R.A. Fisher. In each of the layouts, principles of experimental designs such as randomization, replication are used for analyzing the data with the help of analysis of variance technique. In some designs local control concept is also used besides randomization and replication. These concepts were already discussed in earlier chapter on analysis of variance.

11.2 Completely Randomized Design

This design is generally used in the field when the experimental material such as soil is of uniform nature. In this layout the experimental field is divided into plots of equal size and shape such as rectangular or square in shape and 5 × 4, 6 × 4 etc., sq. metres in size with irrigation channels on borders. The layout is shown below.

1	2	3	.	.
.	.	.	.	n

Each treatment is allotted to the plot in the layout randomly with the help of random number tables as given in many text books. If a particular random number comes in selection then the first treatment is allotted to the plot having serial number equal to the random number selected.

Similarly second treatment is allotted to the plot of second random number selected. This procedure is continued till all the plots are exhausted depending upon the number of replications for each treatment.

The additive model of analysis of variance is

$$Y_{ij} = \mu + \alpha_1 + e_{ij}$$

where Y_{ij} is the response value of j-th plot having i-th treatment for i = 1, 2,....., p; j = 1, 2, .., r_1 and Σr_i = n where i-th treatment is repeated in r_i plots and n is the total number of plots in the experimental field. μ is the overall mean, α_i is the effect of i-th treatment and e_{ij} is the experimental error on (i,j)-th plot.

The analysis of this experiment is same as the analysis of one-way analysis of variance technique described in earlier chapter since treatments are the only one factor used in the experiment.

$$H_0 : \alpha_1 = \alpha_2 = ... = \alpha_p$$

$$H_1 : \alpha_1 \neq \alpha_2 \neq ..... \neq \alpha_p$$

The data are presented in Table 11.1

Table 11.1 Treatment

	1	2	...	i	...	p	
	y_{11}	y_{21}	...	y_{i1}	...	y_{p1}	
	y_{12}	y_{22}	...	y_{i2}	...	y_{p2}	
	$\vdots$	$\vdots$	$\vdots$	$\vdots$		$\vdots$	
	y_{1r1}	y_{2r2}	...	y_{iri}		y_{prp}	
Total	$Y_{1.}$	$Y_{2.}$		$Y_{i.}$		$Y_{p.}$	$Y_{..}$

Correction Factor (C.F) = $\dfrac{Y_{..}^2}{n}$ where n = Σr_i

Total sum of squares (T.S.S) = $\left(y_{11}^2 + y_{12}^2 + ... + y_{prp}^2\right) - \text{C.F.}$

Treatment sum of squares (Tr.S.S) = $\left(\dfrac{Y_{1.}^2}{r_1} + \dfrac{Y_{2.}^2}{r_2} + ... + \dfrac{Y_{p.}^2}{r_p}\right) - \text{C.F.}$

Error sum of squares (within treatment sum of squares)

$$(\text{E.S.S}) = (\text{T.S.S.} - \text{Tr.S.S})$$

The sums of squares are presented in Table 11.2 for carrying out F-test.

Table 11.2 ANOVA

Source	d.f.	S.S.	M.S.	F_{cal}	F_{tab} (d.f.)
Between treatments	$p - 1$	Tr.S.S	Tr.M.S	$\dfrac{Tr.M.S}{E.M.S}$	$(p - 1), (n - p)$
Within treatments (Error)	$n - p$	E.S.S	E.M.S		
Total	$n - 1$				

where Tr.M.S = Tr.S.S/(p – 1) and E.M.S = E.S.S/(n – p)

Conclusion

If F (calculated) value > F (tabulated) value with (p – 1), (n – p) d.f. at chosen level of significance, H_0 is rejected. Otherwise, H_0 is accepted.

If H_0 is rejected, then it can be concluded that there is significant difference between treatment means with respect to character under consideration. In order to know which treatment is superior and which treatment is inferior, the pairwise comparison is done between the treatments with the help of critical difference (C.D) value which is computed as follows when the number of replications are equal. This value is also known as least significant difference (L.S.D.) value.

$$C.D = t_{(n-p)} \times \sqrt{\frac{2(E.M.S)}{r}}$$

where $t_{(n-p)}$ is the value of t-tabulated with error d.f. i.e. (n – p) at chosen level of significance and $r = r_1 = r_2 = \dots r_p$.

The treatment means are arranged in descending order of magnitude and the difference between each pair of them is compared with C.D. value and if the difference is more than C.D. value then different superscripts are placed above the treatment means. Otherwise same superscripts are placed above the treatment means.

When number of replications are unequal for the treatments then student's t-test will be used for each pair of means as follows.

$$t = \frac{|y_{i.} - y_{j.}|}{\sqrt{E.M.S\left(\dfrac{1}{r_i} + \dfrac{1}{r_j}\right)}}$$

where $y_{i.}$ and $y_{j.}$ are the means of i-th and j-th treatments with r_i and r_j replications respectively. If t (calculated) value is greater than t (tabulated) value with (n–p) d.f. at chosen level of significance then there is significant difference between i-th and j-th treatment means. In this way all treatment mean pairs can be compared with t-test.

Example

Five varieties of maize crop were tested in completely randomized design in an experimental field. Each variety is replicated 4 times in the experimental plots of size 6×4 sq.metres. The varieties are denoted as v_1, v_2 .... v_5. These varieties are randomly alloted to 20 plots and are presented in Fig. 11.2.

v_4 (10)	v_3 (22)	v_1 (13)	v_2 (12)	v_4 (16)
v_2 (8)	v_2 (9)	v_4 (13)	v_2 (7)	v_5 (7)
v_3 (20)	v_4 (14)	v_3 (24)	v_1 (10)	v_3 (25)
v_5 (6)	v_5 (10)	v_1 (14)	v_5 (11)	v_1 (15)

Fig. 11.2

The yields (kg) recorded on the net plots where border rows of plants on all the sides of plots are excluded for recording yields. The yields are presented in the plots in parentheses in Fig 11.2 itself.

The yields are taken from Fig 11.2 and reclassified according to varieties and presented in Table 11.3.

Table 11.3 Varieties

	v1	v2	v3	v4	v5	
	13	8	20	10	6	
	14	9	22	14	10	
	10	12	24	13	11	
	15	7	25	16	7	
Total	52	36	91	53	34	266

Correction Factor (C.F.) = $\dfrac{(266)^2}{20}$ = 3537.8

Total sum of squares (T.S.S) = $[(13^2) + (14)^2 + ... + (7)^2] -$ C.F.

$$= 4140 - 3537.8 = 602.2$$

Variety sum of squares (V.S.S.) = $\dfrac{(52)^2}{4} + \dfrac{(36)^2}{4} + \dfrac{(91)^2}{4} + \dfrac{(53)^2}{4} + \dfrac{(34)^2}{4} -$ C.F.

$$= \dfrac{16246}{4} - 3537.8 = 523.7$$

Error sum of squares (E.S.S.) = (T.S.S – V.S.S.)

$$= 602.2 - 523.7 = 78.5$$

The sums of squares obtained are presented in Analysis of Variance (ANOVA) Table 11.4.

H_0 : All varieties means are equal

H_1 : All varieties means are not equal.

Table 11.4 ANOVA

Source	d.f.	S.S.	M.S.	F_{cal}	F_{tab} d.f.
Varieties	5 – 1 = 4	523.7	130.93	25.03	4.89 (4,15)
Error	19 – 4 = 15	78.5	5.23		
Total	20 – 1 = 19	602.2			

Conclusion

Here F (calculated) value i.e., 25.03 > F (tabulated) value 4.89 with (4, 15) d.f. at 1 per cent level of significance. Therefore, H_0 is rejected. Hence, it can be concluded that there is significant difference between the varieties of maize crop with respect to yield.

In order to know which variety is significantly superior or inferior, the varieties means are computed and the difference between each pair of means is compared with C.D. value. The varieties means are arranged in descending order of magnitude and furnished in Table 11.5.

Table 11.5

$\bar{V}_3$	$\bar{V}_1$	$\bar{V}_1$	$\bar{V}_2$	$\bar{V}_5$
22.75[b]	13.25[a]	13.00[a]	9.00[a]	8.5[a]

The C.D. value is obtained as

$$C.D = t_{15} \times \sqrt{\frac{2 \times 5.23}{4}}$$

$$= 2.947 \times 1.62 = 4.77$$

From Table 11.5 it can be observed that the variety 3 is significantly superior to all the remaining varieties.

11.2.1 Advantages

(i) This design can be used whenever experimental material like soil, chemical, patient etc., is of uniform nature. This design is used in pot culture experiment, varietals trials in plant breeding experiments, entomology experiments where insects of some age are used for testing insecticides etc.

(ii) However in conducting experiments in glass-houses care has to be taken with respect to sunshade and air current along and across the bench on which pots are to be kept before proceeding to analyze the experiment.

(iii) In this design any number of treatments and any number of replications for each treatment can be used. In other words complete flexibility is provided in this design.

(iv) Analysis of this design can be carried out even when some values of treatments are missing due to mishaps like grazing by cattle, floods, etc.

11.2.2 Disadvantages

(i) The only disadvantage in using this design is when experimental units are not homogeneous. When experimental units are not homogeneous then within treatment sum of squares will increase and consequently treatments are less precisely compared. The only way to overcome this drawback is to increase the number of replications for each treatment thereby increasing the degrees of freedom for error.

11.3   Randomized Block Design

11.3.1 Introduction

In this design whole experimental field is divided into homogeneous blocks based on soil fertility etc. The blocks are formed in such a way that there will be more homogeneity within blocks and more heterogeneity between the blocks. This is one way of eliminating soil heterogeneity in the experimental field. This design is therefore called as one-way elimination of heterogeneity design. The knowledge of the fertility gradient is known based on the growth of the crop in previous experiments conducted in the same site.

Since the neighbouring plots are expected to be having uniform fertility gradient the blocks are formed in such a way that if the fertility gradient is in the direction of North to South the blocks will be formed perpendicular to the gradient direction i.e., East to West and vice-versa. However in medical experiments the grouping can be formed based on the age group of patients. In animal experiments the grouping will be done based on body weights, age, litter, sex etc.

The additive model of Analysis of Variance is

$$Y_{ij} = \mu + \alpha_i + \beta_i + e_{ij}.$$

where Y_{ij} is the response value on the plot in the j-th block having i-th treatment for i = 1, 2, ..., p, j = 1, 2, ..., r. μ is overall mean, α_i is the effect of i-th treatment, β_i is the effect of j-th block an e_{ij} the experimental error effect of (i, j)-th experimental plot. The procedure of analysis is given as follows. The observational values are furnished in Table 11.6.

Table 11.6

Treatment			Block				
	1	2	...	j	...	r	Total
1.	y_{11}	y_{12}	...	y_{ij}	...	y_{1r}	$Y_{1.}$
2.	y_{21}	y_{22}	...	y_{2j}	...	y_{2r}	$Y_{2.}$
i	$\vdots$	$\vdots$	$\vdots$	$\vdots$	$\vdots$		
i	y_{i1}	y_{i2}	...	y_{ij}	...	y_{ir}	$Y_{i.}$
$\vdots$	$\vdots$	$\vdots$	$\vdots$	$\vdots$	$\vdots$	$\vdots$	$\vdots$
p	yp_1	yp_2	...	yp_j	...	y_{pr}	$Y_{p.}$
Total	$Y_{.1}$	$Y_{.2}$	...	Y_{jj}	...	$Y_{.r}$	$Y_{..}$

$$\text{Correction Factor (C.F.)} = \frac{Y_{..}^2}{pr}$$

where $Y_{..}$ is the grand total p, r are the number of treatments and number of blocks respectively.

Total sum of squares (T.S.S) $= \left(y_{11}^2 + y_{12}^2 + ... + y_{pr}^2\right) - \text{C.F.}$

Treatment squares (Tr.S.S) $= \left(\dfrac{Y_{1.}^2}{r} + \dfrac{Y_{2.}^2}{r} + ... + \dfrac{Y_{i.}^2}{r} + ... + \dfrac{Y_{p.}^2}{r}\right) - \text{C. F,}$

where $Y_{i.}$ is the total of i-th treatment.

Block sum of squares (B.S.S.) $= \left(\dfrac{Y_{.1}^2}{p} + \dfrac{Y_{.2}^2}{p} + ... + \dfrac{Y_{.j}^2}{p} + ... + \dfrac{Y_{.r}^2}{p}\right) - \text{C.F,}$

where $Y_{.j}$ is the total of j-th block.

Error sum of squares (E.S.S) = T.S.S $-$ (Tr.S.S + B.S.S)

The layout of randomized block design (R.B.D) is given in Fig. 11.3.

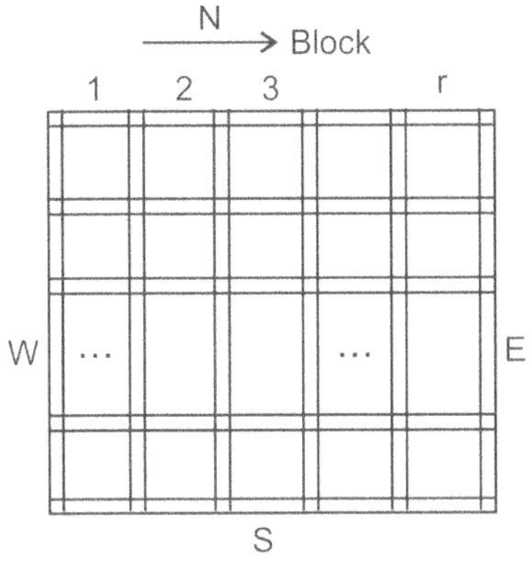

Fig. 11.3

The treatments are randomized in each black separately. In other words treatments are alloted to each plot based on random numbers in each block. Therefore each block is also called as complete replication since each treatment appears once in each block.

The sums of squares computed above are furnished in analysis of variance table given in Table 11.7 for carrying out F- test.

(i) H_0 : $\alpha_1 = \alpha_2 = \ldots = \alpha_p$

      H_1 : $\alpha_1 \neq \alpha_2 \neq \ldots \neq \alpha_p$

(ii) H_0 : $\beta_1 = \beta_2 = \ldots = \beta_p$

      H_1 : $\beta_1 \neq \beta_2 \neq \ldots \neq \beta_p$

Table 11.7

Source	d.f.	S.S.	M.S.	F_{cal}	F_{tab} d.f.
Blocks	$r-1$	B.S.S	B.M.S	$\dfrac{B.M.S}{E.M.S}$	$(r-1),\ (p-1)\,(r-1)$
Treatments	$p-1$	T_r.S.S	Tr.M.S	$\dfrac{Tr.M.S}{E.M.S}$	$(p-1),\ (p-1)\,(r-1)$
Error	$(p-1)\,(r-1)$	E.S.S	E.M.S		
Total	$pr-1$	T.S.S			

where

$$B.M.S = \frac{B.S.S}{(r-1)}, \quad Tr.M.S = \frac{Tr.S.S}{(p-1)} \quad \text{and} \quad E.M.S = \frac{E.S.S}{(p-1)(r-1)}$$

Conclusion

1f F (calculated) value > F (tabulated) value with $(r-1)$, $(p-1)$ $(r-1)$ d.f. for blocks and $(p-1)$, $(p-1)$ $(r-1)$ d.f. for treatments at chosen level of significance, H_0 is rejected. Otherwise H_0 is accepted.

If H_0 is rejected then it can be concluded that there is significant difference between treatments and blocks in each case. Otherwise there is no significant difference between treatments or blocks in each case.

If H_0 is rejected, the treatments are compared with the help of C.D. value. The treatments means are to be arranged in descending order of magnitude. The C.D. formula is given as follows,

$$\text{C.D. (treatments)} = t_{(p-1)(r-1)} \times \sqrt{\frac{2(\text{E.M.S})}{r}}$$

If the difference between two treatments means values is greater than C.D. value then different superscripts will be placed on the corresponding treatments means. Otherwise same superscript is used.

If block means are to be compared then the C.D. value is calculated with the formula given as

$$\text{C.D. blocks} = t_{(p-1)(r-1)} \times \sqrt{\frac{2(\text{E.M.S})}{p}}$$

Example

In an experiment conducted in a pharmacy five drugs are to be compared with respect to their efficacy for patients suffering with arthrritis. The patients are grouped according to their age. The number of days taken to get relief were recorded and presented in Table 11.8. Test whether there is any significant difference between the drugs as well as groups of patients of difference age groups using R.B.D analysis.

Table 11.8

	Age (years)				
Drug	**40**	**50**	**55**	**60**	**Total**
A	4	6	7	10	27
B	6	8	10	9	33
C	8	10	11	13	42
D	7	8	13	10	38
E	3	5	8	11	27
Total	28	37	49	53	167

H_0 : All drugs means are equal

H_1 : All drugs means are not equal

$$\text{Correction Factor (C.F.)} = \frac{(167)^2}{5 \times 4} = 1394.45$$

Total sum of squares (T.S.S) = $[(4)^2 + (6)^2 + \ldots + (11)^2] -$ C.F.

$$= 1537 - 1394.45 = 142.55$$

$$\text{Drug sum of Squares (Dr.S.S)} = \frac{(27)^2}{4} + \frac{(33)^2}{4} + \ldots + \frac{(27)^2}{4} - \text{C.F.}$$

$$= 1438.75 - 1394.45 = 44.3$$

$$\text{Age sum of squares (Ag.S.S.)} = \frac{(28)^2}{5} + \frac{(37)^2}{5} + \ldots + \frac{(53)^2}{4} - \text{C.F.}$$

$$= 1472.6 - 1394.45 = 78.15$$

Error sum of squares (E.S.S.) = T.S.S – (Dr.S.S + Ag.S.S)

$$= 142.55 - (44.3 + 78.15) = 20.1$$

The sums of squares computed are furnished in Table 11.9 for carrying out F-test.

Table 11.9

Source	d.f.	S.S.	M.S.	F_{cal}	F_{tab} d.f.
Drugs	5 – 1 = 4	44.30	11.08	6.60	3.26 (4, 12)
Age Groups	4 – 1 = 3	78.15	26.05	15.51	3.49 (3, 12)
Error	4 × 3 = 12	20.10	1.68		
Total	5 × 4 – 1 – 19				

Conclusion

Here F (calculated) value i.e., 6.60 > F (tabulated) value i.e., 3.26 with (4, 12) d.f. at 5 percent level of significance. Therefore H_0 is rejected. Hence it can be concluded that there is significant difference between drugs with respect to their efficacy.

Similarly F (calculated) value i.e. 15.51 > F (tabulated) value i.e. 3.49 with (3, 12) d.f. at 5 percent level of significance. Therefore H_0 is rejected. Hence it can be concluded that there is significant difference between age groups with respect to efficacy of drugs.

$$\text{C.D. (drugs)} = t_{12} \times \sqrt{\frac{2 \times 1.68}{4}}$$

$$= 2.178 \times 0.92 = 2.00$$

The drugs means are arranged in descending order of magnitude as follows in Table 11.10.

Table 11.10

$\overline{C}$	$\overline{D}$	$\overline{B}$	$\overline{A}$	$\overline{E}$
10.5^c	9.5^{bc}	8.25^{ab}	6.75^a	6.75^a

From Table 11.10 it can be observed that drugs A and E are equally effective compared to other drugs. Drugs C and D are not significantly different from each other and are inferior to other drugs.

$$\text{C.D. (age groups)} = t \times \sqrt{\frac{2 \times 1.68}{5}}$$

$$= 2.178 \times 0.82 = 1.79$$

The age groups means are arranged in descending order of magnitude as in Table 11.11.

Table 11.11

$\overline{60}$	$\overline{55}$	$\overline{50}$	$\overline{40}$
10.6^d	9.8^c	7.4^b	5.6^a

From Table 11.11 it can be observed that there is significant difference between all age groups. The age group of 40 years patients are able to recover from disease in less time compared to other age groups of patients. Age group of 60 years took significantly longer time to recover from suffering compared to other age groups.

11.3.2 Advantages

(i)   This design is widely used in agricultural field experiments since one-way fertility gradient is generally present in fields.

(ii)   Any number of blocks can be used in this experiment.

(iii)   This design is more efficient compared to C.R.D.

(iv)   The analysis is easy.

(v)   Even if some treatment values are missing due to failure of recording or due to any other reasons still analysis can be carried out with the help of missing plot technique.

(vi)   In the glasshouse experiment the blocks will be formed perpendicular to the sunshade on the bench.

(vii)   In animal experiments the characteristics like body weights, age, sex, litter, breed, fat content in milk would be considered in forming blocks.

11.3.3 Disadvantages

The only drawback in this design is when the number of experimental units in each block is more then the heterogeneity within blocks will increase. Consequently the efficiency of the design decreases. For example in agronomy experiments not more than 22 units of size 6 x 4 sq. metres will be generally used.

11.3.4 Missing Plot technique

The data on certain experimental units would not be available due to reasons such as failure to record observations in time by field staff, grazing of cattle in those plots, excessive water due to water logging etc. In such a situation the analysis of the experimental data need not to be abondend. We can still analyze this data using missing plot technique.

If a single value in the experimental plot (i, j) is missing then it can be substituted by the value

$$Y_{ij} = \frac{rY'.j + pY'_i - Y'..}{(p-1)(r-1)}$$

where p, r are the number of treatments and blocks respectively. $Y'_{.j}$ is the total of units in the j-th block in which missing unit occurs, Y'_i is the total of the remaining units of i-th treatment and $Y_{..}$ is the grand total of the units without missing unit.

In the analysis of variance table 1 d.f. would be subtracted from the error d.f. and total d.f. for each missing unit. In substituting the value obtained using the above formula there will be upward bias in treatment sum of squares. The amount of upward bias is computed using the following formula.

$$\text{Bias B} = \frac{\left[Y_{.j} - (p-1)Y_{ij}\right]^2}{p(p-1)}$$

where Y_{ij} is the value obtained for the missing unit occurred in (i, j)th unit, $Y_{.j}$ is the total of jth block without missing unit and p is the number of treatments. The amount 'B' obtained using the above expression will be subtracted from treatment sum of squares before carrying out F-test in analysis of variance table.

The standard error to be used in t-test for comparing treatment mean with missing unit and other treatment mean without missing unit is given as

$$\sqrt{\text{E.M.S}\left[\frac{2}{r} + \frac{p}{r(r-1)(p-1)}\right]}$$

Example

The following (Table 11.12) are the data of number of days taken by patients who were suffering from pneumonia after administering five drugs in 4 age groups. Out of the data the observation on the patient in 40-year age group with drug C was not recorded. Analyze the data using missing plot technique and draw conclusions.

Table 11.12

	Age (years)				
Drug	**35**	**40**	**50**	**60**	**Total**
A	6	8	11	12	37
B	9	12	13	15	49
C	10	X(13)	15	15	41(54)
D	11	14	18	20	63
E	8	10	9	12	39
Total	44	44	66	75	229
		(57)			(242)

(i) H_0 : All drugs means are equal

    H_1 : All drugs means are not equal

(ii) H_0 : All age groups means are equal

    H_1 : All age groups means are not equal

The value in the missing unit of 40-year age group with drug C is estimated using the formula

$$y_{ij} = \frac{rY'_{.j} + pY'_{i.} - Y'_{..}}{(r-1)(p-1)}$$

Here $Y'_{.j} = 44$, $Y'_{i.} = 41$, $p = 5$, $r = 4$, $Y'_{..} = 229$

$$y_{ij} = \frac{4 \times 44 + 5 \times 41 - 229}{(4-1)(5-1)} = 12.67$$

$$\simeq 13.0$$

The upward bias in using this value for missing unit is

$$\text{Bias} = \frac{[44 - (5-1)13]^2}{5(5-1)} = 3.2$$

The value of missing unit is substituted in Table 11.12 in brackets and corresponding age group total, and drug C total and grand total were calculated and presented in brackets in Table 11.12 itself. The analysis is done using this substituted value in the usual way.

$$\text{Correction Factor (C.F.)} = \frac{(242)^2}{5 \times 4} = 2928.2$$

$$\text{Total Sum of Squares (T.S.S)} = (6)^2 + (9)^2 + \dots + (12)^2 - \text{C.F.}$$
$$= 3164.0 - 2928.2 = 235.8$$

$$\text{Age group sum of squares (Ag.S.S)} = \frac{(44)^2}{5} + \frac{(57)^2}{5} + \frac{(66)^2}{5} + \frac{(75)^2}{5} - \text{C.F.}$$
$$= 3033.2 - 2928.2 = 105.0$$

$$\text{Drug sum of squares (Dr.S.S)} = \frac{(37)^2}{4} + \frac{(49)^2}{4} + \dots + \frac{(39)^2}{4} - \text{C.F.}$$
$$= 3044.0 - 2928.2 = 115.8$$

$$\text{Corrected Dr.S.S} = (\text{Dr. S.S} - \text{Bias})$$
$$= 115.8 - 3.2 = 112.6$$

$$\text{Error sum of squares (E.S.S)} = \text{T.S.S.} - (\text{Ag.S.S} + \text{Cor. Dr. S.S.})$$
$$= 235.8 - (105.0 + 112.6) = 18.2$$

The sums of squares obtained above are furnished in the following ANOVA table 11.13 to carry out F-test.

Table 11.13 ANOVA

Source	d.f.	S.S.	M.S.	F_{cal}	F_{tab} d.f.
Age groups	3	105.0	35.0	21.21	3.59 (3, 11)
Drugs	4	112.6	28.15	17.06	3.36 (4, 11)
Error	11	18.2	1.65		
Total	18				

Conclusion

Here F (calculated) value i.e. 21.21 > F (tabulated) value i.e. 3.59 for age groups with (3, 11) d.f. at 5 percent level. Hence H_0 is rejected. Also F (calculated) value i.e. 17.06 > F (tabulated) value i.e., 3.36 for drugs with (4, 11) d.f. at 5 percent level. Therefore H_0 is rejected.

Hence it can be concluded that there is significant difference between age groups as well as drugs with respect to their efficacy.

The two C.D. values are calculated for comparing drugs means due to missing observation for drug C. The second C.D. value will be used whenever drug C is involved in comparison with other drug.

$$C.D.(1) = t_{11} \times \sqrt{\frac{2(E.M.S)}{4}}$$

where t_{11} is the tabulated value of 't' with 11 d.f. at 5 percent level of significance.

$$C.D.\ (1) = 2.20\ 1 \times \sqrt{\frac{2 \times 1.65}{4}}$$

$$= 2.201 \times 0.91 = 2.00$$

$$C.D.\ (2) = t_{11} \times \sqrt{E.M.S\left(\frac{2}{r} + \frac{p}{r(r-1)(p-1)}\right)}$$

$$= 2.201 \times \sqrt{1.65\left[\frac{2}{4} + \frac{5}{4(4-1)(5-1)}\right]}$$

$$= 2201 \times 1.41 = 3.10$$

The drugs means are arranged in descending order of magnitude and present in Table 11.14.

Table 11.14

$\overline{D}$	$\overline{C}$	$\overline{B}$	$\overline{E}$	$\overline{A}$
15.75^c	13.5^{bc}	12.25^b	9.75^a	9.25^a

From Table 11.14 it can be observed that drugs E and A are most effective and drugs D and C are least effective compared to other drugs.

11.4 Latin Square Design

Whenever soil heterogeneity is present in two directions in experimental field this design is used. The heterogeneity of experimental material is eliminated in two ways. This design is also known as two-way elimination of heterogeneity design. If the fertility gradient is present from North to South, the blocks will be formed from East to West and also when the fertility gradient is present from East to West the blocks will be formed from North to South. In other words rows and columns will be blocks in this design. The Latin letters such as A, B, C etc., used as treatments are randomly allotted to rows and columns in such a way that each letter occurs once and only once in each row and column. Each row and each column will be complete replication. The number of rows, number of columns and number of treatments are all equal. Since Latin letters like A, B, C etc are used in the design this design is called as Latin Square design. This design is widely used in animal experiments since animals are effected by minimum two characteristics such as initial body weight, breed, sex, litter, strain, age at first lactation etc. Since the number of treatments, number of rows, and columns are equal if the treatments are 10 then the total number of experimental units will be 10 x 10. Therefore, it is of limited use in agricultural field experiments. However, in pharmaceutical and other clinical trials this design can be effectively used.

The randomization of treatments in each row and column is done by following the given procedure here.

Suppose 4 × 4 Latin square design layout is to be prepared then 4 treatments A, B, C and D are arranged in a square initially as follows.

Row				
1	A	B	C	D
2	B	C	D	A
3	C	D	A	B
4	D	A	B	C

Fig. 11.4

Randomize Rows

The random numbers are (say) 3, 1, 2, 4 then the rows will be rearranged in the order 3, 1, 2, 4 from 1, 2, 3, 4 as follows.

Column	1	2	3	4
	C	D	A	B
	A	B	C	D
	B	C	D	A
	D	A	B	C

Fig. 11.5

Randomize columns

Random numbers are (say) 4, 1, 3, 2. The columns are rearranged from the order 1, 2, 3, 4 to 4, 1, 3, 2 respectively.

B	C	A	D
D	A	C	B
A	B	D	C
C	D	B	A

Fig. 11.6

The arrangement in Fig. 11.6 is the final arrangement which satisfies the properties of randomization, each treatment occurs once and only once in each row and column and number of rows, columns and treatments are equal. This arrangement can be presented in field layout given in Fig. 11.7.

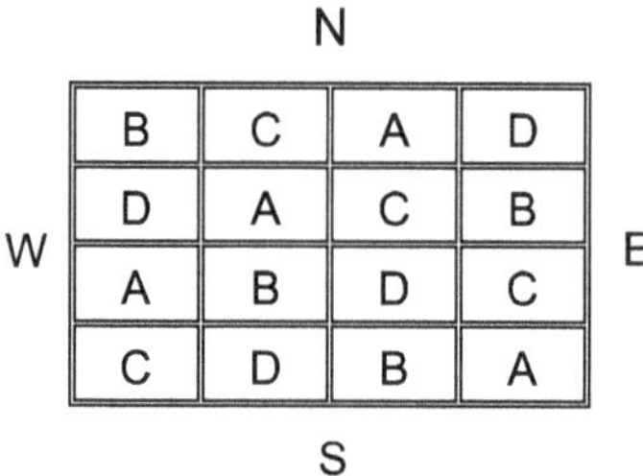

Fig. 11.7

The additive model of analysis of variance for this design is

$$y_{ijk} = \mu + \alpha_i + \beta_j + r_k + e_{ijk}$$

where y_{ijk} is the response value of the i-th treatment which was allotted randomly to the experimental plot in the j-th row of k-th column for i = 1, 2, …., r ; j = 1, 2, …, r and k = 1, 2…., r.

(i) H_0 : $\alpha_1 = \alpha_2 = \ldots = \alpha_r$

  H_1 : $\alpha_1 \neq \alpha_2 \neq \ldots \neq \alpha_r$

(ii) H_0 : $\beta_1 = \beta_2 = \ldots = \beta_r$

  H_1 : $\beta_1 \neq \beta_2 \neq \ldots \neq \beta_r$

(iii) H_0 : $\gamma_1 = \gamma_2 = \ldots = \gamma_r$

  H_1 : $\gamma_1 \neq \gamma_2 \neq \ldots \neq \gamma_r$

The procedure of analysis is given as follows :

Correction Factor (C.F.) = $\dfrac{Y^2_{...}}{r^2}$

where Y... is the grand total and r is the number of treatments, number of rows and also columns.

The sum of squares (T.S.S) = $y^2_{111} + y^2_{112} + \ldots + \ldots + y^2_{rrr} - \text{C.F.}$

Treatment sum of squares (Tr.S.S) = $\dfrac{Y_{1..}^2}{r} + \dfrac{Y_{2..}^2}{r} + ... + \dfrac{Y_{r..}^2}{r}$ – C.F.

Row sum of squares (R.S.S) = $\dfrac{Y_{.1.}^2}{r} + \dfrac{Y_{.2.}^2}{r} + ... + \dfrac{Y_{.r.}^2}{r}$ – C.F.

Column sum of square (C.S.S) = $\dfrac{Y_{.2}^{.1}}{r} + \dfrac{Y_{..2}^{.2}}{r} + ... \dfrac{Y_{....r}^{.2}}{r}$ – C.F.

Error sum of squares (E.S.S) = T.S.S – (Tr.S.S + R.S.S + C.S.S)

These sums of squares are furnished in ANOVA Table 11.15 for carrying out F-test.

Table 11.15 ANOVA

Source	d.f.	S.S.	M.S.	F_{cal}	F_{tab} d.f.
Rows	r–1	R.S.S	R.M.S	R.M.S/E.M.S	(r–1), (r–1) (r–2)
Columns	r–1	C.S.S	C.M.S	C.M.S/E.M.S	-do-
Treatments	r–1	Tr.S.S	Tr.M.S	Tr.M.S/E.M.S	-do-
Erorr	(r–1) (r–2)	E.S.S	E.M.S		
Total	$r^2 - 1$	T.S.S			

Here R.M.S = R.S.S/(r–1), C.M.S = C.S.S/(r–1) and Tr.M.S = Tr.S.S/(r–1).

Conclusion

If F (calculated) value > F (tabulated) value with (r —1), (r — 1) (r — 2) d.f. at chosen level of significance H_0 is rejected for treatments, rows and columns in each case. If H_0 is rejected for treatments then it can be concluded that there is significant difference between treatments means.

Similarly same conclusion can be drawn for rows and columns.

If H_0 is rejected then comparison between treatments means, rows means and columns means can be done by arranging them in descending order of magnitude separately and difference between each pair of means will be compared with C.D.

C.D. (treatments, rows, columns) = $t_{(r-1),(r-2)} \times \sqrt{\dfrac{2(E.M.S)}{r}}$

where $t_{(r-1),(r-2)}$ is the tabulated value of 't' with (r–1) (r–2) d.f. at chosen level of significance.

11.4.1   Advantages

(i) This design is useful whenever two-way heterogeneity of soil fertility gradient is present in field experiments.

(ii) This design is also useful in pharmaceutical experiments since experimental subjects are variants with two or more characteristics.

(iii) It is also useful in animal experiments since animals are varied according to two or more characteristics.

(iv) In general Latin squares of size 5 × 5 to 8 × 8 are used in practice.

(v) This design is superior to R.B.D. whenever the data is having two-way heterogeneity.

(vi) Even if some missing values are present, still analysis can be carried out with missing plot technique.

11.4.2   Disadvantages

(i) This design is useful only when the number of treatments is limited. Otherwise, the total number of experimental units enormously increases involving lot of time and expenditure.

(ii) This design is only of limited use in agricultural field experiments since the experimental fields generally will not have two way soil fertility gradient.

Example 1

The following are the data on number of days required to control typhoid in patients who were classified according to hospitals and age groups by administering different drugs and presented in Table 11.16.

Table 11.16 Age Group (Years)

Hospital	35	40	45	50	60	Total
1	E (10)	C (12)	D (7)	A (24)	B (7)	60
2	B (11)	E (12)	A (23)	C (10)	0 (9)	65
3	D (6)	B (8)	C (13)	E (15)	A (25)	67
4	C (11)	A (20)	B (7)	D (5)	E (17)	60
5	A (21)	D (8)	E (13)	B (6)	C (14)	62
Total	59	60	63	60	72	314

The analysis is given as follows.

(i) H_0 :   All drugs means are equal

         H_1 :   All drugs means are not equal

(ii) H_0 :   All hospitals means are equal

         H_1 :   All hospitals means are not equal

(iii) H_0 :   All age groups means are equal

   H_1 :   All age groups means are not equal.

Correction Factor (C.F.) $= \dfrac{(314)^2}{(5)^2} = 3943.84$

Total sum of squares (T.S.S) $= (10)^2 + (11)^2 + \ldots + (14)^2 - $ C.F.

$$= 4802 - 3943.84 = 858.16$$

Drug sum of squares (Dr.S.S) $= \dfrac{(113)^2}{5} + \dfrac{(39)^2}{5} + \dfrac{(60)^2}{5} + \dfrac{(35)^2}{5} + \dfrac{(67)^2}{5} - $ C.F.

$$= 4720.8 - 3943.84 = 776.96$$

Hospital sum of squares (H.S.S) $= \dfrac{(60)^2}{5} + \dfrac{(65)^2}{5} + \dfrac{(67)^2}{5} + \dfrac{(60)^2}{5} + \dfrac{(62)^2}{5} - $ C.F.

$$= 3951.6 - 3943.84 = 7.76$$

Age group sum of squares (Ag.S.S) $= \dfrac{(59)^2}{5} + \dfrac{(60)^2}{5} + \dfrac{(63)^2}{5} + \dfrac{(60)^2}{5} + \dfrac{(72)^2}{5} - $ C.F.

$$= 3966.8 - 3943.84 = 22.96$$

Error sum of squares (E.S.S) $= $ T.S.S $- $ (Dr.S.S. + H.S.S. + Ag.S.S)

$$= 858.16 - (776.96 + 7.76 + 22.96) = 50.48$$

The sums of squares obtained above are furnished in the following ANOVA Table 11.17 for carrying out F-test.

Table 11.17 ANOVA

Source	d.f.	S.S.	M.S.	F_{cal}	F_{tab} d.f.
Hospitals	4	7.76	1.94	0.46	3.26 (4,12)
Age groups	4	22.96	5.74	1.36	3.26 (4, 12)
Drugs	4	776.36	194.24	46.14	3.26 (4, 12)
Error	12	50.48	4.21		
Total	24	858.16			

Conclusion

Here F (calculated) value i.e. 0.46 < F (tabulated) value i.e., 3.26 for hospitals with (4, 12) d.f. at 5 percent level of significance. Similarly F (calculated) value i.e. 1.36 < F (tabulated) value i.e. 3.26 with (4, 12) d.f. at 5 percent level for age groups. Hence it can be concluded that there is no significant difference between hospitals as well as age groups in controlling the disease. However, F (calculated) value i.e. 46.14 > F (tabulated) value i.e. 3.26 with (4, 12) d.f. at 5 percent level of significance for drugs. Therefore there is significant difference between drugs at 5 percent level.

Since drugs were found significant, drugs were evaluated with respect to their superiority or inferiority in comparison to others.

The critical difference value is obtained as follows.

$$\text{C.D. (drugs)} = t_{12} \times \sqrt{\frac{2(\text{E.M.S})}{5}}$$

$$= 2.179 \times \sqrt{\frac{2 \times 4.21}{5}}$$

$$= 2.179 \times 1.30 = 2.83$$

The drugs means are arranged in descending order of magnitude and presented in Table 11.18.

Table 11.18

$\overline{A}$	$\overline{E}$	$\overline{C}$	$\overline{B}$	$\overline{D}$
22.6^c	13.4^b	12.0^b	7.8^a	7.0^a

From Table 11.18 it can be observed that drug D and drug B are not significantly different from each other and are most effective in controlling the disease compared to other drugs. Drug A is most ineffective in comparison to other drugs.

Example 2

Five doses of fertilizer were tried in paddy crop using Latin Square design layout in experimental field. The yields (kgs) were recorded and presented in the following fig. 11.

1	2	3	4	5	6	Total
1	F_2 (10)	F_1 (8)	F_3 (16)	F_5 (26)	F_4 (20)	80
2	F_4 (18)	F_3 (15)	F_5 (24)	F_2 (12)	F_1 (7)	76
3	F_5 (20)	F_4 (19)	F_1 (9)	F_3 (17)	F_2 (15)	80
4	F_1 (6)	F_5 (22)	F_2 (14)	F_4 (16)	F_3 (14)	72
5	F_3 (20)	F_2 (12)	F_4 (17)	F_1 (10)	F_5 (23)	82
Total	74	76	80	81	79	390

Fig. 11.8

The doses are represented by F_1, F_2, F_3, F_4 and F_5. Analyse the data and draw conclusions :

Analysis

Correction Factor (C.F.) $= \dfrac{Y^2_{...}}{r^2} = \dfrac{(390)^2}{5 \times 5} = 6084$

Where $\qquad\qquad r = 5$

Total sum of squares (T.S.S) $= [\,(10)^2 + (18)^2 + \ldots. + \ldots. + (23)^2\,] - \text{C.F}$

$$= 6800 - 6084 = 716$$

Row sum of squares (R.S.S) $= \dfrac{1}{5}[\,(80)^2 + (76)^2 + \ldots + (82)^2\,] - \text{C.F}$

$$= 6096.8 - 6084.0 = 12.8$$

Column sum of squares (c.s.s) $= \dfrac{1}{5}[\,(74)^2 + (76)^2 + \ldots.. + (79)\,]$

$$= 6090.8 - 6084.0 = 6.8$$

Fertilizer sum of squares (F.S.S)

$$= \frac{1}{5}[\,(40)^2 + (63)^2 + (82)^2 + (90)^2 + (115)^2\,] - C.F$$

$$= 6723.6 - 6084.0 = 639.6$$

Error sum of squares (E.S.S) $= T.S.S - (R.S.S + C.S.S + F.S.S)$

$$= 716 - (12.8 + 6.8 + 639.6) = 56.8$$

The sum of squares are furnished in the Table 11.19 for carrying out F-test.

H_0 :

(i)   All rows means are equal

(ii)   All columns means are equal

(iii)   All fertilizers means are equal

Table 11.19

Source	d.f.	s.s.	M.s.	F_{cal}	F_{tab} (d.f.)
Rows	4	12.8	3.20	0.68	(4, 12)
Columns	4	6.8	1.70	0.36	(4, 12)
Fertilizer	4	639.6	159.90	33.81	(4, 12)
Error	12	56.8	4.73		
Total	24				

Conclusion

Here F (calculated) value i.e. 0.68 for rows, 0.36 for columns < F (tabulated) value i.e., 3.26 at 5 percent level of significance. Therefore H_0 is accepted. Hence it can be concluded that there is no significant difference between rows and columns.

Here F (calculated) value i.e 33.81 > F (tabulated) value i.e. 3.26 with (4, 12) d.f. at 5 percent level of significance. Therefore, H_0 is rejected. Hence it can be concluded that there is significant difference between fertilizer doses. In order to know which fertilizer dose is most effective the fertilizers means are arranged in descending order of magnitude and presented in Table 11 and C,D. value is computed as follows.

Table 11.20

$\overline{F_5}$	$\overline{F_4}$	$\overline{F_3}$	$\overline{F_2}$	$\overline{F_1}$
d	c	c	b	a
23.0	18.0	16.4	12.6	8.0

$$C.D. = t_{12} \times \sqrt{\frac{2(E.M.S)}{r}}$$

$$= 2.179 \times \sqrt{\frac{2 \times 4.73}{5}}$$

$$= 2.179 \times 1.38 = 3.00$$

From Table 11.20 it can be observed that the fertilizer dose F5 gave significantly higher yield than the other doses. The fertilizer dose F1 gave lowest yield compared to other doses.

CHAPTER 12

Statistical Quality Control

12.1 Introduction

In a manufacturing unit quality of product it produces is very important. For example in a pharmaceutical company the quality of product like life saving drug in heart diseases is very important. If the product is not meeting the specific requirements of its composition then so many lives are at stake. Therefore the producer would like to confirm whether the manufacturing unit is producing uniform products without deviating from set standards. This is known as quality control. If the deviation from unit to unit is minor then it can be ignored. If the deviation is major then the manufacturing process has to be stopped and the defect occurred has to be rectified before releasing to the market for sale.

12.2 Chance Variation

The minor variation occurs in products in the manufacturing process is called chance variation. This variation occurs inspite of taking all precautions with respect to raw material, machine, operator etc. This vaiation cannot be completely removed. Further this variation in the product can be tolerable and will not cause significant damage to the producer and consumer.

12.3 Assignable Variation

The variation in the products of same brand or composition is significant or noticeable with respect to quality then, it is due to assignable variation. This variation might have occurred due to raw material, composition, machine, operator or scientist involved etc. The effect of this variation will effect the image of the company in the market and also consumer to a large extent. If the manufacturing company is drug manufacturing company, the major variation in the quality of drug produced causes maximum harm to the patients. Therefore the producer should immediately withdraw the product from the market to arrest the damage to the public at large and also to maintain reputation of its brand name in the market.

12.4 Statistical Quality Control

If the manufactured product varies its quality due to chance variation only then it is said to be under statistical quality control and if it varies its quality due to assignable cause then it is said to be not under statistical quality control. The statistical quality control charts were first developed by Dr. Walter A. Shewart. He used confidence limits for mean, standard deviation and range using normal distribution as control limits for manufactured product. If the means of sample lie within control limits then the manufacturing process is under control. Otherwise the manufacturing process is not under control and check has to be administered with respect to entire process of manufacture at different stages.

12.5 Advantages of Statistical Quality Control

(i)   It can be confirmed that whether the manufacturing unit is producing uniform standard products or not.

(ii) It is useful to the producer since his product gets maximum demand in the market and also maintains his reputation as a producer of quality product.

(iii) It is useful to the consumer that he/she is purchasing quality product with minimum risk.

(iv) Statistical quality control makes low cost of inspection within a shortest time.

(v)   The producer can take remedial measures when the product is lying outside control limits immediately.

(vi) Statistical quality control protects manufacturer from further losses as without it he or she incurs huge losses when the product is released into the market as otherwise it may result in so many loss of lives if it is a drug manufacturing company.

(vii) Statistical quality control is useful especially when the units manufactured are electric bulbs, explosives, life of a battery cell.

Statistical control of products in a production process is administered through statistical control charts. The chart consists of control line at the middle and lines of upper control limit and lower control limits on either side of the middle line. If the measurements of sample units falls within upper and lower control limits then it can be concluded that the production process is under quality control. Otherwise the production process is not under quality control and it requires immediate inspection for taking corrective measures. If the units fall in control limits then they are considered as homogeneous and whatever variation exists amongst them is due to chance variation and which will not effect the quality of the unit or product. For quality control of the product, different samples are taken from the production line and compared with the help of control charts at regular intervals of time. The sampling scheme may be of different types.

12.6 Control Charts

Control charts are of two types (i) for measurement data and (ii) for qualitative characteristics or attributes.

In case of measurement data the statistical control charts were developed based on the assumption that the data follows normal distribution.

The different charts are (i) Mean Chart ($\bar{x}$ – chart) (ii) Range chart (R – chart) and (iii) Standard deviation chart (σ – chart).

12.6.1   Mean Chart ($\bar{x}$ – chart)

In this chart different samples of same size are drawn at random from the production line and their measurements were recorded. Let $\bar{x}_1$, $\bar{x}_2$ .... , $\bar{x}_k$ be the k samples means based on n observations for each sample then

$$\bar{x}_i = \frac{1}{n}\sum_{j=1}^{n} x_{ij}\; \frac{1}{k}\sum_{i=1}^{k} x_i \text{ for i} = 1, 2.... \text{ K Mean of 'k' means of samples.}$$

Let $R_1, R_2, ..., R_k$ be the ranges of k samples where each sample consists of n observations.

$$R_i = Max(x_{ij}) - Min\,(x_{ij}) \qquad\qquad \text{for } j = 1, 2, ..., n$$
$$i = 1, 2, ..., k$$

$$\bar{R} = \frac{1}{k}\;\sum_{i=1}^{k} R_i = \text{Mean of 'k' ranges.}$$

Let 'μ' and 'σ' are the 'mean' and 'standard deviation' respectively of the population of units from which samples are drawn then the control limits are given as $\mu \pm 3\sigma$.

Where $\mu + 3\,\sigma$ is upper control limit and $\mu - 3\sigma$ is lower control limit and 'μ' is middle value. In normal distribution 99.7 percent values lie between $\mu + \dfrac{3\sigma}{\sqrt{n}}$ and

$\mu - \dfrac{3\sigma}{\sqrt{n}}$ limits. Therefore the upper and lower control limits are taken as $\mu + 3\sigma$ and $\mu - 3\sigma$ respectively.

The corresponding control limits in sample are given as $\bar{\bar{x}} \pm \dfrac{3\sigma}{\sqrt{n}}$ where $\dfrac{\sigma}{\sqrt{n}}$ is the standard error of means. Since 'σ' is the standard deviation in the population and it is not known in most of the cases. 'σ' is estimated by standard deviation based on sample.

It may be noted that in control charts the standard deviation is substituted with the range using correction term for simplicity purpose. 'σ' is estimated as $\dfrac{\overline{R}}{d_2}$ where d_2 is a constant depending upon sample size 'n'. The d_2 values are given in table given at the end in Appendix for different values of n.

The control limits are given as

$$\overline{\overline{x}} + \frac{3\overline{R}}{\sqrt{n}\,d_2} = \overline{\overline{x}} + \frac{3}{\sqrt{n}\,d_2}\overline{R}$$

$$\text{Let } A_2 = \frac{3}{\sqrt{n}\,d_2}$$

then control limits are

$\overline{\overline{x}}$ = Control line or central line

$\overline{\overline{x}} + A_2R$ = upper control limit (U.C.L)

$\overline{\overline{x}} - A_2\overline{R}$ = lower control limit (L.C.L).

The values of A_2 are obtained from Table in Annexure based on 'n' the number of observations in each sample. These limits are shown in Fig. 12.1.

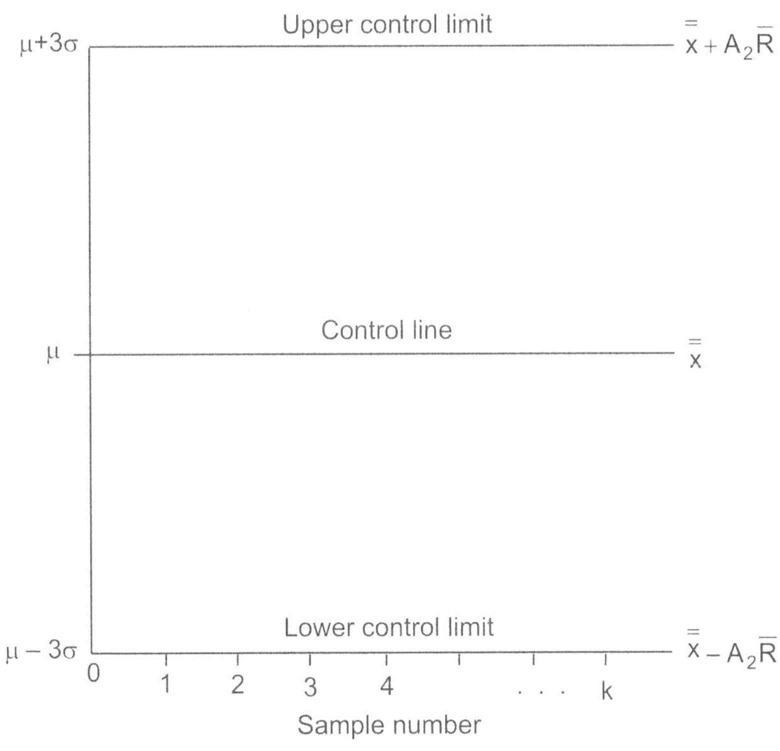

Fig. 12.1

From Fig.12.1 it can be observed that the means of samples should lie on the control line. However the means of samples can vary between upper and lower control limits due to chance causes which are permissible. However if the means of samples fall above upper control limit and below lower control limit then there is a cause for concern and the production process has to be checked for maintaining quality standard.

Example

The following are the Disodium Hydrogen Citrate BP content (gms) in different samples of syrup manufactured by pharmaceutical company. Draw the mean control chart and verify whether the production of syrup is under control.

Table 12.1

Sample	Range	Hydrogen citrate (gm)	Total	Mean
1	0.38	1.50 1.38 1.27 1.65	5.80	1.45
2	0.18	1.48 1.37 1.30 1.45	5.60	1.40
3	0.13	1.39 1.41 1.40 1.52	5.72	1.43
4	0.14	1.50 1.48 1.39 1.36	5.73	1.43
5	0.12	1.51 1.39 1.44 1.46	5.80	1.45
Total	0.95			7.16

$$\bar{\bar{x}} = \frac{7.16}{5} = 1.43$$

$$\bar{R} = \frac{0.95}{5} = 0.19$$

Upper control limit $= \bar{\bar{x}} + A_2 \bar{R}$

$$= 1.43 + 0.729 \times 0.19$$

$$= 1.57$$

where $A_2 = 0.729$ with $n = 4$ from Table

Lower control limit $= \bar{\bar{x}} - A_2 \bar{R}$

$$= 1.43 - 0.729 \times 0.19$$

$$= 1.29$$

The mean control chart is given in Fig. 12.2.

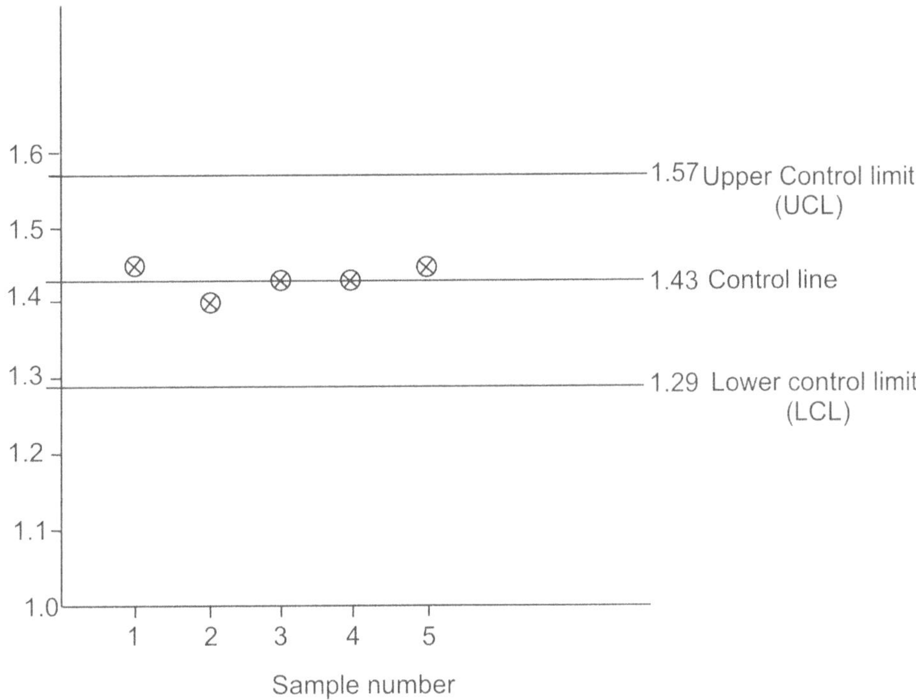

Fig. 12.2

From Fig. 12.2 it can be observed that all sample means are lying within control limits. Therefore it can be concluded that the production process of the company is under quality control with respect to syrup.

12.6.2   Range Control Chart (R – Chart)

Range control chart is used when the data of sample is large in a production process. Range can be computed easily as it depends upon only. The largest and smallest values whereas the mean depends upon the all the observations in the sample. Sometimes both R-chart and $\bar{x}$-chart are obtained in order to study the variation with respect to range as well as with respect to mean in a pharmaceutical company to take extra precaution.

Let R_{ij} = Max. (xij) – Min (xij)   for j = 1, 2...., n and i = 1, 2, ..., k.

$$\overline{R} \;=\; \frac{1}{k}\sum_{i=1}^{k} R_i$$

The upper and lower control limits are given as

$$U.C.L = D_4\,\overline{R}$$

$$L.\,C.\,L = D_3\,\overline{R}$$

where D_3 and D_4 are the table values obtained from Table in Annexure based on 'n' the number of observations in each sample. R-chart can be drawn in the same way as $\overline{x}$ -chart using upper and lower control limits.

Example

The following are the data on Ammonium Chloride content m_g in cough syrup samples produced by pharmaceutical company. Draw the mean and range charts. Each sample is based on 5 observations.

Sample	1	2	3	4	5	6	7	8	9	10
Mean	110	105	108	112	107	106	106	112	104	109
Range	8	10	12	14	10	11	13	9	8	7

$$\overline{\overline{x}} \;=\; \frac{\sum \overline{x}i}{k} \;=\; \frac{1079}{10} \;=\; 107.9 \text{ where } k = 10$$

$$\overline{R} \;=\; \frac{\sum R_i}{k} \;=\; \frac{102}{10} \;=\; 10.2$$

Mean Chart Control limits are

(i) $U.C.L = \overline{\overline{x}} + A_2\,\overline{R} = 107.9 + 0.58 \times 10.2$

$$= 113.82$$

(ii) $L.C.L = \overline{\overline{x}} - A_2\overline{R} = 107.9 - 0.58 \times 10.2$

$$= 101.98$$

(iii) $C.L = \overline{\overline{x}} = 107.9$

The mean chart is given in Fig. 12.3

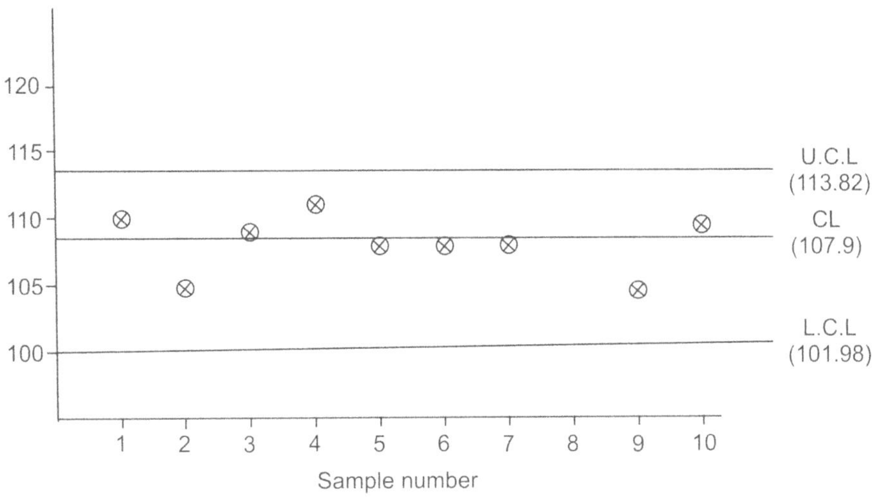

Fig.12.3

From Fig 12.3 it can be seen that the means are falling within control limits. Therefore, it can be concluded that the production process of cough syrup is within quality control limits as far as mean chart is concerned.

Range chart control limits are obtained as follows :

$$U.C.L. = D_4\ \overline{R} = 2.115 \times 10.2 = 21.57$$

$$L.C.L = D_3\ \overline{R} = 0 \times 10.2 = 0$$

$$C.L = \overline{R} = 10.2$$

The Range chart is given in Fig. 12.4

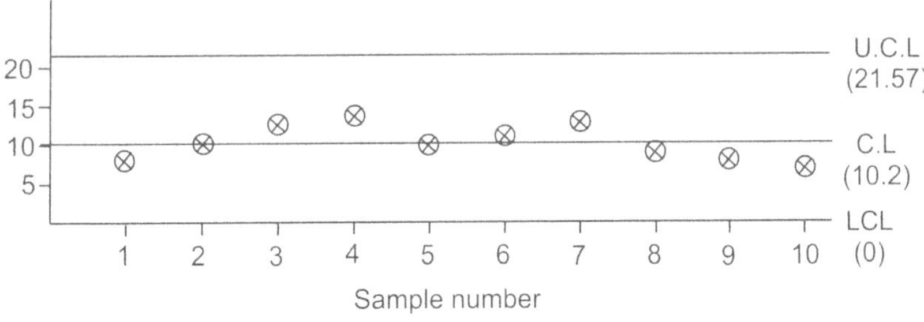

Fig.12.4

From Fig. 12.4, it can be verified that all the sample ranges are lying within control limits. Therefore it can be concluded that the production of syrup samples are under quality control with respect to Ammonium Chloride content.

12.6.3   Standard Deviation Chart (σ – Chart)

Range gives only the rough measure of dispersion of data whereas standard deviation measures the exact measure of dispersion. Though computation of standard deviation takes little more time in comparison to range, the control chart based on standard deviation is more efficient. The upper and lower control limits are given as

$$\text{U.C.L} = B_2 \sigma$$

$$\text{L.C.L} = B_1 \sigma$$

Usually 'σ' the population standard deviation is not known therefore it is estimated by sample standard deviation 's'. The lower and upper control limits based on sample standard deviation are given as.

$$\text{L.C.L} = B_3 \ \bar{s}$$

$$\text{U.C.L} = B_4 \ \bar{s}$$

$$\text{where } \bar{s} = \frac{\sum si}{n} \text{ and } s_i^2 = \frac{1}{ni-1} \sum_j (xij - \bar{x})^2$$

B_1, B_2, B_3 and B_4 are the constant values based on different sample sizes and are given in Table in the Annexure.

The Control Chart is given in Fig. 12.5.

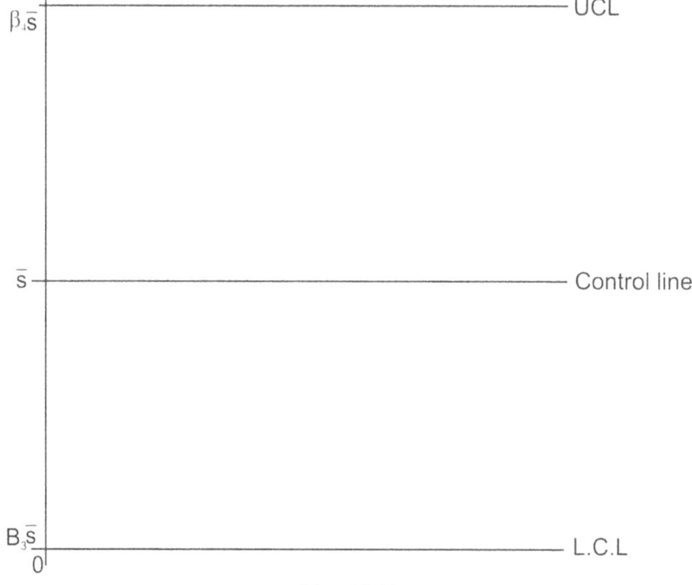

Fig.12.5

12.7 Control Charts for Attributes

So far we have discussed about control charts for products which are measurable. The products which cannot be measured but can be described as attributes or qualitative characteristics. The control charts based on qualitative characteristics are called control charts for attributes.

The following are the types of control charts which are used for attributes.

(i)   Proportion chart (P-chart)

(ii)   Number of defective items chart (np – chart)

(iii)   Number of defective items per unit (C- chart)

12.7.1   Proportion Chart (P – Chart)

In production process the number of defective items will be counted from the total number of items of sample which is selected at random. Let pi be the proportion of defective items for i-th sample.

$$\overline{P} = \overline{P}\frac{\sum Pi}{n}$$ where 'n' is the number of samples selected randomly from the production process.

The standard deviation of $\overline{P}$ is known as standard error. The standard error of $\overline{p}$

is given as $\sqrt{\dfrac{\overline{p}\,\overline{q}}{n}}$ based on Binomial distribution and $q = 1 - \overline{p}$.

The upper and lower control limits for p – chart are given by

$$\text{U.C.L} = \overline{P} + 3\sqrt{\frac{\overline{p}\overline{q}}{n}}$$

$$\text{L.C.L} = \overline{p} - 3\sqrt{\frac{\overline{p}\overline{q}}{n}}$$

The control line for this chart is at $\overline{p}$. If all the pi s lie within control limits then the production process is within quality control limits and otherwise it is not within control limits.

Example

In a pharmaceutical company the proportion of injection bottles found defective were 0.2, 0.1, 0.08, 0.04, 0.06 out of 80, 60, 40, 50 and 80 sample bottles selected respectively. Find the control limits for maintaining quality control of the medicine.

$$\overline{p} = \frac{n_1p_1 + n_2p_2 + n_3p_3 + n_4p_4 + n_5p_5}{n_1 + n_2 + n_3 + n_4 + n_5}$$

Here $n_1 = 80$, $p_1 = 0.2$, $n_2 = 60$, $p_2 = 0.1$, $n_3 = 40$, $p_3 = 0.08$

$n_4 = 50$, $p_4 = 0.04$ and $n_5 = 80$, $p5 = 0.06$ and $n = 80 + 60 + 40 + 50 + 80 = 310$

$$\bar{p} = \frac{80 \times 0.2 \times 60 \times 0.1 \times 40 \times 0.08 + 50 \times .04 + 80 \times .06}{80 + 60 + 40 + 50 + 80}$$

$$\bar{p} = \frac{32}{310} = 0.1032$$

$$\bar{q} = 1 - 0.1032 = 0.8968$$

The control limits are

$$\text{U.C.L} \quad = \bar{p} + \sqrt{\frac{\bar{p}\,\bar{q}}{n}}$$

$$= 0.1032 + 3\sqrt{\frac{0.1032 \times 0.8968}{310}}$$

$$= 0.1032 + 3 \times 0.0173 = 0.1551$$

$$\text{L.C.L} \quad = \bar{p} - 3\sqrt{\frac{\bar{p}\,\bar{q}}{n}}$$

$$= 0.1032 - 3 \times 0.0173 = 0.0513$$

The control line value is $\bar{p} = 0.1032$. From the data given in example it can be observed that the proportion of defective injection bottles 0.04 out of 50 was out of control limits. Therefore the production process should be checked up in the factory.

12.7.2   Number of defectives charts (np – chart)

If the size of the sample is same for inspection in a production process of a pharmaceutical company or any other industry then np-chart can be used instead of p-chart. Here the number of defective items would be counted out of uniform sample size, n. The np becomes average number of defective items for sample size of 'n'. The control limits are given as

$$\text{U.C.L} = np + 3\sqrt{npq}$$

$$\text{L.C.L} = np - 3\sqrt{npq}$$

$$\text{Control line} = np$$

Example

The number of defective injection needles in production process are 20, 28, 16, 34 and 22 out of 1000 needles in each sample. The average number of defective needles for each sample is

$$np = \frac{20 + 28 + 16 + 34 + 22}{5}$$

$$= 24$$

$$p = \frac{24}{1000} = 0.024$$

$$q = 1 - 0.024 = 0.976$$

The control limits are

(i) U.C.L = np + $3 \times \sqrt{npq}$

$$= 24 + 3 \times \sqrt{1000 \times 0.024 \times 0.976}$$

$$= 24 + 3 \times 4.8398 = 38.52$$

(ii) L.C.L = n p $- 3 \times \sqrt{npq}$

$$= 24 - 3 \times \sqrt{1000 \times 0.024 \times 0.976}$$

$$= 9.48$$

(iii) Control line = np = 24

It can be observed from the data of the example that all the values of defective items are falling within upper and lower control limits. Hence it can be concluded that the production process of the factory is under quality control. In other words, the needles produced by the factory are within quality control limits and no correction is necessary.

12.7.3 Number of defective items per unit chart (c-chart)

In this chart the number of defectives are counted per unit instead of number of defective items as in np-chart. Since the number of defectives per unit is generally small the average number of defectives per unit when several units are under consideration is assumed to follow poisson distribution instead of Binomial distribution as in the case of P or np-charts. If the average number of defectives per unit is considered this chart is named as $\bar{c}$ - chart instead of c-chart. If $\bar{c}$ is the mean number of defectives in poisson distribution then the standard error of mean is $\sqrt{c}$. The control limits for this chart are given as.

$$U.C.L = \bar{c} + 3\sqrt{c}$$

$$L.C.L = \bar{c} - 3\sqrt{c}$$

$$C.L = \bar{c}$$

Example

The following are the number of B-complex syrup bottles which are defective with respect to chemical composition observed in sealed packets containing 100 bottles supplied by a pharmaceutical company. Construct control chart for the defective items.

No. of Packets	1	2	3	4	5	6	7	8	9	10
No. of defectives	1	2	3	5	1	4	2	5	6	7

Let c_i be the number of defective items per i-th packet

$$\bar{c} = \frac{\Sigma ci}{n} \text{ where } n = \text{number of packets inspected.}$$

$$\bar{c} = \frac{1+2+3+5+1+4+2+5+6+7}{10} = \frac{36}{10} = 3.6$$

$$\text{S.E} (\bar{c}) = \sqrt{\bar{c}} = \sqrt{3.6} = 1.90$$

$$\text{U.C.L} = \bar{c} + 3\sqrt{\bar{c}} = 3.6 + 3 \times 1.90 = 9.3$$

$$\text{L.C.L} = \bar{c} - 3\sqrt{\bar{c}} = 3.6 - 3 \times 1.90 = 2.1$$

$$\text{C.L} = 3.6$$

It can be verified that all the packets are within control limits except 1st and 5th packets. Therefore the pharmaceutical company has to check the processing of production of B – Complex.

Exercises

1. Construct a control chart for mean and the range for the following data on the basis of fuses samples of 5 being taken every hour (each set of 5 has been arranged in ascending order of magnitude). Comment on whether the production seems to be under control, assuming that these are the first data.

42	42	19	36	42	51	60	18	15	69	64	61
65	45	24	54	51	74	60	20	30	109	90	78
75	68	80	69	57	75	72	27	39	113	93	94
78	72	81	77	59	78	95	42	62	118	109	109
87	90	81	84	78	132	138	60	84	153	112	136

2. The following are the mean and range of 20 samples of size 5 each. The data pertain to the overall length of fragmentation bomb base manufactured during the war by American Store Camp.

Group No	Mean	Range	Group No	Mean	Range
1	0.8372	0.010	11	0.8380	0.006
2	0.08324	0.009	12	0.8322	0.002
3	0.8318	0.008	13	0.8356	0.013
4	0.8344	0.004	14	0.8322	0.005
5	0.8346	0.005	15	0.8404	0.008
6	0.8332	0.011	16	0.8372	0.011
7	0.8340	0.009	17	0.8282	0.006
8	0.8344	0.003	18	0.8346	0.006
9	0.8308	0.002	19	0.8360	0.004
10	0.8350	0.006	20	0.8374	0.006

From the data, obtain the control limits for $\bar{x}$ and R charts to control the length of bomb bases produces in the future.

3. Eight samples each of size 6 are drawn at regular intervals from a manufacturing pharmaceutical company. The sample means $\bar{x}$ and their range are given below.

Sample No.	1	2	3	4	5	6	7	8	9	10
Mean ($\bar{x}$)	25	28	32	40	35	36	29	41	29	25
Range	6	4	7	3	8	5	4	5	8	7

Compute control limits in respect of $\bar{x}$ and R – charts.

4. The values of sample means ($\bar{x}$) and range (R) for 8 samples of size 6 each are given below. Draw mean and range charts and comment on the quality control of production process.

Sample No.	1	2	3	4	5	6	7	8
$\bar{x}$	36	38	40	32	30	43	44	46
R	5	6	7	4	8	3	2	7

5. In a manufacturing company of T.V. sets, lots of 100 items are inspected at a time. The number of defectives in 10 lots are given are given as in the following table. Draw an appropriate chart.

Lot No.	1	2	3	4	5	6	7	8	9	10
No. of defectives	10	8	9	12	14	8	7	6	13	14

6. The following are the number of defective parts observed by inspection of 10 Maruthi cars. Find the control limits for the number of defective parts.

Car No.	1	2	3	4	5	6	7	8	9	10
No.of defective parts	3	5	8	6	10	4	9	11	12	7

7. A manufacturer of computer systems found the number of defectives in 20 sub systems of 40 computer systems

2	5	6	8	3	1	5	8	9	11	5
12	4	6	2	1	4	5	6	7		

Construct a control chart for the fraction defective.

8. Construct a suitable control chart for the following data and draw your conclusions.

Sample each of 50 items	1	2	3	4	5	6	7	8
No. of defectives	4	8	6	7	10	5	9	6

References

1. *Cochran, W.G. (1953) :* Sampling techniques, John wiley and Sons, inc., New York.

2. *Cochran, W.G. and Cox, G.M. (1957) :* Experimental Designs. John Wiley and Sons, Inc., New York.

3. *Croxton and Cowden (1966) :* Applied general statistics, Printice – Hall of India (Pvt.) Ltd., New Delhi.

4. *Federer, W.T. (1967) :* Experimental Design, Oxfor and I.B.H publishing Co., New Delhi.

5. *Fisher, R.A and Yates, F (1948) :* Statistical Tables for Agricultural, Biological and Medical Research. Oliver and Boyd, Edinburgh, 3rd Edition.

6. *Fisher, R.A. (1947) :* The Design of Experiments. Oliver and Boyd, Edinburgh, 11the Edition.

7. *Goulden, C.H. (1939) :* Methods of statistical Analysis – John Wiley and Sons inc., New York.

8. *Hoel, P.G (1947) :* An introduction of Mathematical Statistics, John wiley and Sons Inc., New York.

9. *Kempthorne, O (1966) :* The Design and Analysis of Experiments, wiiley Eastern Pvt. Ltd., New Delhi.

10. *Krus Kal, W.H. (1957) :* Historical notes on the Wilcoxon unpaired two-sample test. Jour, Amer. Stat. Assn., S2 : 356 – 60.

11. **Kruskal, W.H and Wallis, W.A. (1952) :** Use of ranks in one criterion variance analysis. Jour. Amer. Stat. Assn., 47 : 583.

12. *Mann, H.B and Whitney, D.R. (1947) :* On a test of whether, one of two random variables is stochastically larger than the other. Ann. Math. Stat. 18 : 50.

13. *Massey, F.J. Jr. (1951) :* The Kolmogorov Smirnov test for goodness of fit. J. Amer statistics Ass. 46 : 70.

14. *Ostle, (1966) :* Statistics in Research, Oxford and IBH publishing Co., New Delhi.

15. ***Panse, V.G. and Sukhatme, P.V. (1967)** :* Statistical Methods for Agricultural Workers, Indian Council of Agricultural Resarch, New Delhi.

16. ***Rao, C.R. (1952):*** Advanced Statistical Methods in Biometric Research, John wiley and Sons Inc., New York.

17. ***Rao, G. Nageswara (2007)** :* Statistics for Agricultural Sciences, B.S. Publications, Hyderabad, 2nd Edition.

18. ***Siegel, Sydney, (1956):*** Non–Parametric Statistics for the Behavioural Sciences : Mc Graw Hill Book Co. Inc., New York.

19. ***Snedecor, G.W. and Cochran, W.G. (1968)** :* Statistical Methods. Oxford and I.B.H Publishing Co., New Delhi.

20. ***Steel and Torrie (1960):*** Principles and Procedures of Statistics. Mc Graw – Hill Book Co., New York.

21. ***Sukhatme, P.V. (1953)** :* Sampling Theory of Surveys with Applications. Indian Council of Agricultural Research, New Delhi.

22. ***Wilcoxon, F. (1947)** :* Probability tables for individual comparisons by ranking methods. Biometrics, 3 : 119 – 22.

APPENDICES

x		0	1	2	3	4	5	6	7	8	9
0·0	0·	50000	49601	49202	48803	48405	48006	47608	47210	46812	46414
0·1		46017	45620	45224	44828	44433	44038	43644	43251	42858	42465
0·2		42074	41683	41294	40905	40517	40129	39743	39358	38974	38591
0·3		38209	37828	37448	37070	36693	36317	35942	35569	35197	34827
0·4		34458	34090	33724	33360	32997	32636	32276	31918	31561	31207
0·5		30854	30503	30153	29806	29460	29116	28774	28434	28096	27760
0·6		27425	27093	26763	26435	26109	25785	25463	25143	24825	24510
0·7		24196	23885	23576	23270	22965	22663	22363	22065	21770	21476
0·8		21186	20897	20611	20327	20045	19766	19489	19215	18943	18673
0·9		18406	18141	17879	17619	17361	17106	16853	16602	16354	16109
1·0		15866	15625	15386	15151	14917	14686	14457	14231	14007	13786
1·1		13567	13350	13136	12924	12714	12507	12302	12100	11900	11702
1·2		11507	11314	11123	10935	10749	10565	10383	10204	10027	098525
1·3	0·0	96800	95098	93418	91759	90123	88508	86915	85343	83793	82264
1·4		80757	79270	77804	76359	74934	73529	72145	70781	69437	68112
1·5		66807	65522	64255	63008	61780	60571	59380	58208	57053	55917
1·6		54799	53699	52616	51551	50503	49471	48457	47460	46479	45514
1·7		44565	43633	42716	41815	40930	40059	39204	38364	37538	36727
1·8		35930	35148	34380	33625	32884	32157	31443	30742	30054	29379
1·9		28717	28067	27429	26803	26190	25588	24998	24419	23852	23295
2·0		22750	22216	21692	21178	20675	20182	19699	19226	18763	18309
2·1		17864	17429	17003	16586	16177	15778	15386	15003	14629	14262
2·2		13903	13553	13209	12874	12545	12224	11911	11604	11304	11011
2·3		10724	10444	10170	99031	96419	93867	91375	88940	86563	84242
2·4	$0{\cdot}0^2$	81975	79763	77603	75494	73436	71428	69469	67557	65691	63872
2·5		62097	60366	58677	57031	55426	53861	52336	50849	49400	47988
2·6		46612	45271	43965	42692	41453	40246	39070	37926	36811	35726
2·7		34670	33642	32641	31667	30720	29798	28901	28028	27179	26354
2·8		25551	24771	24012	23274	22557	21860	21182	20524	19884	19262
2·9		18658	18071	17502	16948	16411	15889	15382	14890	14412	13949
3·0		13499	13062	12639	12228	11829	11442	11067	10703	10350	10008
3·1	$0{\cdot}0^3$	96760	93544	90426	87403	84474	81635	78885	76219	73638	71136
3·2		68714	66367	64095	61895	59765	57703	55706	53774	51904	50094
3·3		48342	46648	45009	43423	41889	40406	38971	37584	36243	34946
3·4		33693	32481	31311	30179	29086	28029	27009	26023	25071	24151

Table I is adopted from Table II. of Fisher and Yates, *Statistical Tables for Biological, Agricultural and Medical Research*. Published by Longman Group Ltd., London. (Previously Published by Oliver and Boyd, Edinburgh). and by Permission of the authors and Publishers.

PROBABILITY

d.f.	.1	.05	.02	.01	.001
1	6.314	12.706	31.821	63.657	636.619
2	2.920	4.303	6.965	9.925	31.598
3	2.353	3.182	4.541	5.841	12.924
4	2.132	2.776	3.747	4.604	8.610
5	2.015	2.571	3.365	4.032	6.869
6	1.943	2.447	3.143	3.707	5.959
7	1.895	2.365	2.998	3.499	5.408
8	1.860	2.306	2.896	3.355	5.041
9	1.833	2.262	2.821	3.250	4.781
10	1.812	2.228	2.764	3.169	4.587
11	1.796	2.201	2.718	3.106	4.437
12	1.782	2.179	2.681	3.055	4.318
13	1.771	2.160	2.650	3.012	4.221
14	1.761	2.145	2.624	2.977	4.140
15	1.753	2.131	2.602	2.947	4.073
16	1.746	2.120	2.583	2.92	4.015
17	1.740	2.110	2.567	2.898	3.965
18	1.734	2.101	2.552	2.878	3.922
19	1.729	2.093	2.539	2.861	3.883
20	1.725	2.086	2.528	2.845	3.850
21	1.721	2.080	2.518	2.83	3.819
22	1.717	2.074	2.58	2.819	3.792
23	1.714	2.069	2.500	2.807	3.767
24	1.711	2.064	2.492	2.797	3.745
25	1.708	2.060	2.485	2.787	3.725
26	1.706	2.056	2.479	2.779	3.707
27	1.703	2.052	2.473	2.771	3.690
28	1.701	2.048	2.467	2.763	3.674
29	1.699	2.045	2.462	2.75	3.659
30	1.697	2.042	2.457	2.750	3.646
40	2.021	2.423	2.704	3.551	3.551
50	1.671	2.000	2.390	2.660	3.460
60	1.658	1.980	2.358	2.17	3.373
∞	1.645	1.960	2.326	2.576	3.291

TABLE III. DISTRIBUTION OF χ^2

Probability.

n	.99	.98	.95	.90	.80	.70	.50	.30	.20	.10	.05	.02	.01
1	$.0^3157$	$.0^3628$	.00393	.0158	.0642	.148	.455	1.074	1.642	2.706	3.841	5.412	6.635
2	.0201	.0404	.103	.211	.446	.713	1.386	2.408	3.219	4.605	5.991	7.824	9.210
3	.115	.185	.352	.584	1.005	1.424	2.366	3.665	4.642	6.251	7.815	9.837	11.345
4	.297	.429	.711	1.064	1.649	2.195	3.357	4.878	5.989	7.779	9.488	11.668	13.277
5	.554	.752	1.145	1.610	2.343	3.000	4.351	6.064	7.289	9.236	11.070	13.388	15.086
6	.872	1.134	1.635	2.204	3.070	3.828	5.348	7.231	8.558	10.645	12.592	15.033	16.812
7	1.239	1.564	2.167	2.833	3.822	4.671	6.346	8.383	9.803	12.017	14.067	16.622	18.475
8	1.646	2.032	2.733	3.490	4.594	5.527	7.344	9.524	11.030	13.362	15.507	18.168	20.090
9	2.088	2.532	3.325	4.168	5.380	6.393	8.343	10.656	12.242	14.684	16.919	19.679	21.666
10	2.558	3.059	3.940	4.865	6.179	7.267	9.342	11.781	13.442	15.987	18.307	21.161	23.209
11	3.053	3.609	4.575	5.578	6.989	8.148	10.341	12.899	14.631	17.275	19.675	22.618	24.725
12	3.571	4.178	5.226	6.304	7.807	9.034	11.340	14.011	15.812	18.549	21.026	24.054	26.217
13	4.107	4.765	5.892	7.042	8.634	9.926	12.340	15.119	16.985	19.812	22.362	25.472	27.688
14	4.660	5.368	6.571	7.790	9.467	10.821	13.339	16.222	18.151	21.064	23.685	26.873	29.141
15	5.229	5.985	7.261	8.547	10.307	11.721	14.339	17.322	19.311	22.307	24.996	28.259	30.578
16	5.812	6.614	7.962	9.312	11.152	12.624	15.338	18.418	20.465	23.542	26.296	29.633	32.000
17	6.408	7.255	8.672	10.085	12.002	13.531	16.338	19.511	21.615	24.769	27.587	30.995	33.409
18	7.015	7.906	9.390	10.865	12.857	14.440	17.338	20.601	22.760	25.989	28.869	32.346	34.805
19	7.633	8.567	10.117	11.651	13.716	15.352	18.338	21.689	23.900	27.204	30.144	33.687	36.191
20	8.260	9.237	10.851	12.443	14.578	16.266	19.337	22.775	25.038	28.412	31.410	35.020	37.566
21	8.897	9.915	11.591	13.240	15.445	17.182	20.337	23.858	26.171	29.615	32.671	36.343	38.932
22	9.542	10.600	12.338	14.041	16.314	18.101	21.337	24.939	27.301	30.813	33.924	37.659	40.289
23	10.196	11.293	13.091	14.848	17.187	19.021	22.337	26.018	28.429	32.007	35.172	38.968	41.638
24	10.856	11.992	13.848	15.659	18.062	19.943	23.337	27.096	29.553	33.196	36.415	40.270	42.980
25	11.524	12.697	14.611	16.473	18.940	20.867	24.337	28.172	30.675	34.382	37.652	41.566	44.314
26	12.198	13.409	15.379	17.292	19.820	21.792	25.336	29.246	31.795	35.563	38.885	42.856	45.642
27	12.879	14.125	16.151	18.114	20.703	22.719	26.336	30.319	32.912	36.741	40.113	44.140	46.963
28	13.565	14.847	16.928	18.939	21.588	23.647	27.336	31.391	34.027	37.916	41.337	45.419	48.278
29	14.256	15.574	17.708	19.768	22.475	24.577	28.336	32.461	35.139	39.087	42.557	46.693	49.588
30	14.953	16.306	18.493	20.599	23.364	25.508	29.336	33.530	36.250	40.256	43.773	47.962	50.892

Table IV (a) F-distribution

5 per cent points

df_2 \ df_1	1	2	3	4	5	6	7	8	9	10	12	15	20	24	30	40	60	120	∞
5	6.61	5.79	5.41	5.19	5.05	4.95	4.88	4.82	4.77	4.74	4.68	4.62	4.56	4.53	4.50	4.46	4.43	4.40	4.36
6	5.99	5.14	4.76	4.53	4.39	4.28	4.21	4.15	4.10	4.06	4.00	3.94	3.87	3.84	3.81	3.77	3.74	3.70	3.67
7	5.59	4.74	4.35	4.12	3.97	3.87	3.79	3.73	3.68	3.64	3.57	3.51	3.44	3.41	3.38	3.34	3.30	3.27	3.23
8	5.32	4.46	4.07	3.84	3.69	3.58	3.50	3.44	3.39	3.35	3.28	3.22	3.15	3.12	3.08	3.04	3.01	2.97	2.93
9	5.12	4.26	3.86	3.63	3.48	3.37	3.29	3.23	3.18	3.14	3.07	3.01	2.94	2.90	2.86	2.83	2.79	2.75	2.71
10	4.96	4.10	3.71	3.48	3.33	3.22	3.14	3.07	3.02	2.98	2.91	2.84	2.77	2.74	2.70	2.66	2.62	2.58	2.54
11	4.84	3.98	3.59	3.36	3.20	3.09	3.01	2.95	2.90	2.85	2.79	2.72	2.65	2.61	2.57	2.53	2.49	2.45	2.40
12	4.75	3.89	3.49	3.26	3.11	3.00	2.91	2.85	2.80	2.75	2.69	2.62	2.54	2.51	2.47	2.43	2.38	2.34	2.30
13	4.67	3.81	3.41	3.18	3.03	2.92	2.83	2.77	2.71	2.67	2.60	2.53	2.46	2.42	2.38	2.34	2.30	2.25	2.21
14	4.60	3.74	3.34	3.11	2.96	2.85	2.76	2.70	2.65	2.60	2.53	2.46	2.39	2.35	2.31	2.27	2.22	2.18	2.13
15	4.54	3.68	3.29	3.06	2.90	2.79	2.71	2.64	2.59	2.54	2.48	2.40	2.33	2.29	2.25	2.20	2.16	2.11	2.07
16	4.49	3.63	3.24	3.01	2.85	2.74	2.66	2.59	2.54	2.49	2.42	2.35	2.28	2.24	2.19	2.15	2.11	2.06	2.01
17	4.45	3.59	3.20	2.96	2.81	2.70	2.61	2.55	2.49	2.45	2.38	2.31	2.23	2.19	2.15	2.10	2.06	2.01	1.96
18	4.41	3.55	3.16	2.93	2.77	2.66	2.58	2.51	2.46	2.41	2.34	2.27	2.19	2.15	2.11	2.06	2.02	1.97	1.92
19	4.38	3.52	3.13	2.90	2.74	2.63	2.54	2.48	2.42	2.38	2.31	2.23	2.16	2.11	2.07	2.03	1.98	1.93	1.88
20	4.35	3.49	3.10	2.87	2.71	2.60	2.51	2.45	2.39	2.35	2.28	2.20	2.12	2.08	2.04	1.99	1.95	1.90	1.84
21	4.32	3.47	3.07	2.84	2.68	2.57	2.49	2.42	2.37	2.32	2.25	2.18	2.10	2.05	2.01	1.96	1.92	1.87	1.81
22	4.30	3.44	3.05	2.82	2.66	2.55	2.46	2.40	2.34	2.30	2.23	2.15	2.07	2.03	1.98	1.94	1.89	1.84	1.78
23	4.28	3.42	3.03	2.80	2.64	2.53	2.44	2.37	2.32	2.27	2.20	2.13	2.05	2.01	1.96	1.91	1.86	1.81	1.76
24	4.26	3.40	3.01	2.78	2.62	2.51	2.42	2.36	2.30	2.25	2.18	2.11	2.03	1.98	1.94	1.89	1.84	1.79	1.73
25	4.24	3.39	2.99	2.76	2.60	2.49	2.40	2.34	2.28	2.24	2.16	2.09	2.01	1.96	1.92	1.87	1.82	1.77	1.71
26	4.23	3.37	2.98	2.74	2.59	2.47	2.39	2.32	2.27	2.22	2.15	2.07	1.99	1.95	1.90	1.85	1.80	1.75	1.69
27	4.21	3.35	2.96	2.73	2.57	2.46	2.37	2.31	2.25	2.20	2.13	2.06	1.97	1.93	1.88	1.84	1.79	1.73	1.67
28	4.20	3.34	2.95	2.71	2.56	2.45	2.36	2.29	2.24	2.19	2.12	2.04	1.96	1.91	1.87	1.82	1.77	1.71	1.65
29	4.18	3.33	2.93	2.70	2.55	2.43	2.35	2.28	2.22	2.18	2.10	2.03	1.94	1.90	1.85	1.81	1.75	1.70	1.64
30	4.17	3.32	2.92	2.69	2.53	2.42	2.33	2.27	2.21	2.16	2.09	2.01	1.93	1.89	1.84	1.79	1.74	1.68	1.62
40	4.08	3.23	2.84	2.61	2.45	2.34	2.25	2.18	2.12	2.08	2.00	1.92	1.84	1.79	1.74	1.69	1.64	1.58	1.51
60	4.00	3.15	2.76	2.53	2.37	2.25	2.17	2.10	2.04	1.99	1.92	1.84	1.75	1.70	1.65	1.59	1.53	1.47	1.39
120	3.92	3.07	2.68	2.45	2.29	2.18	2.09	2.02	1.96	1.91	1.83	1.75	1.66	1.61	1.55	1.50	1.43	1.35	1.25
∞	3.84	3.00	2.60	2.37	2.21	2.10	2.01	1.94	1.88	1.83	1.75	1.67	1.57	1.52	1.46	1.39	1.32	1.22	1.00

Table IV (b) F-distribution

1 per cent points

df_2 \ df_1	1	2	3	4	5	6	7	8	9	10	12	15	20	24	30	40	60	120	∞
5	16.26	13.27	12.06	11.39	10.97	10.67	10.46	10.29	10.16	10.05	9.89	9.72	9.55	9.47	9.38	9.29	9.20	9.11	9.02
6	13.74	10.92	9.78	9.15	8.75	8.47	8.26	8.10	7.98	7.87	7.72	7.56	7.40	7.31	7.23	7.14	7.06	6.97	6.88
7	12.25	9.55	8.45	7.85	7.46	7.19	6.99	6.84	6.72	6.62	6.47	6.31	6.16	6.07	5.99	5.91	5.82	5.74	5.65
8	11.26	8.65	7.59	7.01	6.63	6.37	6.18	6.03	5.91	5.81	5.67	5.52	5.36	5.28	5.20	5.12	5.03	4.95	4.86
9	10.56	8.02	6.99	6.42	6.06	5.80	5.61	5.47	5.35	5.26	5.11	4.96	4.81	4.73	4.65	4.57	4.48	4.40	4.31
10	10.04	7.56	6.55	5.99	5.64	5.39	5.20	5.06	4.94	4.85	4.71	4.56	4.41	4.33	4.25	4.17	4.08	4.00	3.91
11	9.65	7.21	6.22	5.67	5.32	5.07	4.89	4.74	4.63	4.54	4.40	4.25	4.10	4.02	3.94	3.86	3.78	3.69	3.60
12	9.33	6.93	5.95	5.41	5.06	4.82	4.64	4.50	4.39	4.30	4.16	4.01	3.86	3.78	3.70	3.62	3.54	3.45	3.36
13	9.07	6.70	5.74	5.21	4.86	4.62	4.44	4.30	4.19	4.10	3.96	3.82	3.66	3.59	3.51	3.43	3.34	3.25	3.17
14	8.86	6.51	5.56	5.04	4.70	4.46	4.28	4.14	4.03	3.94	3.80	3.66	3.51	3.43	3.35	3.27	3.18	3.09	3.00
15	8.68	6.36	5.42	4.89	4.56	4.32	4.14	4.00	3.89	3.80	3.67	3.52	3.37	3.29	3.21	3.13	3.05	2.96	2.87
16	8.53	6.23	5.29	4.77	4.44	4.20	4.03	3.89	3.78	3.69	3.55	3.41	3.26	3.18	3.10	3.02	2.93	2.84	2.75
17	8.40	6.11	5.18	4.67	4.34	4.10	3.93	3.79	3.68	3.59	3.46	3.31	3.16	3.08	3.00	2.92	2.83	2.75	2.65
18	4.29	3.01	3.09	2.58	2.25	2.01	2.84	2.71	2.60	2.51	2.37	2.23	2.08	3.00	2.92	2.84	2.75	1.66	1.92
19	8.18	5.93	5.01	4.50	4.17	3.94	3.77	3.63	3.52	3.43	3.30	3.15	3.00	2.92	2.84	2.76	2.67	2.58	2.49
20	8.10	5.85	4.94	4.43	4.10	3.87	3.70	3.56	3.46	3.37	3.23	3.09	2.94	2.86	2.78	2.69	2.61	2.52	2.42
21	8.02	5.78	4.87	4.37	4.04	3.81	3.64	3.51	3.40	3.31	3.17	3.03	2.88	2.80	2.72	2.64	2.55	2.46	2.36
22	7.95	5.72	4.82	4.31	3.99	3.76	3.59	3.45	3.35	3.26	3.12	2.98	2.83	2.75	2.67	2.58	2.50	2.40	2.31
23	7.88	5.66	4.76	4.26	3.94	3.71	3.54	3.41	3.30	3.21	3.07	2.93	2.78	2.70	2.62	2.54	2.45	2.35	2.26
24	7.82	5.61	4.72	4.22	3.90	3.67	3.50	3.36	3.26	3.17	3.03	2.89	2.74	2.66	2.58	2.49	2.40	2.31	2.21
25	7.77	5.57	4.68	4.18	3.86	3.63	3.46	3.32	3.22	3.13	2.99	2.85	2.70	2.62	2.54	2.45	2.36	2.27	2.17
26	7.72	5.53	4.64	4.14	3.82	3.59	3.42	3.29	3.18	3.09	2.96	2.82	2.66	2.58	2.50	2.42	2.33	2.23	2.13
27	7.68	5.49	4.60	4.11	3.78	3.56	3.39	3.26	3.15	3.06	2.93	2.78	2.63	2.55	2.47	2.38	2.29	2.20	2.10
28	7.64	5.45	4.57	4.07	3.75	3.53	3.36	3.23	3.12	3.03	2.90	2.75	2.60	2.52	2.44	2.35	2.26	2.17	2.06
29	7.60	5.42	4.54	4.04	3.73	3.50	3.33	3.20	3.09	3.00	2.87	2.73	2.57	2.49	2.41	2.33	2.23	2.14	2.03
30	7.56	5.39	4.51	4.02	3.70	3.47	3.30	3.17	3.07	2.98	2.84	2.70	2.55	2.47	2.39	2.30	2.21	2.11	2.01
40	7.31	5.18	4.31	3.83	3.51	3.29	3.12	2.99	2.89	2.80	2.66	2.52	2.37	2.29	2.20	2.11	2.02	1.92	1.80
60	7.08	4.98	4.13	3.65	3.34	3.12	2.95	2.82	2.72	2.63	2.50	2.35	2.20	2.12	2.03	1.94	1.84	1.73	1.60
120	6.85	4.79	3.95	3.48	3.17	2.96	2.79	2.66	2.56	2.47	2.34	2.19	2.03	1.95	1.86	1.76	1.66	1.53	1.38
∞	6.63	4.61	3.78	3.32	3.02	2.80	2.64	2.51	2.41	2.32	2.18	2.04	1.88	1.79	1.70	1.59	1.47	1.32	1.00

THE CORRELATION COEFFICIENT

TABLE V: Values of the Correlation Coefficient for Different Levels of Significance

n	·1	·05	·02	·01	·001	n	·1	·05	·02	·01	·001
1	·98769	·99692	·999507	·999877	·9999988	16	·4000	·4683	·5425	·5897	·7084
2	·90000	·95000	·98000	·990000	·99900	17	·3887	·4555	·5285	·5751	·6932
3	·8054	·8783	·93433	·95873	·99116	18	·3783	·4438	·5155	·5614	·6787
4	·7293	·8114	·8822	·91720	·97406	19	·3687	·4329	·5034	·5487	·6652
5	·6694	·7545	·8329	·8745	·95074	20	·3598	·4227	·4921	·5368	·6524
6	·6215	·7067	·7887	·8343	·92493	25	·3233	·3809	·4451	·4869	·5974
7	·5822	·6664	·7498	·7977	·8982	30	·2960	·3494	·4093	·4487	·5541
8	·5494	·6319	·7155	·7646	·8721	35	·2746	·3246	·3810	·4182	·5189
9	·5214	·6021	·6851	·7348	·8471	40	·2573	·3044	·3578	·3932	·4896
10	·4973	·5760	·6581	·7079	·8233	45	·2428	·2875	·3384	·3721	·4648
11	·4762	·5529	·6339	·6835	·8010	50	·2306	·2732	·3218	·3541	·4433
12	·4575	·5324	·6120	·6614	·7800	60	·2108	·2500	·2948	·3248	·4078
13	·4409	·5139	·5923	·6411	·7603	70	·1954	·2319	·2737	·3017	·3799
14	·4259	·4973	·5742	·6226	·7420	80	·1829	·2172	·2565	·2830	·3568
15	·4124	·4821	·5577	·6055	·7246	90	·1726	·2050	·2422	·2673	·3375
						100	·1638	·1946	·2301	·2540	·3211

Table V is reproduced from Table VII, of Fisher and Yates: *Statistical Tables for Biological, Agricultural and Medical Research*. Published by Longman Group Ltd., London. (Previously Published by Oliver and Boyd, Edinburgh), and by Permission of the Authors and Publishers.

TABLE VI : FACTORS USEFUL IN THE CONSTRUCTION OF CONTROL CHARTS.

Sample size	Mean-chart			Factors for central line	Standard deviation chart				Factors for central line	Range chart			
	Factors for control limits				Factors for control limits					Factors for control limits			
n	A	A_1	A_2	c_2	B_1	B_2	B_3	B_4	d_2	D_1	D_2	D_3	D_4
2	2.121	3.760	1.880	0.6642	0	1.843	0	3.267	1.28	0	3.686	0	3.267
3	1.732	2.394	1.023	0.7236	0	1.858	0	2.566	1.693	0	4.358	0	2.575
4	1.500	2.880	0.729	0.7979	0	1.808	0	2.269	2.059	0	4.698	0	2.282
5	1.342	1.596	0.577	0.8407	0	1.756	0	2.089	2.236	0	4.918	0	2.115
6	1.225	1.410	0.483	0.8686	0.026	1.711	0.030	1.970	2.534	0	5.078	0	2.004
7	1.114	1.277	0.419	0.8882	0.105	0.62	0.118	1.888	2.704	2.205	5.203	0.076	1.924
8	1.061	1.175	0.073	0.9027	0.167	1.638	0.185	1.815	2.847	0.387	5.307	0.136	1.864
9	1.000	1.094	0.337	0.9139	0.219	1.609	0.239	1.761	2.970	0.546	5.394	0.184	1.816
10	0.949	1.028	0.308	0.9227	0.262	1.584	0.284	1.716	3.078	0.687	5.469	0.223	1.777
11	0.905	0.973	0.285	0.9300	0.299	1.561	0.321	1.679	3.173	0.812	5.534	0.256	1.744
12	0.866	0.925	0.256	0.9359	0.331	1.541	0.354	1.646	3.258	0.924	5.592	0.284	1.716
13	0.832	0.883	0.249	0.9410	0.359	1.523	0.382	1.618	3.336	1.026	5.646	0.308	1.692
14	0.802	0.848	0.235	0.9453	0.384	1.507	0.406	1.594	3.407	1.121	5.693	0.329	1.671
15	0.775	0.816	0.223	0.9490	0.406	1.492	0.428	1.572	3.472	1.207	5.737	0.348	1.652
16	0.750	0.788	0.212	0.9523	0.427	1.478	0.448	1.542	3.352	1.285	5.279	0.365	1.636
17	0.728	0.762	0.203	0.9551	0.445	1.465	0.466	1.534	3.588	1.359	5.817	0.379	1.621
18	0.707	0.738	0.816	0.9576	0.461	1.454	0.482	1.518	3.640	1.426	5.854	0.404	1.608
19	0.688	0.670	0.187	0.9599	0.477	1.443	0.497	1.503	3.689	1.490	5.888	0.404	1.596
20	0.671	0.697	0.180	0.9619	0.491	1.433	0.510	1.490	3.735	1.548	5.922	0.414	1.585
21	0.655	0.670	0.173	0.9638	0.504	1.424	0.523	1.447	3.778	1.606	5.950	0.425	1.575
22	0.640	0.662	0.167	0.9655	0.516	1.415	0.534	1.466	3.819	1.659	5.979	0.434	1.566
23	0.626	0.647	0.162	0.9670	0.527	1.407	0.545	1.455	3.858	1.710	6.006	0.443	1.557
24	0.612	0.632	0.157	0.9684	0.538	1.399	0.555	1.445	3.895	1.759	6.031	0.452	1.548
25	0.600	0.619	0.153	0.9696	0.548	1.392	0.565	1.435	3.931	1.804	6.058	0.459	1.541

PART - B
Computer Applications

CHAPTER 13

Introduction to Computers

13.1 Introduction

Today computers have an important and widespread influence on our society. Every educated person should study the basic disciplines of computer operation and its applications. A student must study the basics of computers. Wherever there are phenomena of interest to man, there can be a science to describe and explain those phenomena. Computer science is therefore the study of computer and the phenomena requiring their use.

A computer is a device capable of accepting information or data, processing the information, and providing the results as an output. More specifically, a computer can be described as follows:

"Computer is a data processing machine that can perform substantial computation, including numerous arithmetic or logic operations, without intervention by a human operator during the process or it may be defined as" a device capable of solving problems by accepting data, performing described operations on the data, and supplying the results of these operations or."

"A computer is a programmable, multiuse machine that accepts data – raw facts and figures and processes, or manipulates it into information we can use, such as summaries or totals".

A visual representation, or schematic diagram shows how the computer processes the information.

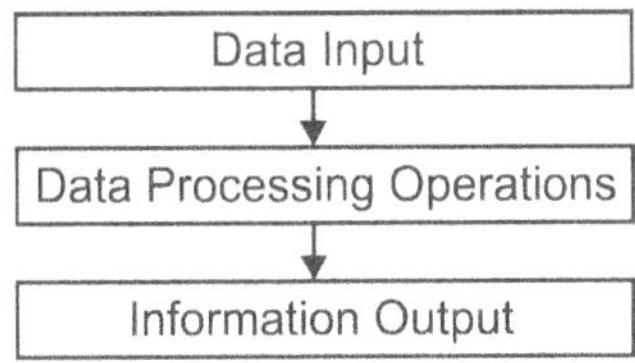

Fig. 13.1 Information processing system.

13.2 Information Processing and the Electronics Digital Computer

The electronic computer allows man to increase his productivity and permits him to do tasks he would be enabling to complete without computer. As we discussed above, the computer is a machine capable of :

- Accepting data
- Performing described operations on the data
- Providing the results of these operations.

Thus computer also permits man to improve his output permit of time, or productivity. We can say that the computer's two most important contributions as a tool are to increase.

I – Speed of the operation

II – Accuracy of the results.

Of course, when we consider these two factors, we realize that the computer enables us to accomplish tasks that we would probably never even attempt manually. For example, if the number of input data is greater than several millions and the time necessary to accomplish a task is more than fifty years, we would probably never attempt it, yet it is just tasks that we can require the computer to accomplish. The term electronic implies that the computer is powered by electrical and electronic devices rather than by mechanical ones or those affected by heat or air pressure. Here digital refers to discrete, non-continuous quantities, as contrasted with continuous quantities.

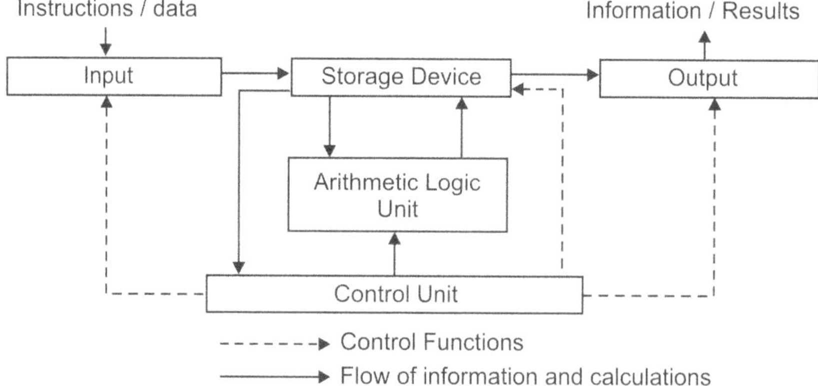

Fig. 13.2 Information processing on electronics digital computer.

Electronics digital computer is an information-processing device that accepts and processes data represented by discrete symbols. It is constructed primarily of electric or electronic devices.

We can use the computer to process the input data by sorting them, or by series of planned actions and operations. This may be illustrated by a common data processing operation which a person usually accomplishes manually, but which is increasing accomplished automatically by data processing service companies. These processing works requires:

- Data input
- Storage and retrieval of data
- Arithmetic steps
- Output of result
- Control of all steps.

A Computer follows a similar process. It is composed of five basic units:

Input unit	– input data and instructions.
Storage or Memory unit	– In which computer instructions and data as well as intermediate results are stored.
Arithmetic logic unit	– In which mathematical operation can be performed and compare the numbers, results.
Output unit	– provides the desired result in a suitable form.
Control unit	– controls the data communication, operations and supervises overall operations of the computer.

The devices accomplish the functions of input, output and storages. The arithmetic and control functions are accomplished by the control-processing unit locates with storage in the pattern.

13.3 Information Technology

Data communication, network and computer have brought a new technology, the information technology (IT). IT is the most powerful synthesis of computers and communications. The Information Technology mainly deals with customers, computers costs and communication. Information is useful only if it is accurate relevant, precise and provides timely information to the users. This would be possible, only when stored information is instantaneously retrievable at the time of need. Time will come when there will be only computer workstation around which will receive data from some sources to do some processing with the data, convert it into information and forward it to some other person or workstation. This is a networking environment.

Computer has become an indispensable tool, helping to shape the society it serves. The banking industry is an integral part of the society, and has grown phenomenally since last three decades with manifold rise in its transactions and area of activities. Thus the role and utility of the computer and Information Technology cannot be over emphasized.

13.4 Comparison of Computer with Human Being

Computer and Human

- Have Memory
- Reading Capability
- Perform arithmetic and logic calculation
- Manipulate symbols
- Make Comparisons

Human

- Make processing based on results at a point
- Remember or read data from file
- Remember instructions for processing
- Write or speak out the output

Computer

- Hold program instruction in internal storage
- Read data in machine readable form and store in the storage device.
- Make processing possible by choosing instruction based on comparison or an examination result at a point
- Retrieve data from internal memory or secondary storage device.
- Exhibits the results on an output device.

Table 13.1 Comparison between Character of Human and Computer.

Character	Human	Computer
Speed of execution	Slow	Extremely fast
Continuous work	Poor	Excellent
Memory retrieval	Inaccurate	Accurate
Accuracy	Make errors	No errors
Follow instructions	Perfect / Imperfect	Consistency
Ability to innovate new situation	Good	Lacking

13.5 Characteristics of Computers

The vital characteristics of the computers are as follows :

Speed

Computer works on electrical pulses, which travel at incredible speeds and because the computer is an electronic device, its internal speed is instantaneous. An arithmetic calculation can be performed in a thousandth, millionth, billon things even in a trillionth seconds. It is capable of executing over ten thousand instructions in a second.

Milli. Sec. (ms)	-	1/1000 of a second
Micro. Sec (ms)	-	1/1000000 of a second
Nano sec (ms)	-	1/1000000000 of a second
Pic sec (ps)	-	1/1000,000,000,000 of a second.

Storage

This is very important character of the computer, which separates it from other machine. The basic unit of storage is bit (acronym for binary digit). The speed with which computer can perform, i.e. to input data and the instructions for processing, is humanly impossible. The storage space available in the central processing unit, being limited, large quantity of data and entire introductions of all the required programs cannot be stored in it. These are stored outside and read into the memory of CPU at the time of processing.

BIt	-	Smallest unIt of storage
Byte	-	8 Bits
KB	-	1024 bytes
MB	-	1024 KB
GB	-	1024 MB

Accuracy

Accuracy of the computers is consistently high. Errors in computing are due to machine failure, imprecise programming logic, inaccurate data, poorly designed systems. Precision is the degree of accuracy to which the computer gives the result. The precision of computers is phenomenal.

Versatility

Computers seem capable of performing almost any task, provided the task can be reduced to series of logical steps. It performs numeric and non-numeric tasks equally well. An algorithm, a step-by-step procedure, which applied to the problem, leads to solution. Programming is to convert this computer language to solve the problem.

Automation

Once a program is in the computers memory, CPU follows the instructions until it meets the last instruction once the process begins; It would continue without human intervention until completion.

Diligence

Being a machine, a computer does not suffer from the human tracts of tiredness and lack of concentration. If five million calculations are to be performed, computer performs all these calculations with the same speed and accuracy.

13.6 Limitations of Computers

The computer also has certain limitations. It works at a very high speed and is extremely accurate. This very characteristic becomes its limitation when a mistake over, occurs because when a wrong instruction is fed, it excuses it with the same speed and accuracy that it would have executed with a right instruction. As a result, there is hardly any scope or time to recover.

The computers understand only instructions and cannot distinguish between suspicious and genuine customers. It does not posses intelligence and cannot take up even a simple action unless instructed to do so. It does not posses any morals or and therefore can be easily misused in the hands of a wrong individual. However, the computers never make any mistake or error. Errors, whenever found in the computer-based processing, are due to human errors.

13.7 Components of a Computers

Computer is an electronic data processing machine. It is made up of various devices, which help you to interact. Process it and output is the result. A computer system has three essential parts :

- Keyboard
- Central Processing Unit (CPU)
- Monitor.

Block Diagram of a Computer

The computer consists of three parts: Input device, CPU and output device. Keyboard, which is the input device, is connected to the central -processing unit. Central processing unit consists of three sections memory, control unit and arithmetic logic unit

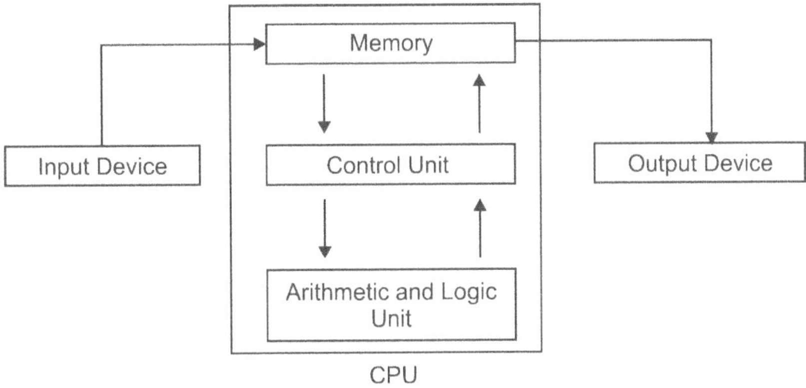

Fig. 13.3 Block diagram of computer.

Key Board

Programs and data are entered into a computer through a keyboard, which is attached to a microcomputer or the terminal of a mini or large computer. A keyboard is similar to the keyboard of a typewriter. It contains alphabets digits special characters and some control keys. When a key is pressed, an electronic signal is produced which is detected by an electronic circuit called keyboard encoder. A keyboard encoder may be special IC or a single chip microcomputer used as encoder. The function of an encoder is to detect which key has been pressed and send a binary code

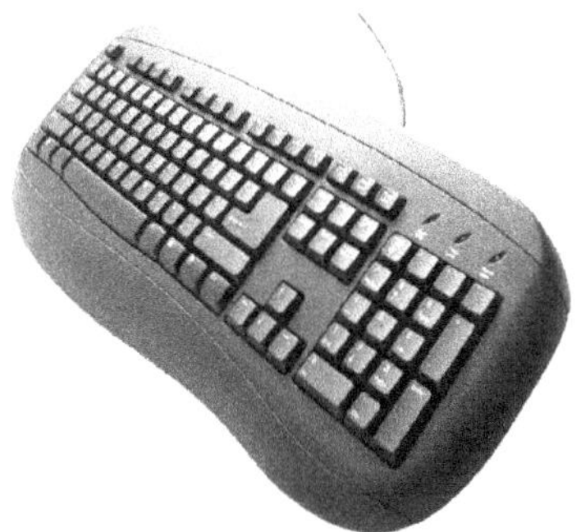

Central Processing Unit (CPU)

This is also called System unit, which is a Technically known as Microprocessor. CPU is the brain of computer. It is made of three units:

1. Control unit
2. Arithmetic logic unit
3. Memory

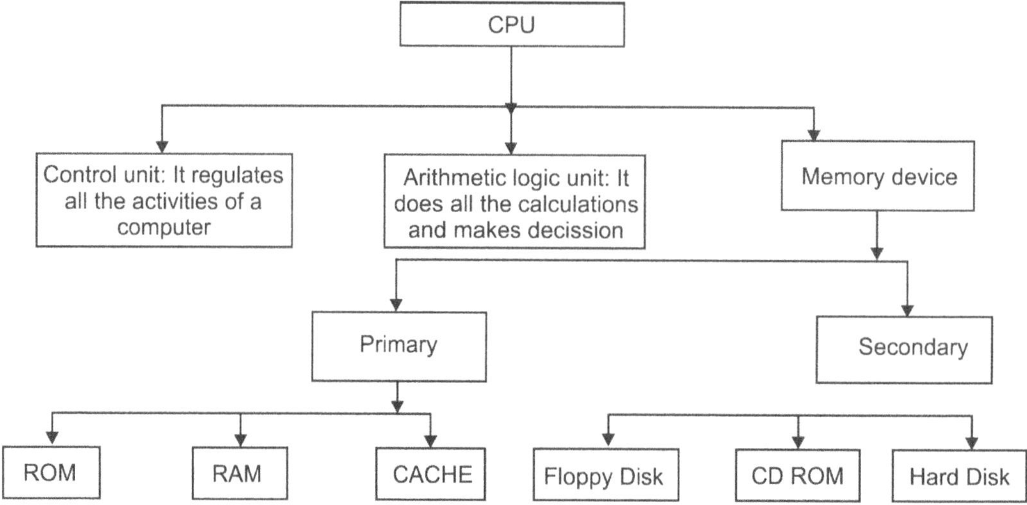

Fig. 13.4 Central Processing Unit with different devices.

- **Control unit**

  The control section of the CPU maintains and directs the operations of the entire system. It acts like the central nervous system for all the components, through it does not process any data.

- **Arithmetic and Logic Unit (ALU)**

  ALU processes the data entered. All types of processing, mathematical calculation, comparison decision making and processing of non numeric information takes place in ALU and data is once again moved to RAM.

- **Memory**

  Memory refers to the storage space in computer. Memory stores the data entered as well as the results given by the computer. Memory works on the application of binary system. The basic unit of memory is byte. Memory units can be divided into two sub-parts :

  (a) Primary storage   (b) Secondary storage

Monitor

Monitor is also called video display unit. It accepts programming instructions. Sometimes a monitor is also referred to as a video display terminal (VDT).

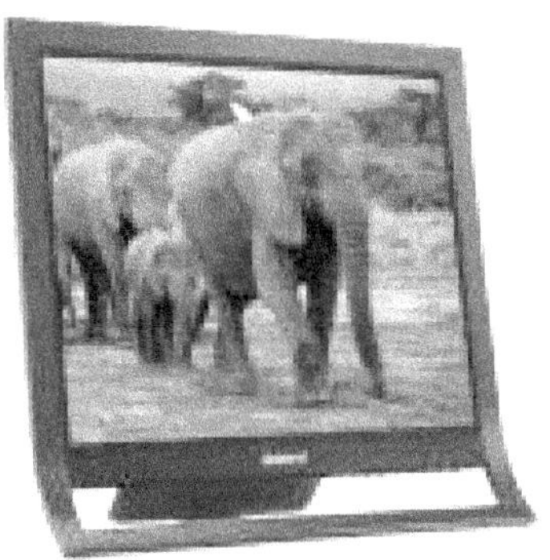

CHAPTER 14

History of Computers

In the previous chapter we understood what computer is? In this chapter we discuss the history of the computers and how this machine came into being over the years.

The computers started from the development of a counting system. Therefore we start with the very early ages.

14.1 Early Methods of Calculation

Today we do all calculations using computers. How were calculations done in olden days? The simplest calculating device was the finger. Even today we begin to learn calculations with the fingers but it has many limitations. You can only do simple additions and subtraction.

14.2 Abacus

In olden days, people learnt to do calculations by marking lines on the walls. This slowly development into a device called the abacus.

The abacus was probably the first calculating device. It was invented over 3000 years ago and still used in some countries including India. An abacus consists of a row of wires held in wooden frame, which have balls or beads strung on them. Calculations are done on an abacus by sliding the beads along the wires. An abacus in skilled hand can work almost as fast as an electronic calculator. There are three different kinds of abacus.

14.2.1   The Russian Abacus

It has ten beads on each wire. Beds on the first wire present single units, beads on the second wire 10s beads on the third wire 100s and so on. Calculations are done by sliding the beads along the wires.

The Russian Abacus is shown in the Fig 14.1 represents the number **1,24,00,23,070**

14.2.2   The Chinese Abacus

In a Chinese abacus, a beam is passed into two regions, known as heaven and earth, dividing the frame. There are two beads on one side of the beam and five on the other. A bead in heaven has a value of five and a bead in earth a value of one.

Moving the beads away from or towards the beam did calculations. The bead has numerical value only when it is adjacent to the beam. The Fig. 14.2 shows a Chinese abacus presenting the number **1215235020**

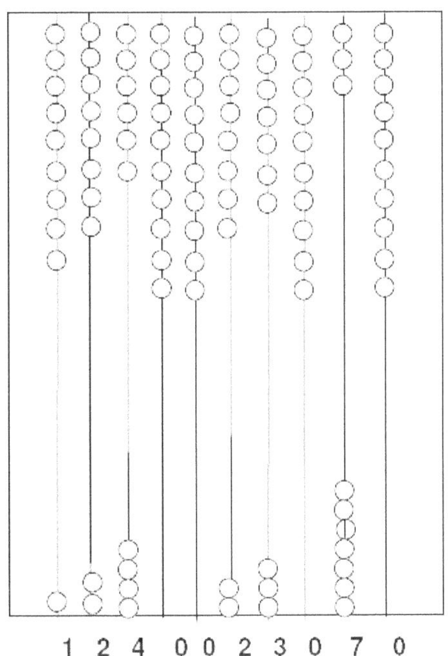

Fig. 14.1 Russian abacus.

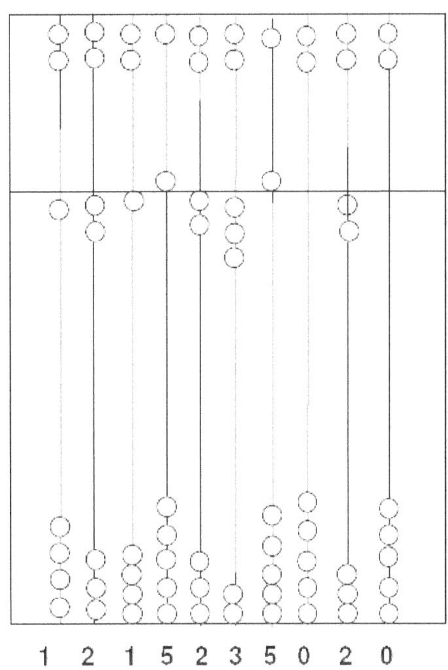

Fig. 14.2 Chinese abacus.

14.2.3   The Japanese Abacus

In a Japanese abacus, one bead is in the heaven side and 4 beads in the earth are placed for calculations. The value of the beads in heaven was considered to have a value of five and a bead in the earth, a value of one. This abacus are called SOROBAN. The Figure 14.3 shows a Japanese abacus presenting the number **1115235025**

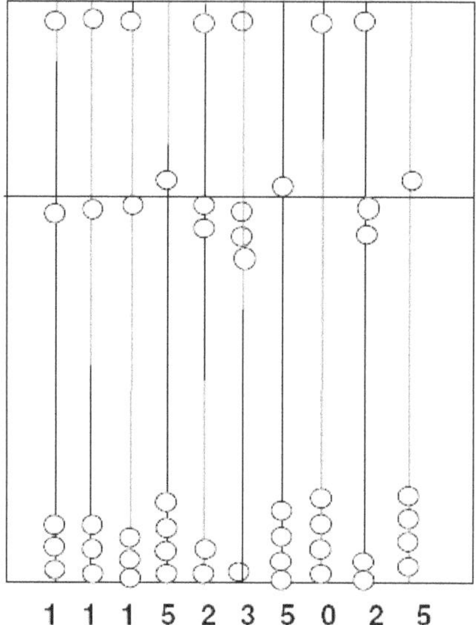

Fig. 14.3 Japanese abacus.

14.3 Napier's Bones

In the seventeenth century, John Napier, a mathematician from Scotland, did a considerable amount of work on calculations. He devised a set of even rods each having four faces, which were used as multiplication trolls. These rods were carved from bones and were called Napier's bones.

The rods have number marked an them in such a way that, by placing them on a side, products and quotients of large numbers can be obtained.

14.4 Pascal's Mechanical Calculating Machine

In 1642, Blaire Pascal, a French mathematician, invented the machine; dialing a series of numbered wheels and entering numbers. A series of toothed wheels transferred the movements to a deal, which showed the results. This machine also had limitation. It could be used for addition and subtraction only.

14.5 Leibnitz's Machine

1671, Goff pride Ven Leibnitz, a German mathematician, invented a calculating machine which could perform multiplications and divisions. This machine was an improved version of Pascal's machine.

14.6 Babbage Analytical Engine

In 1821, Charles Babbage designed a machine called the difference engine to calculate and print mathematical tables. Again in 1833-34 Babbage designed his a programmed analytical engine which was mechanical calculator.

The Analytical Engine had many features similar to modern computers. But it was too complicated to be built at that time. But for these ideas Charles Babbage is rightfully known as the FATHER OF COMPUTERS. Lady Ada Augusta developed ideas for Babbages machine. She is considered to be first programmer.

14.7 Hollerith's Card Machine

Herman Hollerith, an American statistician in 1887-1890 developed a punch card reading machine. He used punch cards as input and output devices. This machine was used for tabulating and calculating data.

This machine was also known as Tabulating machine. It was used in 1890 as census process and proved to be very successful. Till recently punch cards were used in some computers.

14.8 The Analytical Engine by Babbage

It was a general purpose-computing device, which could be used for performing any mathematical operation automatically. It consisted of the following components.

The Stone : A mechanical memory unit consisting of sets of center wheels.

The Mill : An arithmetic unit which is capable of performing the four basic arithmetic operations.

Cards : There are basically two types of cards.

    (a) *Operation Cards :* Selects one for arithmetic operations by activating the mill to perform the selected function.

    (b) *Variable Cards :* Selects the memory locations to be used by the mill for a particular operation.

Output : Could be directed to a printer or a cardpunch device.

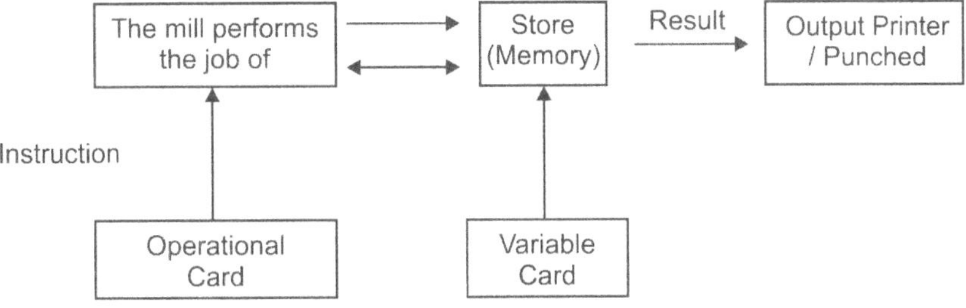

Fig. 14.4 Logical structure of Babbage analytical engine.

14.9 Basic Features of Analytical Engine

- It is a general-purpose programmable machine.
- It had the provision of automatic sequence control, thus enabling programs to ablerits its sequence of operations.
- The Prussian of sign checking of result assessed.
- Mechanism for a changing or reversing of control card was permitted thus enabling execution of any desired instruction.

The Babbage machine is fundamentally the same as a modern computer. Unfortunately Babbage work could not be completed. However as a tribute to Charles Babbage his analytical engine was completed in the last decade and it is now on display at the Science Museum at London.

14.10   Prehistoric and Early Calculating Devices

When the electronic computer was introduced man has apparently always had a need to process data and calculate it. The history of computers and calculating devices in western civilisation reaches back a thousand years before the birth of Christ, when abacus was used.

14.11   First Electro Mechanical Computer

Howard Aiken, A Harvard professor with the help of some IBM engineers, developed the first electro mechanical computer "MARKET". This, computer used Hollerith's punch cards. The principles of Charles Babbage were first time used practically in this computer.

This was huge machine, which occupied a large space. The inside of the machine had several miles of electrical wires, many electro-mechanical relays and mechanical counters for arithmetic calculations with all these circuits the machine looked like a monster.

14.12   First Electronic Computer: ENIAC

ENIAC was the first general-purpose electronic computer, produced around 1943 for the US Army. It used 18,000 vacuum tubes, weighted 30 tons and occupied about 5000 square feet of space. It could perform 300 multiplications per second and was the fastest machine at the time of its development. In this machine, instructions were given by external Plug boards or switches. The US Army used this computer until 1955.

14.13   EDSAC

Research work continued to make computers faster and smaller. John Van Nuemam a mathematician suggested that Computers could be used not only for storing data calculations but could be used in development of program. In 1949, the first Electronic Delay Storage Automatic Calculator (EDSAC) was made and used at Cambridge University, London.

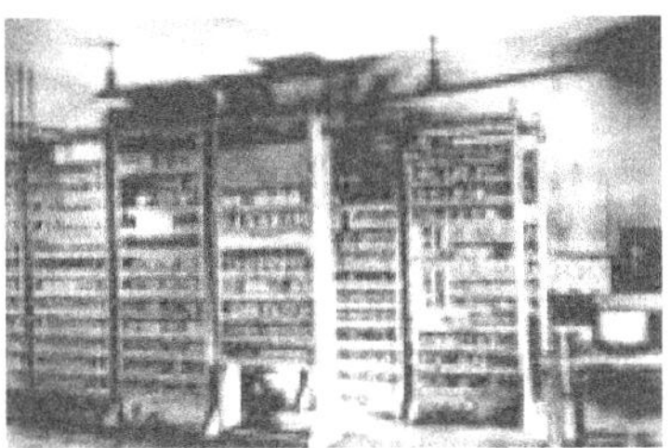

14.14   EDVAC

In 1949, Eckert and Mauchly developed the first stored program electronic computer and named it EDVAC. EDVAC stands for electronic discreet variable automatic computer. This was the first commercial data processing machine used to store data and program instructions in its memory through the binary number system.

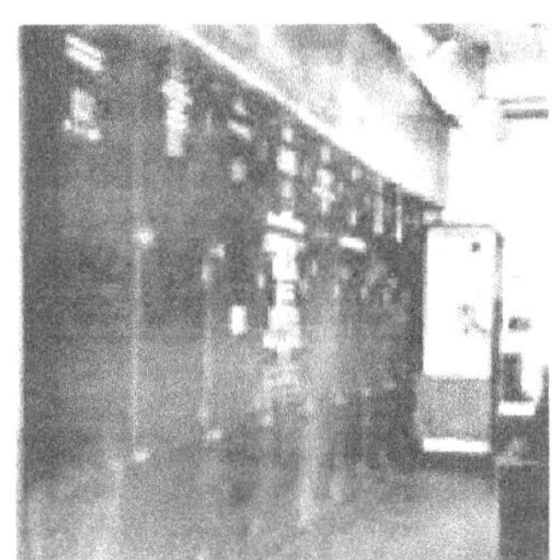

14.15   UNIVAC

Eckert and Mauchly developed universal Automatic Computer in 1951 in their own company. In 1954 UNIVAC was developed which was the computer used for business applications.

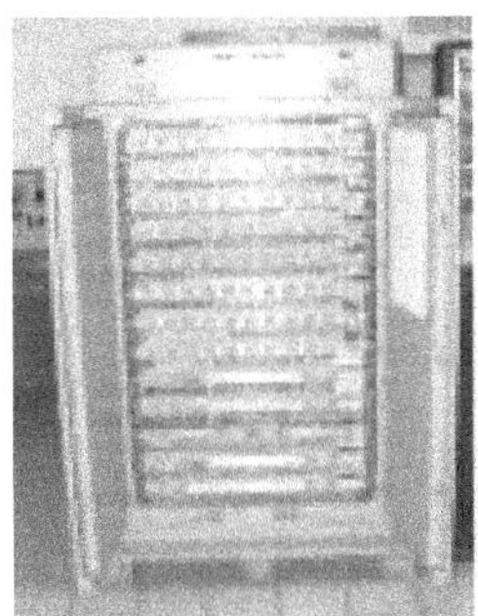

IBM 650

In the year 1955, Thomas Walton Jr, son of IBM's founder was introducing this computer. This computer had a memory capacity of 2000 words. IBM 650 computer was widely accepted and became very popular which led IBM becaming the leader in computer production. The other computers produced by IBM were IBM 1401 and RAMAC 350.

14.16   From Vacuum Tube to Microprocessor

Computers used to be made from vacuum tubes. Then the small transistor came followed by integrated circuit (IC), made from the common mineral silicon and followed by the micro processor.

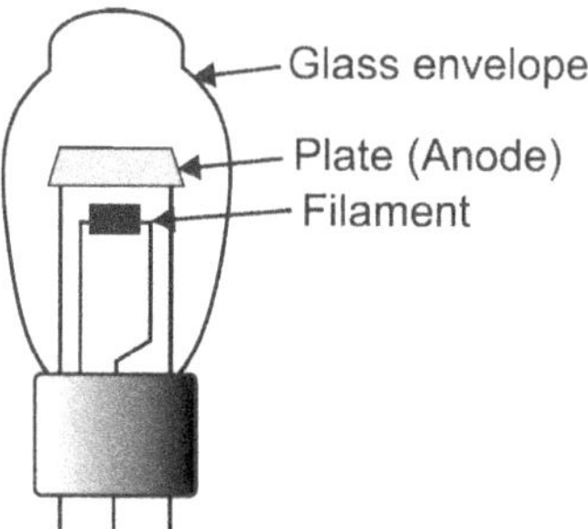

14.17   First Generation Computers

The computers produced and used between 1940-1955 were called first generation of computers.

The first generation computers were characterized by vacuum tube (valve) circuitry. Hence they were very large, they were placed in large air-conditioned rooms had small internal storage and were relatively very slow. The first generation machines used punched paper tape, punched card, magnetic wire, magnetic tape and printers as input / output devices.

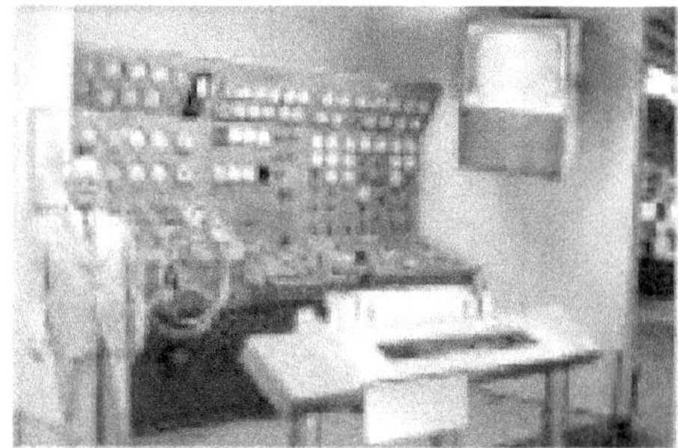

The trends, which were encountered during the era of first generation computers, were :

- The first generation computer control was centralized in a single CPU, and all the operations required a direct intervention of the CPU.
- Use of finite-care main memory was started during this time.
- Concerts such as use of virtual memory and endure register started.
- Punched cards were used as input device.
- Magnetic tapes and magnetic drums were used as secondary memory.
- Binary coder or machine language was used as secondary memory.
- Towards the end, the use of symbolic language, which is now called assembly language started.
- Assembler was a program that translated assembly language program to machine language.
- Computer was accessible to only one programmer at a time.
- Advent of von Neumann architecture.

14.18   Second Generation Computers

The computer produced after 1955 are called second generation of computers. They had faster access and were more reliable than first generation of computers. Transistors replaced vacuum tubes of first generation in this period. By this time a wide range of input/output devices such as higher performance magnetic tapes, magnetic drums and early magnetic disks were available. During the second generation, computer languages such as FORTRAN and ALGOL were introduced. The second generation of computers started with the advent of transistorized computers.

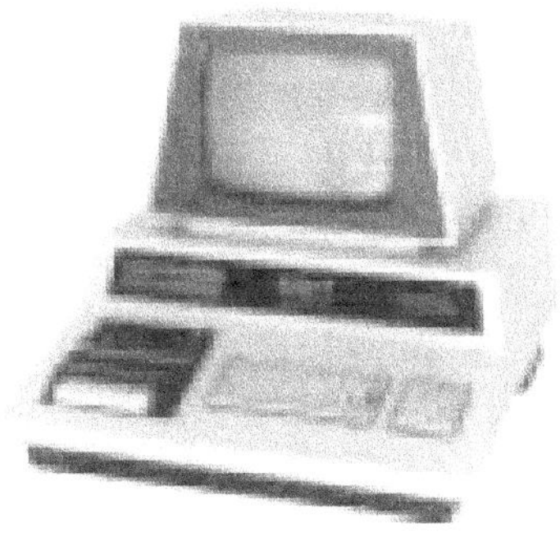

The generation of computers is basically differentiated by a fundamental hardware technology. Each new generation of computer is characterized by greater speed, large memory capacity and smaller size than the previous generation. Thus, second generation computers were more advanced in terms of arithmetic, logic unit and control unit than their counterparts of first generation. Another feature of second generation was that by this time high-level languages were beginning to be used and the transmission for system software were starting.

The first of the IBM 7090 was delivered in 1959, which was followed by the CDC 1604, Philco 2000 and Remington Rand's UNIVAC LARC. Other widely used second generation Computers were IBM 1620, IBM 1401 and IBM 7094.

14.19   Third Generation Computers

IBM announced the third generation of computers in 1964 with its 360 line of computers. They were used integrated circuits in the hardware. It also had the provision of facilities for time-sharing and multi programming. The speed and storage capacity of their computers were much higher than the previous generation computers and the size was much reduced.

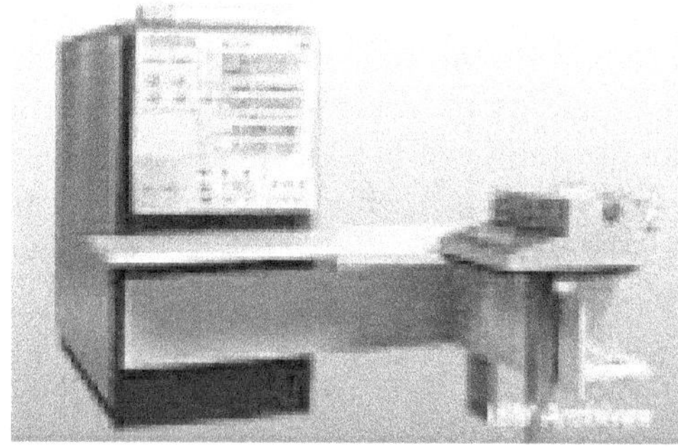

In the third generation of computer, more than one user could work with the computer at the same time, whereas the first and second generation of computer worked on a one-to-one basis. Almost all computers introduced after 1960 were said to be third generation computers. Most of the mainframe computers used in India till the early 1980s were third generation computers only.

In integrated circuit a components such as transistors, resistors and conductors are fabricated on a semi conductor material such as silicon. Thus, a desired circuit can be fabricated in a tiny piece of silicon rather than assembling several discrete components into the same circuit. Hundreds or even thousands of transistors could be fabricated on a single wafer of silicon. In addition, these fabricated transistors can be connected with a process of metallisation from logic circuits on the same chip on which they have been produced.

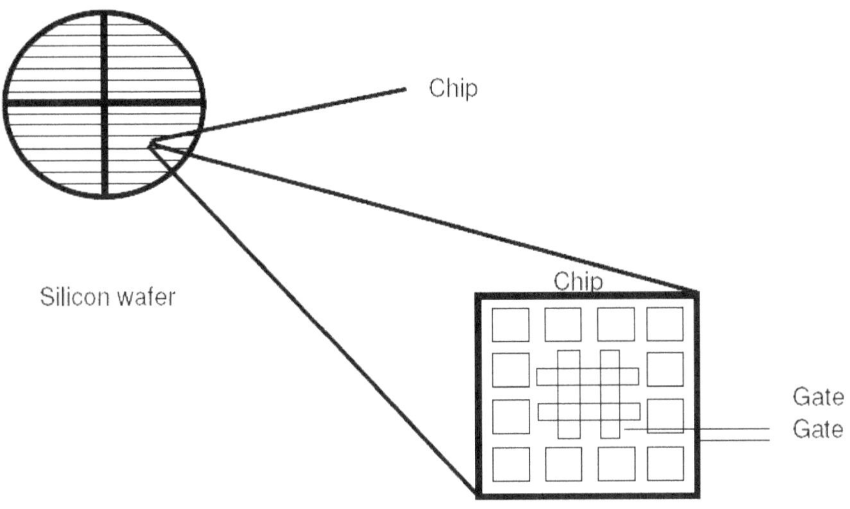

Fig. 14.5 Wafer, chip and gate.

Integrated circuits are constructed on a thin wafer of silicon which is divided into a matrix of small area. An identical circuit pattern is fabricated on each of their areas and the wafer is then broken into chips. Each of these chips consists several gates, which are made using transistors and a number of input and output connection points. Each of these chips then can be packaged separately in a housing to protect it. In addition, this housing provides a number of pins for connecting these chips with other clerics or circuits. The pins of these packages can be provided in two ways in two parallel rows with 0.1 inch spacing between two adjacent pins is each row. This package is called dual in line package (DIP) (Fig.14.6a)

In case more than hundred pins are required then pin grid array (PGA), is used, where pins are arranged in arrays of rows and columns, with spacing between two adjacent pins of 0.1 inch (Fig. 14.6b)

Different circuits can be constructed on different wafers, all these packaged circuits chips then can be inter connected on a printed circuit board to produce several complier electronic circuits such as computers

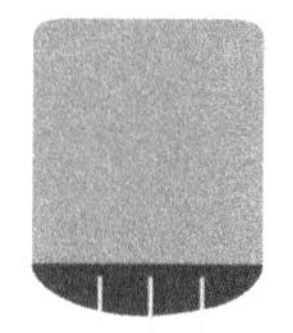

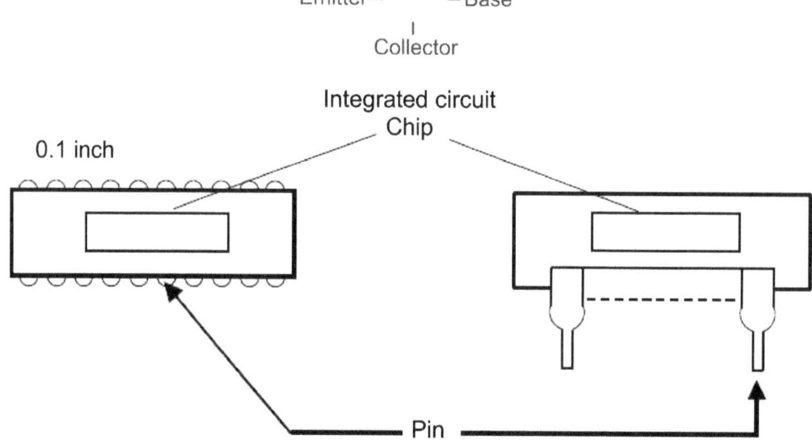

Fig. 14.6 (a) A 24 pin dual in line package (DIP).

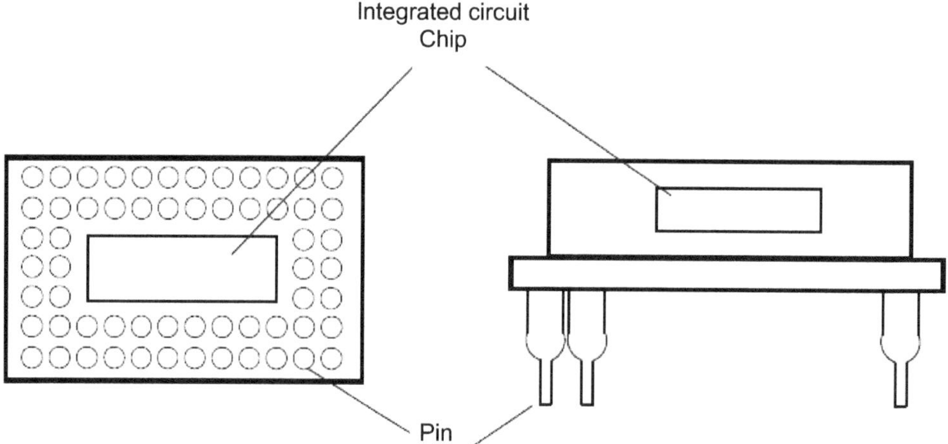

Fig. 14.6 (b) 144 Pin-grid array (PGA) package.

Densely packed Inspected circuit has following advantage

- **Low cost** : The cost of a chip has remained almost constant while the chip density is ever increasing. It implies that the cost of computer logic and memory circuitry is reducing rapidly.
- **Fast Speed** : The more is density, the closer are the logic or memory elements, which implies shorter electrical paths and hence the higher operating speed.
- **Size Smaller**
- **Better portability**
- **Reduction in power and cooling requirements**
- **Reliability**

Some of the examples of third generations computers are IBM system 360 family and DEC PDPI System. The third generation computers mainly used SSI chips.A family of computer consist of several models. Each model is assigned a model number, for example, the IBM system 360 family model 30, 40, 50, 65 and 75. As we go from lower model number to higher model number in this family, the memory capacity processing speed and cost increase.

The main characteristics of the family are :

- The instructions set on a family are of similar type.
- The operating system used in family members is the same. In certain case some features can be added in the operating system for the higher members.
- The speed of execution of instruction increases from low-end family members to upper number end family members.
- The number of I/o ports interfaces increases as we move to higher members.
- Memory size increases as we move towards higher members.

The major developments, which took place in third generation, can be summarised as follows :

- IC circuits were starting to find their applications in the computer hardware replacing the discrete transistor circuits. This resulted in reduction in the cost and physical size of the computer.
- Semi-conductor memories were starting to augment finite core memory in main memory.
- The CPU design was made simple and more flexible using a technique called microprogramming.
- Certain new techniques were introduced to increase the effective speed of program execution. These techniques were pipelining and multi processing.
- The operating systems of computers were incorporated with the efficient method of sharing the facilities or resources such as processor and memory space, automatically.

14.20   Fourth Generation Computers

The fourth generation computers were produced after 1970. The term fourth generation computer is used to designate microcomputers which use large-scale integrated circuits (LSI) and very large integrated, had greater input / output capacity and system reliability.

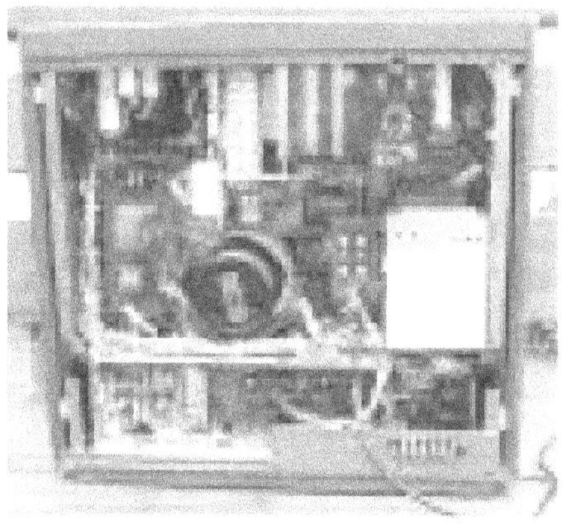

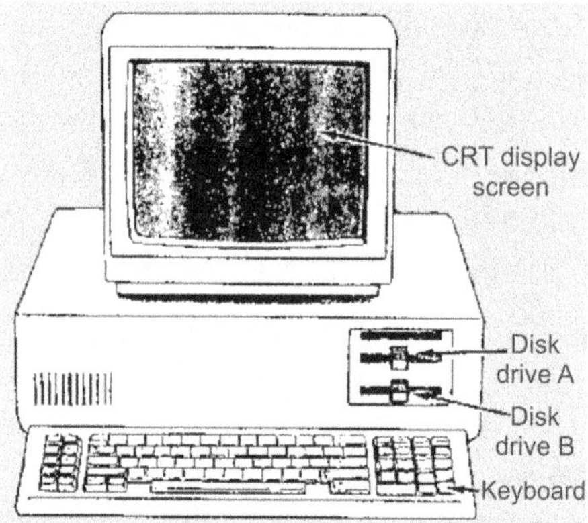

The most important criterion that can be used to separate them from third generation computers is that they have been designed work efficiently with the current generation of high-level languages.

Other developments that took place during 1975-1980 include: Package programs, word processing, voice response units and microprocessors. A microprocessor is a single "Chip" which by itself can perform the control, arithmetic and logical functions of a computer. A microcomputer is a collection of a small number of memory chips and some input / output devices.

Semiconductor Memories

Initially the IC technology was used for constructing processor, but soon it was realised that same technology can be used for construction of memory. The first memory chip was constructed in 1970 and could hold 256 bits. The cost of this chip is high, but gradually the cost of semi conductor memory is going down. The memory capacity per chip has increased as 1K, 4K, 16K, 64K, 256K, and 1M bits.

Microprocessors

Keeping pace with electronics more and more component were fabricated on a single chip. Fewer chips were needed to construct a single processor. Intel in 1971 chirred the breakthough of putting all the components on a single chip. The single chip processors are known as microprocessor. The Intel 4004 was the first microprocessor. It was a primitive microprocessor designed for a specific application. Intel 8080, which came in 1974, was the first general-purpose microprocessor. It was an 8-bit microprocessor. Motorola is another manufacture in this field. At present 32, 64-, 128-bit general-purpose microprocessors are available in the market. Figure 14.7 shows the families of INTEL & MOTOROLA microprocessor.

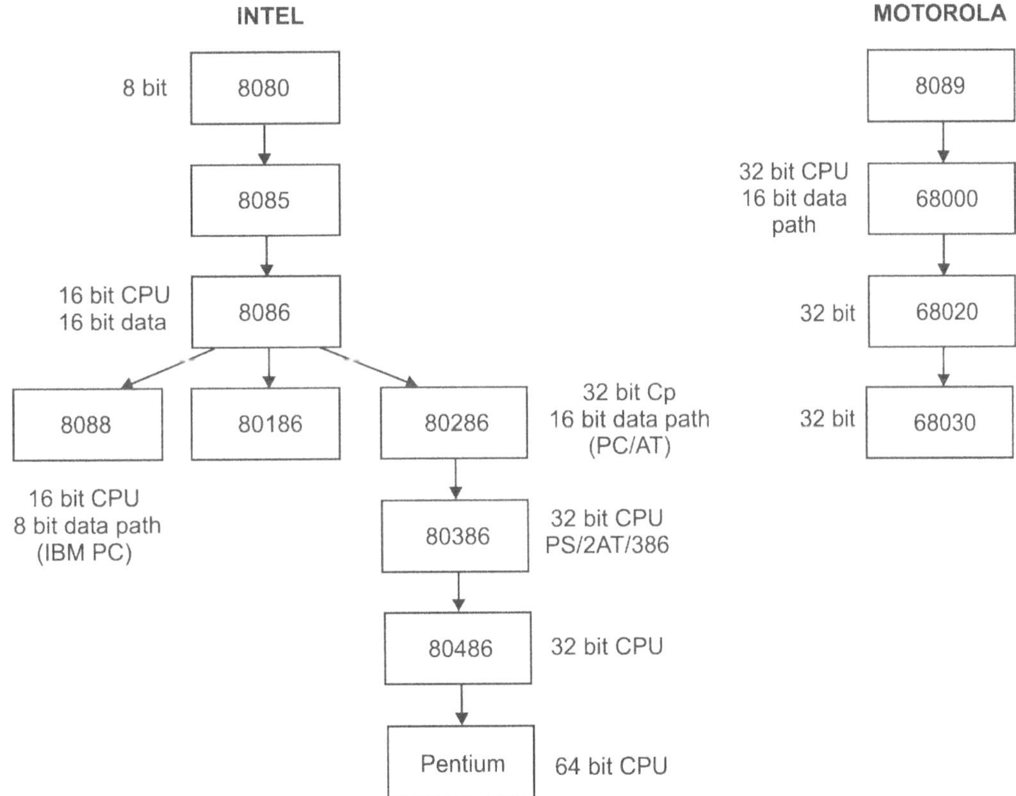

Fig. 14.7 Families of INTEL & MOTOROLA Microprocessor.

14.21   Fifth Generation Computers

In October 1981, a conference of 300 computer scientists and engineers from fourteen countries was held in Japan to discuss the features of the fifth generation computers.

These machines will incorporate artificial intelligence, which will not be far different from that of human intelligence. They will use stored reservoirs of knowledge to make expert judgment and decisions. They will process non-numerical information such as pictures and graphs.

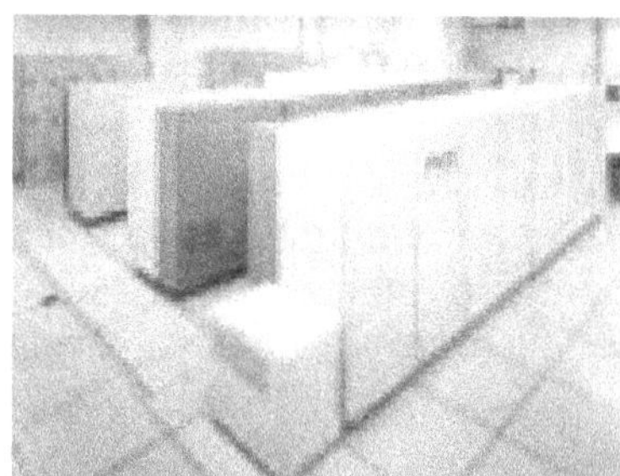

In these machines, intelligence will be greatly improved and the man-machine interface will be closes to the human systems. Progress on these has not been as fast as originally planned although same significant advances have been made.

CHAPTER 15

Classification of Computers

15.1 Analog, Digital and Hybrid Computers

Computers, which are use today, are digital computers they manipulate numbers. They operate on binary digits 0 and 1. They understand information composed of only 0_s and 1_s. In the case of alphabetic information, the alphabets are coded in binary digits. Computers do not operate on analog quantities directly. If in any analog quantity is to be processed, it must be converted into digital quantity before processing. The output of a computer is also converted into analog quantity. The components, which convert alphanumeric characters to binary format and binary output to alphanumeric characters, are the essential parts of a digital computer.

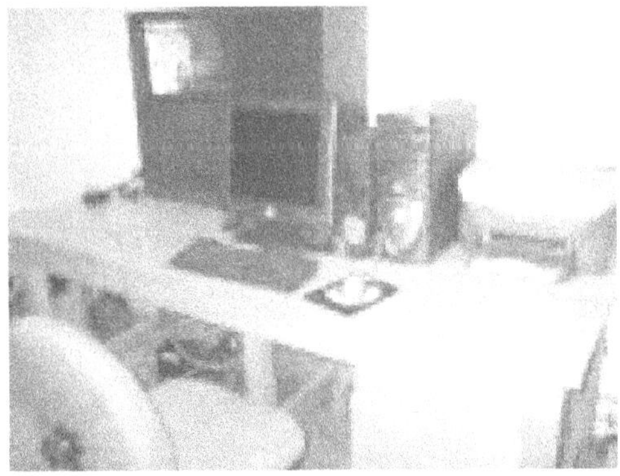

Digital computer

The computer, which can process analog quantities, is called analog computers, today analogy computers are rarely used. Earlier analog computers were used to simulate certain systems. They were used to solve differential equations.

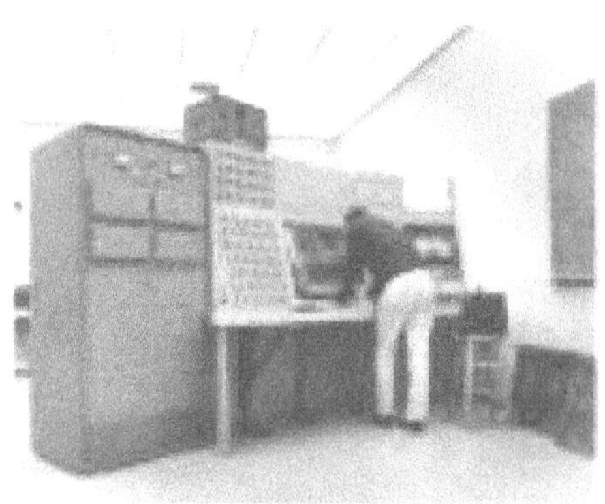

Analog computers

Hybrid computers are combination of digital and analog. Hybrid computer is mainly used in medical field.

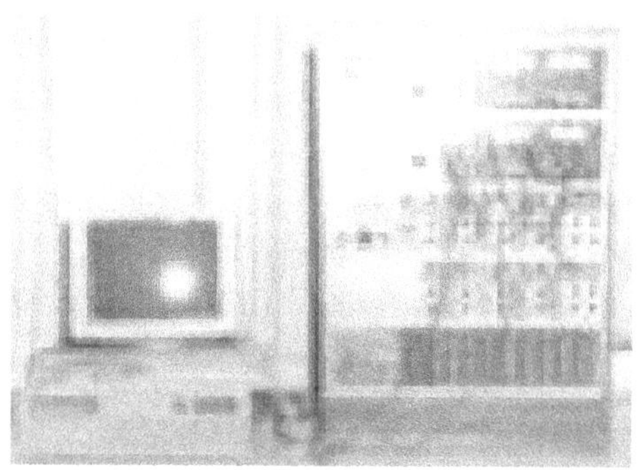

Hybrid computers

15.2 Classification of Computers Based on Size

Computers can be classified in various ways depending upon its size, memory capacity, processing speed etc. Here were going to discuss the broadly accepted classification of computer. The criteria of this classification is as discussed above. Computers are classified into four categories.

1. Main frame computers
2. Mini Computers
3. Micro Computers
4. Super Computers

15.2.1   Mainframe Computers

Mainframe computers are generally 32 bit machines or on the higher side. These are suited for organization, to manage high volume applications. Few of popular mainframe series are MEDHA, SPERRY, DEC, IBM, HP, ICL etc. Mainframes are also used are just below super computers. In some ways mainframes are more powerful than super computers because they support more simultaneous programs. But supercomputers can execute a single program faster than mainframe.

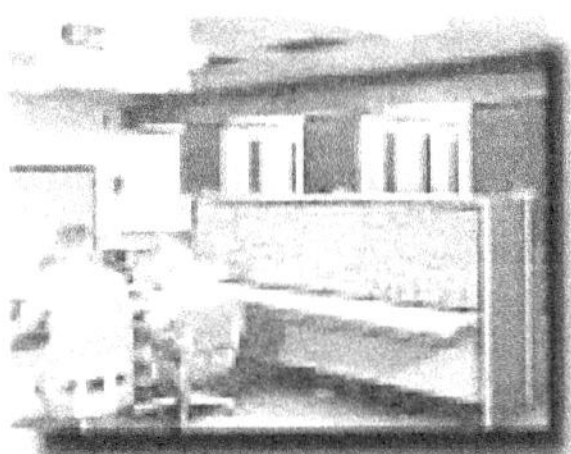

Mainframe Computers

The Important features of mainframe are :

- They are big computer systems, sensitive to temperature, humidity, dust etc.
- Qualified trained operators are required to operate them.
- They have a wide range of peripherals attached.
- They have a wide storage capacity.
- They can use wide variety of software.
- They are not user-friendly.
- They can be used for more mathematical calculations.
- They are installed in large commercial places or government organization.

15.2.2   Mini Computers

The term mini computer originated in 1960 when it was realised that many computing task do not require an expensive contemporary computers but can be solved by a small, inexpensive computer. Initial mini computers were 8 bit and 12 bit machines but by 1970s almost all mini computers were 16 bit machines.

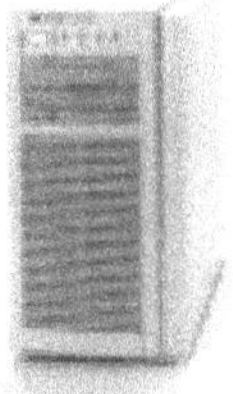

Mini frame

The 16 bit mini computers have the advantage of large instruction set and address field, and efficient storage to handling of text in comparison to lower bit machines. Thus, 16-bit mini computer was more powerful machine, which could be used in variety of applications and could support business applications, along with the scientific application.

With the advancement in technology the speed, memory size and other characteristics developed and the minicomputer was than used for various stand alone or dedicated applications. The mini computer was also used as a multi-user system, which can be used by various users at the same time. Gradually the architectural requirement of mini computers grew and a 32 bit mini computer, which was called super mini, was introduced. The super mini had more peripheral devices, larger memory and could support more users working simultaneously on the computer in comparison to previous mini computers. A mini computer has a multiprocessing system capable of supporting 4 to about 200 users simultaneously.

Traditionally, mini computers have been used to cater to the needs of medium sized companies or departments within large companies, open for accounting or design and manufacturing (CAD / CAM). Mini computers are also becoming more important as 'servers' A server is a computer on a network that manages network resources. The entire network is called client server network.

Characteristics of mini computer are

- They have less memory and storage capacity.
- They offer limited range of peripherals
- They can use limited range of software.
- End users can directly use it.
- They are not very sensitive to the external environment and hence are more generalized.
- They are used for data processing.

15.2.3   Micro Computers

A micro computer's CPU has a microprocessor. The microcomputer originated in late 1970's. The first microcomputers were built around 8-bit microprocessor chips. 8 bit chip means that the chip can retrieves instruction/data from storage, manipulate, and process an 8-bit data at a time or we can say that the chip has a built in 8-bit data transfer path.

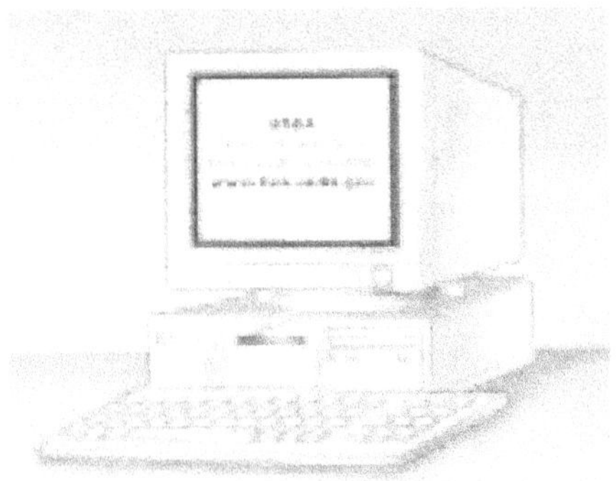

Micro Computer

An improvement on 8-bit chip technology was seen in early 1980s when a series of 16 bit chips namely 8086 and 8088, were introduced by Intel corporation, each one with an advancement over the other.

8088 is an 8116-bit chip i.e. an 8 primary storage, but processing is done within the chip using a 16-bit path at a time. 8086 is a 16116-bit chip i.e. the internal and external paths both are 16 bits wide and these chips can support a primary storage capacity of upto 1 mega byte. Intel 80286 is 16/32-bit chip and it can support up to 16 MB of primary storage.

Similar to Intel chip series, exists another popular chip series of Motorola. The first 16-bit microprocessor of this series is MC 68000. It is a 16/32 bit chip and can support up to 16 MB of primary storage. An advancement over 16/32 bit chips and the 32/32 chips some of the popular 32 bit chips are Intel's 80386 and MC 68020 Chip.

A small, relatively inexpensive computer is designed to test a few thousand rupees to over fifty thousand rupees. Personal computers first appeared in the late 1970. One of the most popular and first personal computers was the Apple II, Introduced in 1977 by Apple computer during the late 1970s and early 1980s. New models and competing operating system seemed to appear daily. Then, in 1981, IBM entered the fray with its first processor computer, known as the IBM PC. The IBM PC, quickly became the personal computer of choice. In general, microcomputers are considered to be of two types:

(a) Personal computer   (b) Workstations.

(a) Personal Computer (PC)

The first personal computer produced by IBM was called IBMPC, and increasingly the term PC come to mean IBM or IBM – compatible personal computer, to the exclusion of other types of personal computers, such as Macintoshes. Microcomputers or PC comes in various sizes.

Desktop models

A computer designed to fit comfortably on top of a desk, typically with the monitor sitting on top of the computer. Desktop model computers are broad and flat, whereas tower models computers are norms and tall. Based on their shape, desktop model computers are generally limited to three internal mass storage devices. Desktop model designed to be very small are sometimes referred to as slim line models.

Portable or luggable

Portable means small and lightweight. A portable computer is a computer small enough to carry. Portable computers include notebook and sub notebook computers, hand-held computers, palmtops and PDAS.

Laptop computers

A small, portable computer, small enough that can be sit on your lap. Nowadays, laptop computers are more frequently called notebook computers. It is extremely lightweight personal computer. Notebook computers typically weight less then 6 pounds and are small enough to fit easily in a briefcase. A side from size, the principal difference between a notebook computer and a personal computer is the display screen. Notebook computers use a variety of techniques, known as flat panel technologies, to produce a lightweight and non-bulky display screen. Notebook computers come with battery packs that enable you to run them without plugging them in electric socket. However, the batteries need to be recharged every few hours. The most common substances used in computer battery packs are nickel cadmiums (Nickel), Nickel metal hydride (NiMH) and Lithium gun.

Pocket or hand-held computer

A portable computer is small enough to be held in one's hand. Although extremely convenient to carry, hand held computers have not replaced notebook computers because of their small keyboards and screens. Some manufacturers are trying to solve the small keyboard problems by replacing the keyboard with an electronic pen. However, these pen-based devices rely on handwriting recognition technologies, which are still in their infancy.

Pocket computers may be classified into three types :

1.   Electronic Organizers

Electronic organizers or electronic diary are specialized pocket computers that mainly store appointments addresses, and ' to-do' lists.

2. Palmtop

A small computer that literally fits in your palm is called palmtop. Compared to full-size computers, palmtops are severely limited, but they are practical for certain functions such as phone books and calendars. Palmtops that use a pen rather than a keyboard for input are often called hand held computer or PDA's.

3. PDA

PDA stands for Personal Digital Assistant, a handheld device that combined computing, telephone, face and networking features. A typical PDA can function as cellular phone, fare sender and personal organizer. PDAs are pen based, using a stylus rather than a keyboard for input. Some PDAs can also react voice input by using voice recognition technologies.

(b) Workstation

Workstation are those computers which are used for engineering application, desktop publishing, software development and other type of applications that require a moderate amount of computing power and relatively high quality graphics capabilities.

Workstations generally come with a large, high-resolution graphics screen, at least 64 MB of RAM, built-in network support, and a graphical user interface. Most workstation also have a mass storage device as a disk drive, but a special type of workstation, called a diskless workstation comes with out a disk drive. The most common operating systems for workstation are UNIX, LINUX and Windows 2000, The leading manufacturers of workstations are SUN Micro systems, Hewlett packars, Silicon Graphics Incorporated and Compaq.

Summarized features of Micro Computers are :

- They brought revolution in the history of computers.
- They are also known as personal computers.
- They are cheap and user-friendly.
- This type of computer used wide range of software.

CHAPTER 16

The System Concept

16.1 Introduction

You might have observed by now that we have been referring to a computer as a system (computer system). To know the answer let us first consider the definition of a system.

A system is group of integrated parts that have common purpose of achieving some objective (s). So, the following three characteristics are key to a system

1. A system has more than one element.
2. All the elements of a system are logically related.
3. All the elements of a system are controlled in such a way that the system goal is achieved.

Since a computer is made up of integrated components (input and output devices, storage, CPU) that work together to process the data when the program is executed, it is a system. The input or output units cannot function until they receive signals from the CPU. Similarly, the storage unit or the CPU alone is of no use. So the usefulness of each unit depends on other units and can be realized only when all units are put together (integrated) to form a system.

A computer system can also be said to be consisting of:

1. Hardware   2. Software

16.2   Hardware

Hardware is a general term used to represent the physical components of the computer itself i.e. those components, which can be seen or touched. In computer system the hardware includes devices, like keyboards, monitor, printer and the central processing unit:

1.   Input devices   2. Output devices   3. Central processing unit
4.   Memory devices   5. Communication devices

The electronic circuits consist of resistors, capacitors; ICs etc. inside a computer's cabinet are all examples of computer hardware. All input and output devices connected to computer are collectively known as peripherals we can define peripheral as any piece of hardware that is connected to a computer." examples are the keyboards, mouse, monitor and disk drives.

16.3   Software

Software is defined as sets of instructions stored as programs that govern the operation of a computer system and make the hardware run. "Software or computer programs are the step by step instructions that tell the computer what to do. In general software can be classified as "System Software" and "Application Software".

16.3.1   System Software

The user of a computer has at his disposal a large amount of software provided by the manufacturer. Most of this software contribute to the control and manage its internal resources and give optimum performance from the system.

A more detailed subdivision of such software is as follows:

Operating systems and control programs

Translators

Utilities and service programs

16.3.2   Application software

Application software is defined as software that can be used to perform a general purpose or specific task. Word processing software is used to create a text document. Database software is used to create a database for a specific purpose, DTP software is used to create a document for electronic publishing. Application software may be either customized or packaged.

Customized software is that software which is designed for a particular customer for particular use. Packaged software is the kind of program developed for sale for general-purpose applications. These software are more commonly used in organisation & business applications.

We will discuss software in great detail. In this chapter we concentrate on hardware.

16.4   Input Devices

Data and instructions are entered into a computer through input devices. An input device converts input data and instructions into a suitable binary form accepted by the computer. The most commonly used input device is a keyboard. A number of other input device have also been developed which do not require typing for inputting information, for Example: mouse, light pen, graphic tablet, joystick, track ball, touch screen etc. Each of these devices permits the user to select something on CRT screen by pointing to it. Therefore, these devices are called pointing devices. Voice input systems have also been developed. A microphone is used as a voice input device.

Input devices are categorised as keyboard entry and direct entry devices: In keyboard entry we use keyboard to enter the information into the computer readable form. Direct entry refers to many forms of data entry devices that do not use keyboard. Such devices create machine-readable data. These include pointing devices, scanning devices, smart and optical cards, voice recognition devices etc.

Often keyboard and direct entry devices are combined in a single computer system. A Desk Top Publishing (DTP) system for example uses a keyboard, a mouse and a image scanner.

16.4.1   Keyboard

Programs and data are entered into a computer through a keyboard, which is attached to a microcomputer of the terminal of a mini or large computer. A keyboard is similar to the keyboard of a typewriter. It contains alphabets, digits, special characters and some control keys. When a key is pressed, an electronic signal is produced which is detected by an electronic circuit called keyboard encoder. A keyboard encoder may be a special IC or a single-chip microcomputer used as encoder. The function of an encoder is to detect which key has been pressed and send a binary code (corresponding to the pressed key) to the computer. The binary code may be an ASCII, EBCDIC or HEX code.

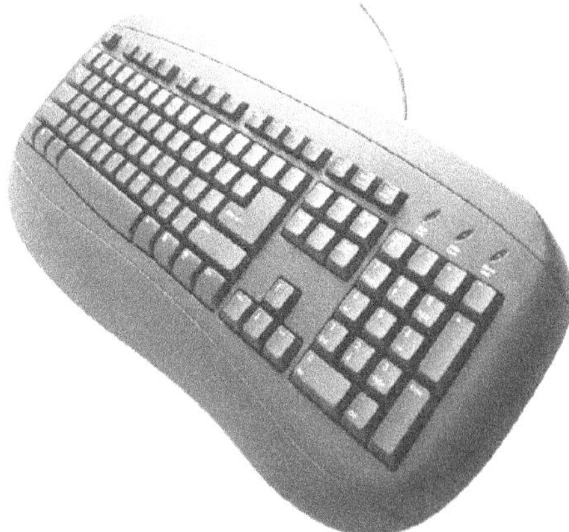

Conventional computer keyboards have all the keys that typewriter keyboards have plus others keys unique to computers. Actually, computer keyboards are easier to use than most typewriter keyboards because you can easily rectify your typing mistakes.

Standard typewriter keys *:* Typewriter keys are the same familiar QWERTY arrangement of letter, number, and punctuation keys found on any typewriter. QWERTY refers to the order of alphabet keys in the top left row on a standard typewriter keyboard.

The space bar, Shift, Tab, and Caps Lock Keys do the same things on the computer that they do on a typewriter. (When you press the Caps Lock Key, a light on your keyboards shows you are typing ALL CAPITAL LETTERS until you press the Caps Lock key again.)

An exception is the Enter (bent left arrow) key, which occupies the place where a carriage – return key would be on a typewriter. The Enter key, sometimes called the Return key, is used to enter commands into the computer.

Cursor-movement keys *:* The cursor is the symbol on the display screen that shows where data may be entered next. The cursor-movement keys, or arrow keys, are used to move the cursor around the text on the screen. These keys move the cursor left, right, up or down.

The keys labeled PgUp stands for page up and the key labeled PgDn stands for page down. These keys move the cursor one page or one screen at a time up (backward) or down (forward). Some software lets you use the Home key to move the cursor to the top of the document and the End key to move to the bottom of the document.

Numeric Keys *:* A separate set of keys, 0 - 9, known as the numeric keypad, is laid out like the keys on a calculator. The numeric keypad has two purposes.

Whenever the Num Lock key is off, the numeric keys may be used as arrow keys for cursor movement. When the Num Lock key is on, the keys may be used for typing numbers, as on a calculator. A light is illuminated on the keyboard when the Num Lock key is pressed once and goes off when the Num Lock key is pressed again.

For space reasons, portable computers often lack a separate numeric keypad or the numeric keys may be superimposed on the typewriter letter keys and are activated by the Num Lock key.

Function Keys *:* Function keys are the keys labeled with an F and a number, such as F1 and F2 that are used for tasks that occur frequently. Desktop microcomputers usually have 12 function keys.

The software you are using defines the purpose of each function key. For example, pressing F2 may print your document in one program but save your work to disk in another. Special-purpose keys include Backspace, Del, Ins, Esc, Ctrl, and Alt. The uses of these special purpose keys are as follows:

Backspace (indicated by a left pointing arrow) erases as you move left over the preceding text you have typed.

Del (Delete) erases text to the right (on Macintoshes, to the left).

Ins (insert) allows you to type over (or push right) existing text, inserting new next.

Esc (Escape) may be used to cancel whatever task you are currently performing.

The purposes of Ctrl (Control) and Alt (Alternate) are defined be the software you are using. Some computers may have other special-purpose keys.

Light Pen : A light pen is a pointing device used to select a displayed menu option on the CRT. It is a photosensitive pen-like device. It is capable of sensing a position on the CRT screen when its tip touches the screen. When its tip is moved over the screen surface, its photocell-sensing element detects the light coming from the screen and the corresponding signals are sent to the processor. The menu is a set of programmed choices offered to the user. The user indicates his choice by touching light pen against a desired description of the menu. The signals sent by the light pen to the processor identify the menu option.

16.4.2   Mouse

A device that controls the movement of the cursor or pointer on a display screen. A mouse is a small object you can roll along a hard, flat surface. Its name is derived from its shape, which looks a bit like a mouse. Its connecting wire that one can imagine to be the mouse's tail, is in the fact that one must make it scroll along a surface. As you move the mouse, the pointer on the display screen moves in the same direction. Mouse contains at least one button and sometimes as many as three, which have different functions depending on what program is running. Some new mouse also includes a scroll wheel for scrolling through long documents.

Invented by Douglas Engel Bart of Stanford Research Center in 1963, and pioneered by Xerox in the 1970s, the mouse is one of the great breakthroughs in computer ergonomics because it frees the user to a large extent from using the keyboard. In particular, the mouse is important for graphical user interfaces because you can simply point to options and objects and clicks a mouse button. Such applications are often called point-and-click programs. The mouse is also useful for graphics programs that allow you to draw pictures by using the mouse like a pen, pencil, or paintbrush.

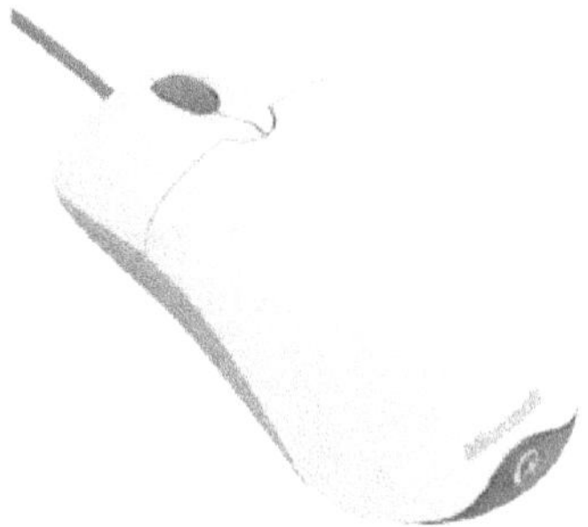

There are three basic types of mouse:

***Mechanical** :* Has a rubber or metal ball on its underside that can roll in all directions. Mechanical sensors within the mouse detect the directed ball is rolling and move the screen pointer accordingly.

***Opt mechanical** :* Same as a mechanical mouse, but uses optical sensors to detect motion of the ball.

***Optical** :* Uses a laser to detect the mouse movement. You must the mouse along a special mat with a grid so that the optical mechanism has a frame or reference. Optical mouse has no mechanical moving parts. They responds more quickly and precisely than mechanical and opt mechanical mouse but they are more expensive.

16.4.3   Joystick

A joystick is also a pointing device. It is just like a lever that moves in all directions and controls the movement of a pointer or some other display symbol. A joystick is similar to a mouse, except that with a mouse the cursor stops moving as soon as you stop moving the mouse. With a joystick, the pointer continues moving in the direction the joystick is pointing. To stop the pointer, you must return the joystick to its upright position. Most joysticks include two buttons called triggers.

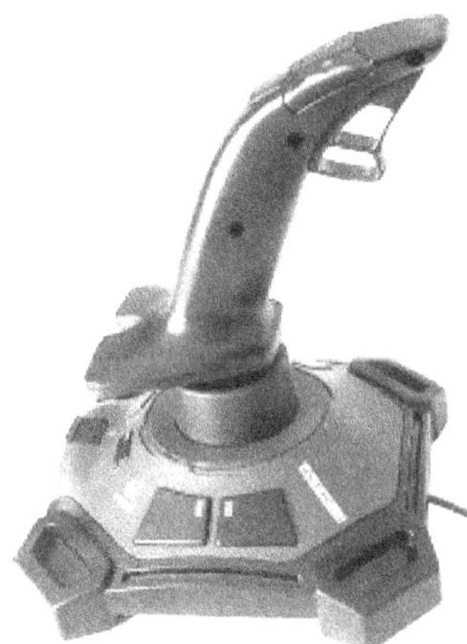

Joysticks are used mostly for computer games, but they are also used occasionally for CAD / CAM systems and other applications.

16.4.4   Trackballs

Trackball is also a pointing device. Essentially, a trackball is a mouse lying on its back. To move the pointer, you rotate the ball with your thumb, your fingers, or the palm of your hand. There are usually one to three buttons next to the ball, which you use just like mouse buttons.

The advantage of trackballs over mouse is that the trackball is stationary so it does not require much space to use it. In addition, your can place a trackball on any type of surface, including your lap. For both these reasons, trackballs are popular pointing devices for portable computers.

16.4.5   Scanners

Scanning device translates images of text, drawings, photos into digital form. Scanners are a kind of input devices. They are capable of entering information directly into the computer. The main advantage of direct entry of information is that users do not have to key the information. This provides faster and moves accurate data entry. Important types of scanners are optical scanners and magnetic-ink character readers.

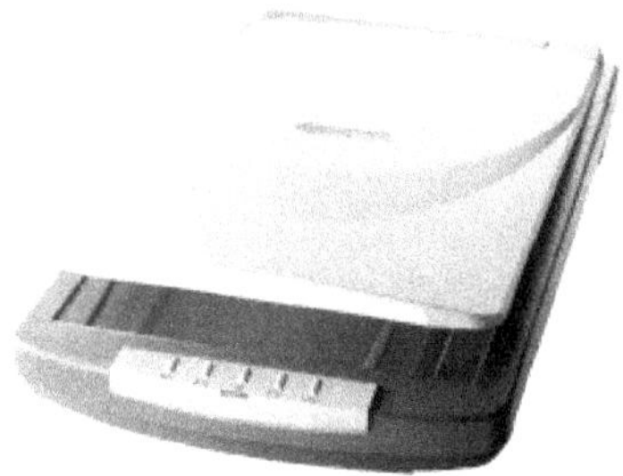

Optical Scanners : The optical scanners are capable of reading information recorded on paper, employ light source and light sensors. The information to be scanned is typewritten information, information is coded as ink or pencil marks or bars.

16.4.6   Optical Character Reader (OCR)

An optical character reader detects alphanumeric character printed or typewritten on paper. The text which is be scanned is illuminated by a low frequency source. The light is absorbed by the dark areas and reflected from the lighted areas. The reflected light is received by photocells or (CCD) charged coupled devices, which provide binary data corresponding to dark and lighted areas. An OCR can scan several thousands of printed or typewritten characters per second. Optical character technology finds use in areas like office automation and electronic documentation.

16.4.7   Optical Mark Readers (OMR)

Special marks such as squares or bubbles are prepared on examination answer sheets or questionnaires. The users fill in these squares with soft pencil or ink to indicate their choice. An optical mark reader detects these marks and the corresponding signals are sent to the processor. If a mark is present, it reduced the amount of reflected light. If a mark is not present, the amount of reflected light is not reduced. This change in the amount of reflected light is used to detect the presence of a mark. This method is used for analysis of objective type questions, for example, market survey, population survey, etc., where choice is restricted to one out of a few choices available.

16.4.8 Optical Bar Code Readers

This method uses a number of bars (lines) of varying thickness and spacing between them indicates the desired information. Bar codes are used on most manufactured retails products. An optical bar reader can read such bars and convert them into electrical pulses to be processed by a computer. The most commonly used bar code is Universal Product Code (UPC). The UPC code uses a series of vertical bars of varying widths. These bars are detected as ten digits. The first five digits identify the supplier or manufacturer of the item. The second five digits identify the product. The code also contains a check digit to ensure that the information read is correct.

16.4.9 Magnetic Ink Character Readers (MICR)

MICR is widely used by banks in advanced countries to process large volumes of cheques and deposit forms written by customers every day. Special ink called magnetic ink (i.e. an ink which contains iron oxide particles) is used to write characters on cheques and deposit forms, which are to be processed by an MICR. MICR is capable of reading characters written with magnetic ink on paper. The magnetic ink is magnetized during the input process. The MICR reads the magnetic patterns of the written characters. To identify the characters these patterns are compared with special patterns stored in the memory. When a cheque is entered into an MICR, it passes through a magnetic field. The iron oxide particles are magnetized under the magnetic field. The read head reads the characters written with magnetic ink on cheque. It interprets the character and sends the corresponding data directly to the computer for processing. An MICR processes upto 2,600 cheques per minute.

16.4.10 CCD Camera

In many applications it is desired that a computer should be able to see its environment. For example, a robot must be able to see to perform its job; a computer-controlled security system must be able to see its environment etc. To provide vision to computers, sensors like video cameras, CCD cameras, OPTICRAM cameras, etc. are employed. These cameras act as sensors to provide signals proportional to the intensity of light falling on various sports of the image of an object. The computer can process these signals and recognize, and display the image of the object.

16.4.11 Sensors

A sensor is a type of input device that collects specific kinds of data directly from the environments and transmits it to a computer. Although you are unlikely to see such input devices connected to a PC in an office, they exist all around us, often in invisible form. Sensors can be used for detecting all kinds of things: speed, movement, weight, pressure, temperature, humidity, wind, current, fog, gas, smoke, light, shapes, images, and so on.

For example, in metro highways there are sensors that detect the speed and volume of traffic. These sensors send data to computers that can adjust traffic lights to keep cars and trucks away from grid locked areas. In aviation, sensors are used to detect ice buildup on airplane wings or to alert pilots to sudden changes in wind direction. Government regulators to monitor whether companies are complying with air-pollution standards also use sensors.

16.5   Output Devices

16.5.1   Softcopy Vs. Hardcopy

Output devices translate information processed by the computer into a form that humans can understand. The two principal kinds of output are hardcopy, which is printed, and softcopy, such as material shown on a display screen. Output devices include display screens; printers, plotters, and multi function devices; audio-output devices; video-output devices; and virtual reality.

Output devices translate information processed by the computer into a form that humans can understand. The principal outputs are hardcopy and softcopy.

Hardcopy : Hardcopy refers to printed output., whether text or graphics, which are printed from printers. Film is also considered as hardcopy output.

Softcopy : Softcopy refers to data that is shown on a display screen or is in audio or voice form. This kind of output is not tangible; it cannot be touched.

There are several types of output devices. We will discuss the following ones.

- Display screens
- Printers, plotters, and multifunction devices
- Audio-output devices
- Video-output devices
- Virtual-reality devices

16.5.2   Display Screen or Monitor

The term monitor usually refers to the display screen. There are many ways to classify monitors. The most basic is in terms of colour capabilities, which separate monitors into three classes:

Monochrome : Monochrome monitors actually display two colours, one for the background and one for the foreground. The colour can be black and white, green and black, or amber and black.

Gray – Scale : A gray scale monitor is a special type of monochrome monitor capable of displaying different shades of gray. The use of many shades of gray to represent an image is called gray-scalling. Continuous-tone images, such as black-and-white photographs, use an almost unlimited number of shades of gray. Conventional computer hardware and software, however, can only represent a limited number of shades of gray (typically 16 or 256). Gray-scaling is the process of converting a continuous-tone image to an image that a computer can manipulate.

Colour : Colour monitors can display anywhere from 16 to over 1 million different colours. Colour monitors are sometimes called RGB monitors because they accept three separate signals—red, green, and blue.

After the classification, the most important aspect of a monitor is its screen size. Like televisions, screen sizes are measured diagonally in inches, the distance from one corner to the opposite corner diagonally. A typical size for small VGA monitors is 14 inches. Monitors that are 16 or more inches diagonally are often called full-page monitors. In addition to their size, monitors can be either portrait (height greater than width) or landscape (width greater than height). Larger landscape monitors can display two full pages, side by side. The screen size is sometimes misleading because there is always an area around the edge of the screen that can't be used. Therefore, monitor manufactures must now also state the viewable area-that is, the area of screen that is actually used.

The resolution of a monitor indicates how densely packed the pixels are. In general, the more pixels (often expressed in dots per inch), the sharper is the image. Most modern monitors can display 1024 by 768 pixels, the SVGA standard. Some high-end models can display 1280 by 1024, or even 1600 by 1200.

Another common way of classifying monitors is in terms of the type of signal they accept: analog or digital. Nearly all-modern monitors accept analog signals, which is required by the VGA, SVGA, 8514/A, and other high-resolution colour standards.

A few monitors have fixed frequency, which means that they accept input at only one frequency. Most monitors, however, are multi-scanning, which means that they automatically adjust themselves to the frequency of the signals being sent to it. This means that they can display images at different resolutions, depending on the data being sent to them by the video adapters.

Other factors that determine a monitor's quality include the following :

Bandwidth : The range of signal frequencies the monitor can handle. This determines how much data it can process and therefore how fast it can refresh at higher resolution.

Refresh Rate : How many times per second the screen is refreshed (redrawn). To avoid flickering, the refresh rate should be at least 72 Hz.

Interlaced or no interlaced : Interlacing is a technique that enables a monitor to have more resolution, but it reduces the monitor's reaction speed.

Dot pitch : The amount of space between each pixel. The smaller the dot pitch, the sharper is the image.

16.5.3   Video Display Unit (VDU)

Video Display Unit also called monitors, or CRTs, are output devices showing programming instructions and data as they are input after they are processed. Sometimes a monitor is also referred to as a VDT (Vide display terminal), although technically a VDT includes both screen and keyboard.

Display screens are of two types: cathode-ray-tubes and flat-panel display.

Cathode-Ray Tubes (CRTs) : The most common form of display screen is the CRT. A cathode-ray tube is a vacuum tube used as a display screen in a computer or video display terminal. This same kind of technology is found not only in the screen of desktop computers but also in television sets. Images are represented on the screen (whether CRT or flat-panel display) by individual dots or "picture elements" called pixels. A pixel is the smallest unit on the screen that can be turned on and off. A stream of bits defining the image is sent from the computer (from the CPU) to the CRT's electron gun, where the bits are converted to electrons. The inside of the front of the CRT screen is coated with phosphor. When a beam of electrons from the electron gun (deflected through a yoke) hits the phosphor, it lights up selected pixels to generate an image on the screen.

Flat-panel Displays : Flat panel display is much thinner and is less in weight and consumes less power and thus they are more useful in portable computers. There are three types of technology used in flat panel display-liquid-crystal display, electro luminescent display and gas plasma display.

Clarity of Picture on a screen : Whether for CRT or flat-panel, screen clarity depends on three qualities: resolution, dot pitch, and refresh rate.

Resolution : It refers to the sharpness and clarity of an image. The term is most often used to describe monitors, printers, and bit-mapped graphic images. For graphics monitors, the screen resolution signifies the number of dots (pixels) on the entire screen. For example, a 640-by-480-pixel screen is capable of displaying 640 distinct dots on each of 480 lines, or about 300,000 pixels. This translates it into different dpi measurements depending on the size of the screen. For example, a 15-inch VGA monitor (640 x 480) displays about 50 dots per inch.

Monitors, scanners, and other I/O devices are often classified as high resolution, medium resolution, or low resolution. The actual resolution ranges for each of these grades is constantly shifting as the technology improves. In the case of dot matrix and laser printers, the resolution indicates the number of dots per inch. For example, a 300-dpi (dots per inch) printer is one that is capable of printing 300 distinct dots in a line 1 inch long. This means it can print 90,000 dots per square inch.

Dot Pitch : Dot pitch is the amount of space between pixels; the closer the dots, the crisper the image. This is a measurement that indicates the diagonal distance between like-coloured phosphor dots on a display screen. Measured in millimeters, the dot pitch is one of the principal characteristics that determine the quality of display monitors. The dot pitch of colour monitors for personal computers ranges from about 0.15 mm to 0.30 mm. Another term for dot pitch is phosphor pitch.

Refresh Rate : Refresh rate is the number of times per second the pixels are recharged so that their glow remains bright. The refresh rate for a monitor is measured in hertz (Hz) and is also called the vertical frequency, vertical scan rate, frame rate or vertical refresh rate. The old standard for monitor refresh rates was 60Hz, but a new standard developed by VESA sets the refresh rate at 75Hz for monitors displaying resolutions of 640 x 480 or greater. This means that the monitor redraws the display 75 times per second. The faster the refresh rate is the image sharper the image.

Monochrome Versus Colour Screens : Display screens can be either monochrome or colour.

Monochrome : Monochrome display screens display only two colours-usually black and white, amber and black, or gray and black.

Colour : Colour display screens can display between 16 and 16.7 million colours, depending on their type. Most software today is developed for colour, except for some pocket PCs.

Text Versus Graphics : Character-Mapped versus Bitmapped Display : Another distinction in display screens relates to their capacity to display graphics. A screen lacking this capacity is referred to as character-mapped. A bitmapped screen can display graphics.

Character-Mapped : Character-mapped display screens display only text-letters, numbers, and special characters. They cannot display graphics unless a video adapter card is installed. Text is displayed in rows and columns, with rows measuring the height of the screen and columns measuring the width. Most computer screens display 25 rows and 80 columns, which means that a row or line can have up to 80 characters of text.

Bitmapped : A representation, consisting of rows and columns of dots, of a graphics image in computer memory. The value of each dot (whether it is filled in or not) is stored in one or more bits of data. For simple monochrome images, one bit is sufficient to represent each dot, but for colours and shades of gray, each dot requires more than one bit of data. The more bits used to represent a dot, the more colours and shades of gray can be represented.

The density of the dots, known as the resolution, determines how sharply the image is represented. This is often expressed in dots per inch (dpi) or simply by the number of rows and columns, such as 640 by 480.

To display a bit-mapped image on a monitor or to print it on a printer, the computer translates the bit map into pixels (for display screens) or ink dots (for printers). Optical scanners and fax machines work by transforming text or pictures on paper into bit maps.

Video Display Adapters

To display graphics, a display screen must have a video display adapter. A video display adapter, also called a graphics adapter card, is a circuit board that determines the resolution, number of colours, and how fast images appear on the display screen. Video display adapters come with their own memory chips, which determine how fast the card processes images and how many colours it can display. A video display adapter with 256 kilobytes of memory will provide 16 colours; one with 1 megabyte will support 16.7 million colours.

The video display adapter is often built on the motherboard, although it may also be an expansion card that plugs into an expansion slot. Video display adapters embody certain standards. New computer displays tend to favor VGA, SVGA or XGA standards.

VGA : Abbreviation of video graphics adapter, a graphics display system for PCs developed by IBM. VGA has become one of the *de facto* standards for PCs. In text mode, VGA systems provide a resolution of 720 by 400 pixels. In graphics mode, the resolution is either 640 by 480 (with 16 colours) or 320 by 200 (with 256 colours). The total palette of colours is 262, 144.

Unlike earlier graphics standards for PCs MDA, CGA and EGA, VGA uses analog signals rather than digital signals. Consequently, a monitor designed for one of the older standards will not be able to use VGA.

Since its introduction in 1987, several other standards have been developed that offer grater resolution and more colours but VGA remains the lowest common denominator. All PCs made today support VGA, and possibly some more advanced standard.

SVGA : Short for Super VGA, a set of graphics standards designed to offer greater resolution than VGA. There are several varieties of SVGA, each providing a different resolution:

- 800 by 600 pixels
- 1024 by 768 pixels
- 1280 to 1024 pixels
- 1600 by 1200 pixels

All SVGA standards support a palette of 16 million colours, but the number of colours that can be displayed simultaneously is limited by the amount of video memory installed in a system. One SVGA system might display only 256 simultaneous colours while another displays the entire palette of 16 million colours. Monitor and graphics manufacturers called VESA develop the SVGA standards.

XGA *:* Short for extended graphics array, a high-resolution graphics standard introduced by IBM in 1990. XGA was designed to replace the older 8514/A video standard. It provides the same resolutions (640 by 480 or 1024 by 768 pixels), but supports more monitors to be non-interlaced.

For any of these displays to work, video display adapters and monitors must be compatible. Your computer's software and the display adapter must also be compatible. Thus, if you are changing your monitor or your video display adapter, be sure the new one will still work with the old.

16.5.4   Paper Output Devices : Printers, Plotters and Multifunction Devices

Printers, plotters and multifunction devices produce printed text or images on paper. Printers may be desktop or portable, impact or non-impact. Impact printers include daisywheel and dot matrix printers. Non-impact printers include laser, ink-jet, and thermal printers. Plotters are pen, electrostatic, and thermal. Multifunction devices combine capabilities, such as printing, scanning, copying, and faxing.

Printers are most popular output devices. They provide information in a permanent readable form. They produce printed outputs of results, programs and data. Printers used with computers can be classified as follows:

(a) Character printers (b) Line printers and (c) Page printers

A character printer prints one character of the text at a time. A line printer prints one line of the text at a time. A page printer prints one page of the text at a time.

The above classification of printers is based on as to how they print. There is one more classification based on the technology used in their manufacture.

Impact printers *:* An electro-mechanical that causes hammers or pins to strike against a ribbon and paper to print the text. Non-impact printers do not use any electro-mechanical printing head to strike against ribbon and paper. They use thermal, chemical, electrostatic, laser beam or inkjet technology for printing the text. Usually a non-impact type printer is faster than an impact type. The disadvantage of non-impact type printers is that they produce only a single copy of the text whereas impact printers produce multiple copies of the text.

Character Printers *:* Characters printers print one characters at a time. They are low speed printers. Their printing speed lies in the range of 60-600 characters per second. Two types of impact character printers are available: dot-matrix printers and letter quality printers.

Dot Matrix Impact Type Character Printers *:* A character is printed by printing the selected number of dots from a matrix of dots. The print head contains a vertical array of 9, 18 or 24 pins. A character is printed in a number of steps. One dot-column of the dot matrix is taken up at a time. The selected dots of a column (i.e. the column of dot-matrix) are printed by the print head at a time as it moves across a line.

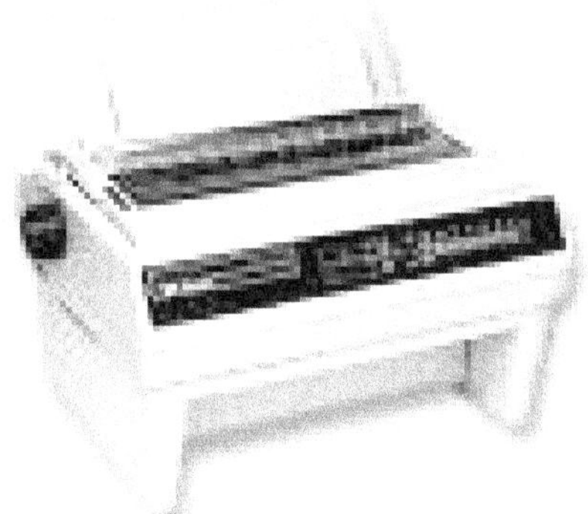

A dot-matrix printer is faster than a letter quality printer. Its printing speed lies in the range of 80-600 cps (character per second). Such printers operate at two or three speeds. The lower the speed, the better the printing quality. Higher speed is for draft printing and the lower speed is for near-letter quality (NLQ) printing, i.e. printing is as good as that of a letter quality printer. Many dot-matrix printers are bi-directional. A bi-directional printer prints one line a text from left to right and then it prints the next line from right to left.

Dot-matrix printers are very flexible. They do not have fixed character fonts. The term font is used to refer to a character set of a printer. As fonts are not fixed, a dot-matrix printer can print any shape of a character by software. This permits printing special characters such as @, Ω, $\sqrt{}$, Θ, Φ, β, ∞, $\subseteq$, $\Leftrightarrow$, Ψ etc; various sizes of print, bold or expanded characters, italics characters of any languages and ability to print graphics.

Letter Quality Impact Character Printer (Daisy Wheel Printers) : An impact type letter quality printer is used where good quality of printing is needed. Such printers also called Daisy Wheel Printers. It is much slower compared to a dot-matrix printer. Its speed is in the range of 20-75 CPS. It is costlier than dot-matrix printer. Its font is of fixed type. It cannot print graphics; Two-to-three types of fonts are available with Daisy Wheel. One can select a font having the desired style of characters.

A daisy wheel printer has a removable print wheel, the flower-like daisywheel consisting of spokes. Each spoke ends with a raised character, which is turned to align the desired letter, and then with a hammer.

Non-impact Character Printers

This type of printers uses thermal, electrostatic, chemical and inkjet technologies. They are briefly described below.

Thermal Character Printers : This type of printers use special heat-sensitive paper. Such papers have a special heat sensitive coating. When a spot on the special paper is hearted, it becomes dark. A character is printed with a matrix of dots. A print head consists of 5 x 7 or 7x9 matrix of tiny heating elements. Electric current heats the heating element. To print a character the printing head is moved first to the correct character position. Then the heating elements for the desired character are turned on. After a short time they are turned off. Therefore the print head is moved to the next Character position. Such printers have a speed of about 200 characters per second (cps).

For people who want the highest quality colour printing available with desktop printers, thermal prints are the answer. However they are expensive and they require expensive paper. Thus they are not generally used for jobs requiring a high volume of output.

Ink-jet Character Printers : It uses dot-matrix approach to print text and graphics. Earlier ink-jet printers used one or more nozzles in print head that emit a steady stream of tiny ink drops. Each droplet is charged when it passes rough a valve. Then it passes through horizontal and vertical deflecting plates. These plates deflect ink drops to direct them to the desired sports on the paper to form the impression of a character. In this type of printers the continuous stream of ink-jet approach is used. The speed of inkjet printers lies in the range of 40-300 cps. The average life of an ink-jet print head is about 10 billion characters, which is 5 times more than that of the print head of an impact type dot-matrix printer.

Inkjet printer's uses ink cartridges containing a column of tiny heaters. The print quality of such printers in very near letter-quality. Speed of such printers is in the same range as that of slow dot-matrix printers. Most colour printing is done on ink-jet because the nozzles can hold four different colours.

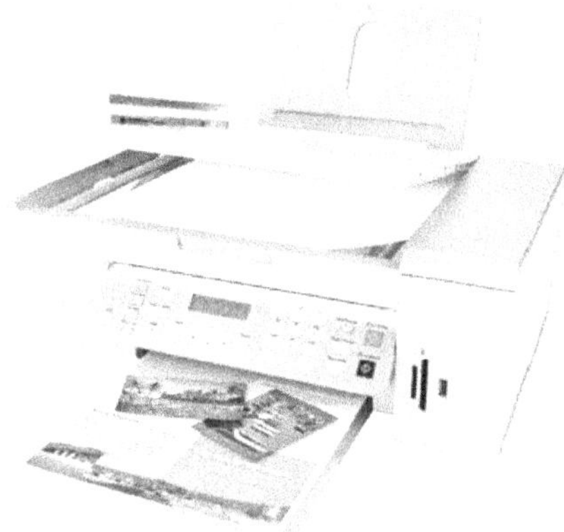

Line Printers

The line printer prints one line of the text at a time. Its printing speed lies in the range of 300-3000 lines per minutes. It is used for large-volume printing jobs. It may be used with mini and mainframe computers.

   (a)   Drum Printer   (b)   Chain Printer   (c)   Band Printer

Drum Printer : A drum printer uses a rapidly rotating drum (cylinder) which contains a complete set of raised characters in each band around the cylinder. Each character position along the text line contains a band of raised character set. There is a magnetically driven hammer in each character position of the line. The printer receives all characters to be printed in one line of the text from the processor. The hammers hit the ribbon and paper against the desired character on the drum when it comes in the printing position. Its noise level is high. Its speed varies from 200 to 2000 lines per minute.

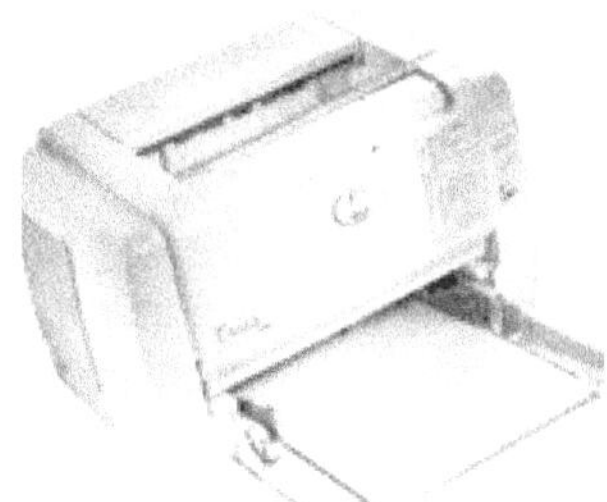

Chain Printer : Chain printer uses a rapidly rotating chain, which is called print chain. The print contains characters each link of the chain is character font. Magnetically driven hammers are located in each print position. The printer receives all the characters to be printed in one line from the processor. The printer prints one line at a time. A chain may contain more than one character set. when desired character comes in the print position the hammer strikes the ribbon and paper against the character. The noise level of the printer is high. Its speed lies in the range of 400-2400 lines/mm.

Band Printer : Band printer is just like a chain printer. It contains fast rotating steel print bands in place of chains. The print band contains a raised character set. Hammers strike the ribbon and the paper against the character to print the character. Some printers can print up to 3000 lines/mm.

Laser Printers : This is a type of printer that utilizes a laser beam to produce an image on a drum. The light of the laser alters the electrical charge on the drum wherever it hits. The drum is then rolled through a reservoir of toner, which is picked up by the charged portions of the drum. Finally, the toner is transferred to the paper through a combination of heat and pressure. This is also the used as a copy machines.

Because an entire page is transmitted to a drum before the toner is applied, laser printers are sometimes called page printers. There are two other types of page printers that fall under the category of laser printers even though they do not use lasers at all. One uses an array of LEDs to expose the drum, and the other uses LCDs. Once the drum is charged, however, they both operate like a real laser printer.

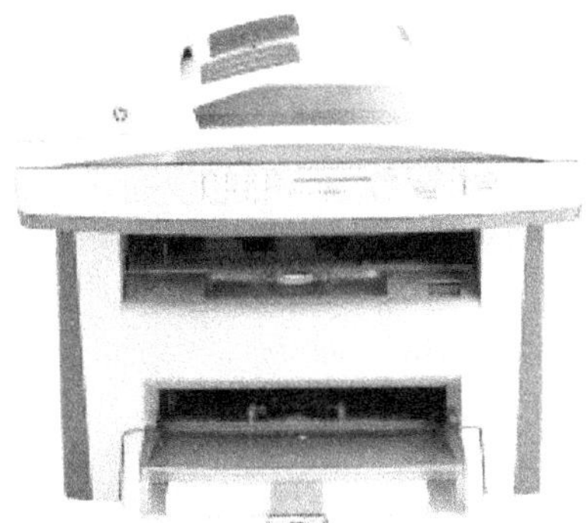

One of the chief characteristics of laser printers is their resolution i.e., how many dots per inch (dpi) they lay down. The available resolution range is from 300 dpi at the low end to 1,200 dpi at the high end. By comparison, offset printing usually prints at 1,200 or 2,400 dpi. Some laser printers achieve higher resolutions with special techniques known generally as resolution enhancement.

16.6   Units of Measurement for Storage

We will discuses the meanings of kilobytes, megabytes, gigabytes, and terabytes as unit of data storage. The same terms are also used to measure the data capacity of storage devices.

Bit : Short for binary digit, the smallest unit of information on a machine. A single bit can hold only on of two values: 0 or 1. More meaningful information is obtained by combining consecutive bits larger units. For example, a byte is composed of 8 consecutive bits.

Byte : To represent letters, numbers, or special characters (such as $ or *), bits are combined into groups. A group of eight bits is called a byte and a byte represents one character, digit, or any other value. (For example, in Binary scheme, 01001000 represents the letter P.) The capacity of a computer's memory of a floppy disk is expressed in terms numbers of bytes.

Kilo Byte : In decimal systems, kilo stands for 1,000, but in binary systems, a kilo is 1,024 (2 to the 10th power). Technically, therefore, a kilobyte is 1,024 bytes, but it is often used loosely as a synonym for 1,000 bytes. For example, a computer that has 256 KB main memory can store approximately 256,000 bytes (or characters) in memory at one time.

Mega Byte : Megabyte is frequently abbreviated as MB. This is equal to 1,048,576 (2 to the 20th power) bytes or 1024 kilo bytes.

Gigabyte : Gigabyte is often abbreviated as GB. One gigabyte is equal to 1,024 megabytes, or 2 to the 30th power (1,073,741,824) bytes.

Terabyte : This is approximately 1 million bytes. 2 to the 40th power (1,099,511,627,776) bytes. A terabyte is equal to 1024 Gigabytes.

Petabyte : 2 to the 50th power (1,125,899,906,842,624) bytes. A petabyte is equal to 1.024 terabytes.

Exabyte : 2 to the 60the power (1,152,921,504,606,846,976) bytes. An exabyte is equal to 1,024 petabytes.

Zettabyte : 2 to the 70th power bytes, which is approximately 10 to the 21st power (bytes. A zettabyte is equal to 1,024 exabytes. The name zeta was chosen because it's the last letter of the Latin alphabet and also sounds like the Greek letter Zeta.

Yottabyte : 2 to the 80the power bytes, which is approximately 10 to the 24th power bytes. A yottabyte is equal to 1,024 zettabytes. The name yotta was chosen because it's the second-to-last letter of the Latin alphabet and also sounds like the Greek letter iota.

16.7   Primary Storage

Storage is categorized as primary or secondary. Primary storage is main memory-working storage or temporary storage. Secondary storage is permanent storage. Examples are floppy disk, hard disk, optical disks, flash memory cards, and magtietic tape.

16.7.1   Primary Storage

Refers to physical memory that is internal to the computer. The word primary, internal or main is used to distinguish it from external mass storage devices such as disk drives. Another term for main memory is RAM.

The computer can manipulate only data that is in main memory. Therefore, every program you execute and every file you access must be copied from a storage device into main memory. The amount of main memory on a computer is crucial because it determines how many programs can be executed at one time and how much data can be readily available to the program.

Because computers often have too little main memory to hold all the data they need a technique called swapping, in which portions of data are copied into main memory when they are needed. Swapping occurs when there is no room in memory for the existing data. When one portion of data is copied into memory, its equal-sized portion is copied (swapped) out to make that memory block vacant.

Primary storage is the computer's small storage capacity, determining the total size of the programs and data files it can work with at any given moment. Primary storage, which is contained on RAM chips, is temporary. Once the power to the computer is turned off, all the data and programs within memory simply vanish. For this reason, primary storage is said to be volatile. Volatile memory is temporary memory; the contents are lost when the power is turned off. If you accidentally kick out the power cord underneath your desk, or a storm knocks down a power line to your house, whatever you are currently working on will immediately washout.

RAM

A RAM is an acronym for random access memory, a type of computer memory that can be accessed randomly; that is, any byte of memory can be accessed without touching the preceding bytes. RAM is the most common type of memory found in computers and other devices.

There are two basic types of RAM :

- Dynamic RAM (DRAM)
- Static RAM (SRAM)

Dynamic RAM : A type of physical memory used in most personal computers. The term dynamic indicates that the memory must be constantly refreshed or else it will lose its contents.

Static RAM : Static RAM pronounced ess-RAM. SRAM is faster and less volatile than dynamic RAM, but it requires more power and is more expensive.

ROM

ROM is an acronym for read only memory. Once data has been written onto a ROM chip, it cannot be removed and can only be read. Unlike main memory, ROM retains its contents even when the computer is turned off. Rom is referred to as being non-volatile, whereas RAM is volatile. Rom stores critical programs such as the program that boots the computer.

Types of ROM

PROM : Pronounced prom, is acronym for programmable Read-Only Memory. A prom is a memory chip on which data can be written only once. Once a program has been written onto a PROM, it remains there forever. The difference between RAM and PROM is that a ROM is programmed during the manufacturing process, whereas a PROM is manufactured as blank memory.

EPROM : Erasable programmable read only memory is a special type of memory that retains its contents until is not exposed to ultraviolet light. The ultraviolet light clears its contents, making it possible to program the memory write and erase an EPROM, you need a special device called a PROM burner.

EEPROM ; Electrically erasable programmable read only memory is a special type of PROM that can be erased by exposing it to an electrical charges.

Cache

Cache pronounced cash is a special high-speed storage mechanism.It can be either a reserved section of main memory or an independent high-speed storage device. Two types of caching are commonly used in personal computers memory caching and disk caching.

16.7.2   Secondary Memory or Secondary Storage

Refers to various techniques and devices used for storing large amounts of data. The earliest storage devices were punched paper cards, which were used as early as 1804 to control silk-weaving looms. Modern mass storage devices include all types of disk drives and tape drives. Mass storage is distinct from memory, which refers to temporary storage areas within the computer. Secondary storage is non-volatile i.e., is, data and programs are permanent, or remain intact, when the power is turned off.The main types of secondary storages are:

Floppy Disks

Floppy disk is round pieces of flat plastic that store data and programs as magnetized spots. The two principal sizes are $3^{1/2}$-inch and $5^{1/4}$-inch. A disk drive copies or reads, data from the disk and writes, or records data to the disk. Components of a floppy disk include tracks and IESors; disks come in various densities. All have writer protect features. Card must be taken to avoid data corruption on disks and users are advised to back up, or duplicate, the data on their disks.

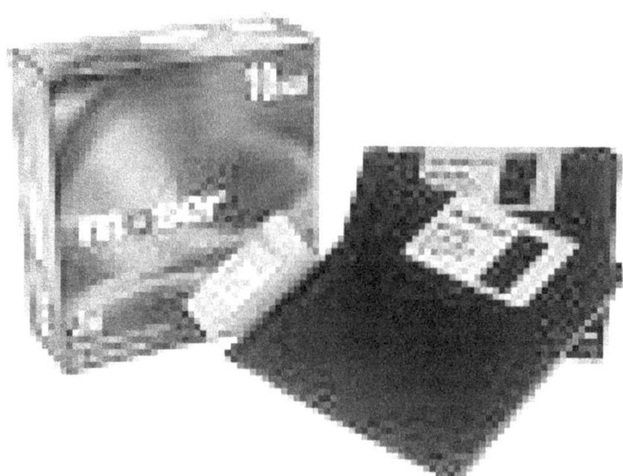

A floppy disk is a soft magnetic disk. It is called floppy because it flops if you wave it (at least, the 5¼-inch variety does). Unlike most hard disks, floppy disk (often called floppies or diskettes) is portable, because you can remove them from a disk drive. Disk drives for floppy disks are called floppy drives. Floppy disks are slower to access than hard disks and have less storage capacity, but they are cheaper and portable.

Floppies come in two basic sizes

5¼ inch : It is common size for PCs made before 1987. This type of floppy is generally capable of storing between 100K and 1.2MB (megabytes) of data. The most common sizes are 360K and 1.2MB.

3½ inch : Despite their small size, microfloppies have a larger storage capacity than their cousins (from 400K to 1.4MB of data). The most common sizes for PCs are 720K (double-density) and 1.44MB (high-density). Macintoshes support disks of 400K, 800K, and 1.2MB.

Floppy disk drive

To use floppy disk we use a machine that reads data from and writes data onto a disk called Floppy Disk Drive. A disk drive rotates the disk very fast and has one or more heads that read and write data. Disk drives can be either internal (housed within the computer) or external (housed in a separate box that connects to the computer). The process of READ and WRITE means the following:

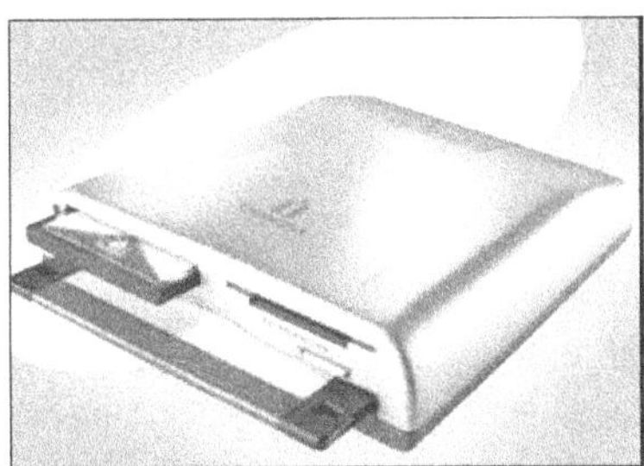

READ : to copy data to a place where it can be used by a program. The term is commonly used to describe copying data from a storage medium, such as a disk to main memory for the purpose of using the data for processing.

WRITE : to copy data from main memory to a storage device, such as a disk. i.e. the data recorded onto the disk from the main memory for later use.

Characteristics of Floppy Disks : Both 5 ¼ inch and 3 ½ inch disks work in similar ways, although there is some difference. The characteristics of floppy disks are as follows:

Tracks and sectors : Once a floppy disk data is recorded in rings it is called tracks. These tracks are not visible. A typical floppy disk has 80 (double density) or 160 (high-density) tracks. Each track is further divided into a number of sectors. Sector is the smallest unit that can be accessed on a disk. The tracks are concentric circles around the disk and sectors are segments within each circle. For example, a floppy disk might have 40 tracks, with each track divided into 10 sectors. The operating system and disk drive keep tabs on where information is stored. They are measured in terms of tracks per inch (TPI). For example, double-density 5.25-inch floppies have a TPI of 48, while high density floppies record 96 TPI. High-density 3.5-inch diskettes are formatted with 135 TPI.

Formatting : formatting means to prepare a storage medium, usually a disk, for reading and writing. When you format a disk, the operating system erases all book keeping information on the disk, tests the disk to make sure all sectors are reliable, makes bad sectors (that is, those that are scratched), and creates internal address tables that it later used to locate information. You must format a disk before you can use it.

Note that reformatting a disk does not erase the data of the disk. It only erases the address tables. Do not panic, therefore, if you accidentally reformat a disk that has useful data. A computer specialist should be able to recover most, if not all, of the information on the disk. You can also buy programs that enable you to recover a disk yourself.

The previous discussion, however, applies only to high-level formats, the type of formats that most users execute. In addition, hard disks have a low-level format, which sets certain properties of the disk such as the interleave sector. The low-level format also determines what type of disk controller can access the disk (e.g. RLL or MFM)

Data capacity – sides and density : Density means how tightly information is packed together on a storage medium (tape or disk). A higher density means that data are closer together, so the medium can hold more information. Floppy disks can be single-density, double-density, high-density, or extra-high-density. To use a double-density, high-density, or extra-high-density disk, you have a disk drive that supports the density level. Density, therefore, can refer both to the media and the device.

Write protect feature : 'Write-Protect' means to mark a file or disk so that its contents cannot be modified or deleted. When you want to make sure that neither you nor user can destroy data, you can write–protect it. Many operating systems include a command to write protect files. You can also write–protect 5¼ inch floppy disks by covering the write protect files. 3½-inch floppy diskettes have a small switch that you can set to turn on write protection. Write protected files and media can only be read; you cannot write to them, edit them, append data to them, or delete them.

Backup of important data : Backup means to copy files to a second medium (a disk or tape) as a precaution in case the first medium fails. One of the cardinal rules in using computer is:

Back up your files regularly.

Even the most reliable computer is apt to break down eventually. Many professionals recommend that you make two, or even three, backups of all your files. To be especially safe, you should keep one backup in a different location from the others.

You can back up files using operating system commands, or you can buy a special-purpose backup utility. Backup programs often compress the data so that backups require fewer disks.

Hard Disk : Hard disk is a magnetic disk on which you can store computer data. The term hard is used to distinguish it from a soft, or floppy disk. Hard disks hold more data and are faster than floppy disks. A hard disk can store data from MB to TB whereas most floppies have a maximum storage capacity of 1.4 MB.

A single hard disk usually consists of several platters. Platter is a round magnetic plate that constitutes part of a hard disk. Each platter requires two read/write heads, one for each side. All the read/write heads are attached to a single access arm so that they cannot move independently. Each platter has the same number of tracks, and a track location that cuts across all platters and is called a cylinder.

Removable Hard Disk

A type of disk drive system in which hard disks are enclosed in plastic or meta cartridges so that they can be removed like floppy disks. Removable disk derives combine the best aspects of hard and floppy disks. They are nearly as capacious and fast as hard disks and have the portability of floppy disks. Their biggest drawback is that they're relatively expensive.

Some Important terms related to Hard / Floppy Disk

Cylinder : A single-track location on all the platters makes up a hard disk. For example, if a hard disk has four platters, each with 600 tracks, then there will be 600 cylinders, and each cylinder will consist of 8 tracks (assuming that each platter has tracks on both sides).

Track : A ring on a disk where data can be written. A typical floppy disk has 80 (double density) or 160 (high-density) tracks. For hard disks, each platter is divided into tracks, and a single-track location that cuts through all platters (and both sides of each platter) is called a cylinder. Each track is further divided into a number of sectors. The operating system and disk drive remembers where information is stored by noting its track and sector numbers.

The density of tracks (how close together they are) is measured in terms of tracks per inch (TPI).

CD-ROM

CD-ROM abbreviation is Compact Disc-Read-Only Memory. This is a type of optical disk capable of storing large amounts of data – up to 1GB, although the most common size is 650 MB (megabytes). A single CD-ROM has the storage capacity of 700 floppy disks, enough memory to store about 300,000 text pages.

The vendor stamps CD-ROM, and once stamped, they cannot be erased and filled with new data. To read a CD, you need a CD-ROM player. All CD-ROMs conform to a standard size and format, so you can load any type of CD-ROM into any CD-ROM player. In addition, CD-ROM players are capable of playing audio CDs, which share the same technology.

CD-ROMs are particularly well-suited to information that requires large storage capacity. This includes software applications, graphics, sound, and especially video.

CD-ROM Player

Also called a CD-ROM drive, a device that can read information from a CD-ROM. CD-ROM players can be either internal, or external, which generally connect to the computer's SCSI interface or parallel port. Parallel CD-ROM players are easier to install, but they have several disadvantages: They're somewhat more expensive than internal players. They use up the parallel port which means that you can't use that part for another device such as a printer, and the parallel port itself may not be fast enough to handle all the data pouring through it.

There are a number of features that distinguish CD-ROM players, the most important of which is probably their speed. CD-ROM players are generally classified as single-speed or some multiples of single-speed. For example, a 4X player access data at four times the speed of a single-speed player.

Constant Linear Velocity, or CLV is a method used by older CD-ROM player to access data. With CLV, the rotation speed of the disk changes based on how close to the center of the disk the data is. For tracks near the center, the disk rotates faster and for data outside the disk it rotates slower. The purpose of CLV is to ensure a constant data rate, regardless of where on the disk the data is being accessed. Because less data can fit on the inside tracks, the disk needs to rotate faster for these areas. An alternative technology, which is becoming increasingly popular, is CAV Constant Angular Velocity.

Constant Angular Velocity, is a technique for accessing data of rotating disks. With constant speed regardless of what area of the disk is being accessed. This differs from constant linear velocity (CLV), which rotates the disk faster for inner tracks. Disk drives use CAV, whereas CD-ROMs generally use CLV, though some new drives use a combination of CAV and CLV. The advantage of CAV is that it is much simpler to design and produce because the motor doesn't need to change speed. In addition, CLV runs into problems for very high-speed CD-ROMs because there's a brief latency whenever the drive needs to change the rotational speed.

CD-R drive : Short for compact Disk-Record able drive, a type of disk drive that can create CD-ROMs and audio CDs. This allows users to "master" a CD-ROM or audio CD for publishing. Until recently, CD-R drives were quite expensive, but prices have dropped dramatically.

A feature of many CD-R drives, called multi session recording, enables you to keep adding data to a CD-ROM over time. This is extremely important if you want to use the CD-R drive to create backup CD-ROMs.

To create CD-ROMs on audio CDs, you'll need not only a CD-R drive, but also a CD-R software package. Often, it is the software package, not drive itself that determines how easy or difficult it is to create CD-ROMs.

CD-R drives can also read CD-ROMs and play audio CDs.

CD-RW DISK *:* Short for CD-Re-Writ able disk, a type of CD disk that enables you to write onto it in multiple sessions. One of the problems with CD-R disks is that you can only write to them once. With CD-RW drives and disks, you are treating the optical disk just like a floppy or hard disk, writing data onto it multiple times.

WORM *:* Short for write once read many, an optical disk technology that allows you to write data onto a disk just once. After that, the data is permanent and can be read any number of times. WORM is also called CD-R.

Erasable optical disk *:* A type optical disk that can be erased and loaded with new data. In contrast, most optical disks, called CD-ROMs are read-only.

Digital Video Disk (DVD) *:* Short for digital versatile disc or digital video disc, a new type of CD-ROM that holds a minimum of 4.7GB (gigabytes), enough for a full-length movie. CD-ROMs, as well as VHS videocassettes and laser discs.

The DVD specification supports disks with capacities of from 4.7 GB to 17 GB and access rates of 600 KBps to 1.3 MBps. One of the best features of DVD drives is that they are backward compatible with CD-ROMs. This means that DVD players can play old CD-ROMs, CD-I disks, and video CDs, as well as new DVD-ROMs. Newer DVD players can also read CD-R disks. DVD uses MPEG-2 to compress video data.

DVD-RAM *:* A new type of re-writable compact disc that provides much grater data storage than today's CD-RW systems. The DVD Consortium is still hammering out the specification for DVD-RAMs. Meanwhile, a competing group of manufactures led by Hewlett-Packard, Philips and Sony, have come up with a competing standard called DVD+RW. Whereas the DVD-RAM standard supports 2.6 GB per disk side, DVD+RW supports 3 GB per side.

DVD-ROM *:* A new type of read-only compact disc that hold a minimum of 4.7 GB (gigabytes), enough for a full-length movie. Many experts believe that DVD-ROMs will eventually replace CD-ROMs, as well as VHS videocassettes and laser discs. Currently, however, DVD-ROMs are more promise than reality. There are only a few DVD-ROM devices that can play old CD-ROMs, CD-I disks, and video CDs, as well as new DVD-ROMs. Newer DVD players can also read CD-R disks.

DVD-ROMs use MPEG-2 to compress video data.

Magnetic Tape

It is a magnetically coated strip of plastic on which data can be encoded. Tapes for computers are similar to tapes used to store music. This is the oldest storage media used till today.

Storing data on tapes is considerably cheaper than storing data on disks. Tapes also have large storage capacities, ranging from a few hundred kilobytes to several gigabytes. Accessing data on tapes is slower than accessing data on disks. Tapes are sequential-access media, which means that to get to a particular point. The tape must go through all the preceding points. In contrast, disks are random-access media because a disk drive can access any point at random without passing through intervening points.

Pen Drive

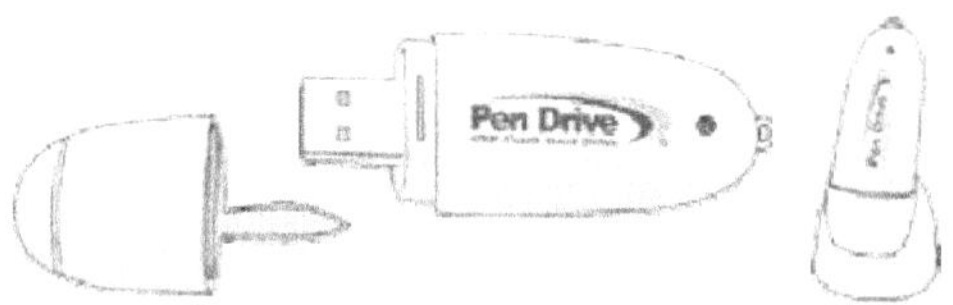

USB Pen Drive is a small key ring-sized device that can be used to easily transfer files between USB-compatible systems. Available in a range of capacities (and in some cases, with an MP3 player built-in) this handy little device can save all those data-transfer hassles.

Simple. Plug it into the USB port* of your PC (or Mac!) and watch the system automatically detects the new device. Take at look at your system drives... a new drive has been created! The operating system can now access your USB Pen Drive just like any ordinary Hard Disk Drive.

Copy across all the files you want to the 'new' drive, wait for the Read/Write LED on the USB Pen Drive to stop flashing then disconnect it. That's it. Your files are now safely stored on your USB Pen Drive. If you want to copy those files to another PC/Mac, just plug it in the new machine, wait for it to be detected and copy them off again.

* If you don't want to reach round to the back of your PC every time to plug it in, you can use the handy Docking Bay to give you USB Pen Drive access right from your desktop.

USB

USB - Universal Serial Bus, is a 'standard' developed by the computer industry to allow a vast number of different devices to be easily attached to one machine with the minimum requirement for extra drivers and software and still operate at an efficient speed.

Put simply, this means: We can plug a USB device in without switching the PC off. It will be automatically detected by the Operating System and will be ready for use in a few seconds. The USB Pen Drive *is* one of those devices.

CHAPTER 17

Fundamentals of Operating System

17.1 Definition and Need of Operating System

The operating system is the link between the hardware and software. An operating system (usually known as the OS) is an organised set or collection of software programs that control the overall operation of the computer system. It controls and directs the flow of data and instruction from one part of the computer to another.

A computer itself is nothing but a collection of various hardware devices such as the keyboard, the visual display unit, Central Processing Unit (CPU). It is the operating system that makes these independent hardware devices, although interconnected by cables, a single entity which is both easy to use and manage. Operating system acts as an interface between the user and the computer system. It is only due to presence of the operating system that the user doesn't have to bother about the technical details and functional aspects of each of the hardware components of the system. All that the user needs to do is to present the problem to the operating system in a language that can be understood by the operating system and get the results. The computer hardware provides the raw processing power or ability. It is the job of the operating system to make this ability conveniently available to the users.

17.2 Function of Operating System

An operating system (OS) is an integrated set of programs that is used to manage the various resources and overall operations of a computer system. It is designed to support the activities of computer Installation. Its prime objective is to improve the performance and efficiency of a computer system and increase facility with which a system can be used. Thus, like a manager of a company, an operating system makes the computer system user friendly. That is, it becomes easier for people to interact with and make use of the computer.

Operating system is known by many different names, depending on the manufacture of the computer. Other terms used to describe the operating system are executive, supervisor, controller and master control programs. Operating System performs the following functions.

1. ***Process Management :*** That is assignment of processors to different tasks being performed by the computer system.

2. ***Memory Management :*** That is, allocation of main memory storage to the system programs.

3. ***Input/Output management :*** That is coordination and assignment of the different input and output devices while one or more programs are being executed.

4. ***File management :*** The storage of files on various storage devices and the transfer of these from one storage device to another. It also allows all files to be easily changed and modified through the use of text editors or some other file manipulation routines.

5. ***Setting Priority :*** It determines and maintains the order in which jobs are to be executed in the computer system.

6. Automatic transition from job to job, directed by special control statements.

7. Interpretation of commands and instructions.

8. Coordination and assignment of compilers, assemblers, utility programs, software.

9. Production of dumps, traces, and error message and other debugging and error detection aids.

10. Facilitates easy communication between the system and the computer operator.

17.3   Useful Terms of Operating System

17.3.1   Multi-Programming

Overlapped or interleaved execution of two or more processes is terms as multiprogramming. In other words, multiprogramming implies that two or more processes are active at the same time and are available for execution. The operating system may select one of these active programs for allocation to CPU or processor on the basis of some selection technique. The next process in the queue is allocated to the CPU, when either of the following takes place.

(i)   The executing process issues an I/O request,

(ii)   The executing process completes execution, or,

(iii)   The time allocated to the executing process is over.

In this way, the CPU or the processor can be kept busy by the operating system, which switches from one process to a waiting process, whenever the first process either terminates or requests an I/O activity or its allocated time is over, while the I/O is outputting the data. All active processes that are not executing are kept on the secondary storage and when one of these is to be executed, it is loaded from there along with the intermediate results that it had computed when the CPU was allocated to it last time. Note that at any time one and only one process is executing.

17.3.2 Multi-Processing

Multiprocessing is a term used with the processing on a system which contains more than one CPUs. In a system with more than one CPU, more than one instruction can be executed by the system at the same time. Thus more than one process can be simultaneously executed in such systems.

A Multiprocessing operating system is an operating system that has been designed for a Multiprocessor system, that is, a system having more than one CPUs output from system. It is the job of the multiprocessing operating system to schedule and balance the input, output and the processing capabilities of a system to schedule processors. Since scheduling and coordinating the activities of multiple CPUs is a very complex task, a multiprocessing operating system is a very complex and sophisticated operating system.

17.3.3 Time Sharing Technique

A real–time operating system is one in which the input data is to be processed and the result produced within a stipulated time period. That is, the processing of data should take very small amount of time. Real time operating systems are generally used in industry as monitors. Such systems are very useful in places where a close watch is kept on the surroundings of the system and some corrective action is to be taken in case one particular thing happens. For examples consider a heat furnace whose temperature is to be kept constant for 30 hours at 300^0 Centigrade and that the maximum allowable temperature variation is $\pm 1^0$ centigrade. In such a situation, manual monitoring is virtually impossible. Here a real-time system can be used very conveniently. Such a system (that is the one that can be used in such a situation) will have heat sensors, which will provide the input, that is the temperature of the furnace, to the system. The system will process this input and accordingly try to adjust the temperature of the furnace.

17.3.4 Real Time

In the manner in which processors working with higher speed were developed, the technique of batch processing proved to be unproductive in view of the use of processing capacity. On the one hand, input and output applications work with a very slow speed and the time taken to read any information from the memory forces the processor to remain free. On the other hand, as all programmes are not of one size the main memory is not utilized and the capacity of the main memory also cannot be fully utilized. After doing other work and after sometime, it again starts doing the first job from where it had left earlier. In this way the time of the processor can be fully utilized. The activities are assessed by the operating system.

If 16 terminals are attached with one system and if work is going on all terminals, then for sometime the computer does the work of one user and then serial wise of other users. It works with such high speed that every one fee that the computer is working and in which you don't have to wait. It is called online processing technique. The method in which computer does work of many users together and distributes it in time slices is known as time–sharing technique.

17.4 Various Types of Operating System

Types of operating system :

On the basis of the number of users working on the system, O.S. can be classified into the following types.

17.4.1 Single-User O.S

The O.S. on which one user can work at a time is known as single operating system. DOS belongs to this category.

17.4.2 Multi-User O.S

When two or more users can work on the same O.S. simultaneously it is known as multi-user O.S. Unix is a multi-user O.S, as two or more persons can work at a time in this type of O.S.

On the basis of the mode of working the O.S. are again classified into following types.

17.4.3 Character User Interface (CUI)

When the user operates the system by means of characters it is known as CUI. Ex DOS. Here the USER gives command to the system by means of characters i.e. in order to copy a file we have to give exact syntax of copy command in DOS ex: Copy A: FILE 1 B: FILE1

17.4.4 Graphical User Interface (GUI)

When the user operates the system by means of pictorial or graphical representations it is known as GUI. Windows is an operating environment, which provides the feature of GUI. i.e. in order to copy a file in windows we have to select the option of copy and it will be copied.

17.5 (Disk Operating System) (DOS)

DOS can support a wide range of disk. At the lower end of the range are the disks with storage capacity of a few hundred bytes and at the higher end, are the disks having enormous storage capacity of the order of tens of mega bytes.

DOS organizes these disks depending on their storage capacities. Each disk surface is divided into tracks. The number of tracks on the disks surface depends upon the type of the disk. These circular tracks are further subdivided into sectors. A sector is the basic unit of storage for disks. Even the number of sectors contained in a track is dependent on the type of disks.

Most floppy disks have 40/80 tracks per surface. Floppy disks with 40 tracks are called the double disks and those with 80 tracks are known as the quad-density disks. On a double density disk, track is divided into 9 sectors. On a quad density disk too, a track contains 9 sectors. Each sector can store up to 512 bytes of information on any type of disk. Even in a hard disk the number of bytes a sector can have the same, that is, 512 bytes.

MS-DOS

MS-DOS stand for Microsoft Disk Operating System developed by the Microsoft Ltd.

Most of the DOS programs are stored in two files, namely IO.SYS and MSDOS.SYS. Another file, which contains DOS routines, is the COMMAND.COM. The IO.SYS and MSDOS.SYS are hidden files and are not visible to ordinary user. These are all present in the boot sector of the system.

The IO.SYS file contains the extensions to the ROM-BIOS. These may be additions to the exiting set of elementary routines stored in ROM and can be changed in already existing routines stored in ROM.

The MSDOS.SYS file contains the MS-DOS service routines. These routines provide better control over various peripheral devices. But these routines are not as flexible as the ROM-BIOS routines.

The COMMAND.COM files are the third part of the DOS. It contains the command interpreter of the DOS. This command interpreter first accepts any command that we give to the system. If what we have entered is correct and it exists as a command by the name then COMMAND.COM invokes the specified command. In case of an error, COMMAND.COM gives an appropriate error message. So any interaction that a user may have with the system or DOS can only be through COMMAND.COM.

17.6   Explanation of DOS Terminology

File

File is a collection of data, instruction or programs. Every set of program and data is given specific name to identify it. There are various types of files as;

Date file : Collection of Characters, letters etc.

Program file : Collection of Instructions.

File naming rules in DOS

In DOS, a file name consists of two parts :

(i) *First Name or Primary file Name :*

It can be 1 to 8 characters long. There should not be any space in between the characters of first name. The characters in primary file name can be A to Z, 0 to 9 and any special characters like &, # % etc.

(ii) *Second name or extension name :*

This is optional and can be 0 to 3 characters long. It can also include any alphabet, digit or special character. The primary and extension name of the file is always separated by a dot (.).

Ex.   PAYROLE.EXE

IES.COM

Ram.TXT

Directory : A directory is an index of the files stored on the disk. This includes a file name that primary name, extension name, memory occupied, date of creation and date of last updating. For ex: -2 directories are created in DOS for storing the 2 different types of files. USER directory stores all files of various users. Another directory is meant for storing system files.

(a)   Subdirectory

Subdirectory is a directory within a directory. It is just like a child directory of parent directory made for maximum use of disk and maintains the records & files properly. With the help of subdirectory we can recognize our files in such a way that the files related to one person are in one place and those related to second are at other place. Thus using subdirectories we can organize the disk in a better way. For ex. :- User1, User2 and User3. 3 subdirectories are created under the directory user, to organize the files for each user specifically in his own directory .

(b)   Default Directory

This directory in which working presently is the default directory. For example, after loading DOS the default directory is C:/ (In Hard Disk) or A:/ (In floppy disk).

(c)   Root Directory

The main directory or the topmost directory is called the root directory. All other directories are branches of the directory, like the roots of a tree. Root directory can include files, programs, other directories or subdirectories. It is designation by a backslash (\).

(d)   Parent Directory

The directory one level above the current working directory is known as parent directory. For ex: The user directory is parent directory for the 3 subdirectories user1, user2 and user3.

Wild card characters

When you want to work with a group of files, you can use wild cards. There are two types of wild cards: asterix (*) and a questions mark (?). That is abc. * means a file has any extension whose name is abc, ? Used only for one word while * used for many words.

(a)   FAT

FAT stands for File Allocation Table. It is a table, which contains mappings of physical locations of all the clusters or files on the disk storage.

(b)   Special files

There are certain files, which have special meaning for DOS.

When you first start DOS, it looks for a file called AUTOEXEC.BAT. This file is nothing but a series of DOS commands which you have to execute every time you start your computer. This file must be stored in the root directory. When DOS starts, it finds the file, and executes it. This file may include commands that control different settings. For example, you might include a command that controls different programs.

17.6.1   File Arrangement in DOS

In DOS files are arranged in hierarchical manner i.e. an inverted tree structure. For example It there are 4 users working on a system such as, USER1, USER2, USER3 and USER4 and they have 16 files as follows.

		ROOT	
USER1	**USER2**	**USER3**	**USER4**
FILES1	FILES2	FILES10	FILES3
FILES12	FILES5	FILES11	FILES4
FILES13	FILES6	FILES114	FILES8
FILES16			FILES15

17.7 Booting Process

The process of starting your computer is called booting. Typically, we will start your computer at the beginning of the day and leave it on until you're done at the end of the day. At that time, you'll exit any programs you're running, return to the DOS command prompt, and turn off the power.

17.7.1   Warm booting

If we reboot our system, we have two options: a warm boot or a cold boot. A warm boot is "gentler" and often quicker because the computer stays powered on during the procedure. To perform a warm boot, press the key combination CTRL+ALT+DEL. To use this key combination, hold down the Ctrl Key, then hold down the Alt key, then hold down the Del key. Release all three keys after the screen clears and the computer restarts.

17.7.2   Cold booting

If a warm boot doesn't seem to clear up the problem completely, you can perform a cold boot. To do so, turn off the power, preferably using the switch on your computer's surge protector. Wait until the computer's hard disk has stopped rotating (counting to 30 slowly should do it!), then turn the power on again.

17.8 DOS Commands

Types of Dos Commands

Dos commands are basically of two types.

17.8.1   Internal DOS Commands

Internal DOS commands are stored in the COMMAND.COM file, which is loaded into the memory, when you start your system. They include the simpler; you need on a regular basis. Because internal commands are part of COMMAND.COM, you never get to see their names in a directory listing. These commands remain resident in memory and are available to you at all times.

17.8.2   External DOS Commands

External Dos Commands exist as separate files on your disk. When you use the dir command to view the files on your MS-DOS system disk, you see the external command in the list of filenames and directory names. The filename of an external command is COM, EXE or BAT extension. External commands need special DOS files for execution.

17.8.3   Switches available in the commands

A switch is a forward slash (/) usually followed by a single letter or number you use Switches are used to modify the way a command performs a task. For example, suppose you want to use the dir command to view a listing or a directory. That contains a large number of files. When you type the dir command by itself, the /p switch, you can view the list of files on screen at a time.

MS-DOS commands do not have any switches, whereas others have several. If a command has more than one switch, you type them one after the other. You can separate switches with a space but the space is optional.

Internal Commands

To create a file

COPY CON

COPY CON < file name >. txt >

This command creates a file in the specified directory. Pressing ENTER would take the cursor to the next line. Now we can type the data we want to feed into the file. Once this is done. Press Ctrl+Z. The following message appears.

1. File (s) copied

Directory : There might be times when you want to keep some related files together and at the same time separate it from other files. To help this situation, directories can be made to hold these files.

A directory is a collection of files or in other words, it is a folder that contains related files.

To create a directory

Make Directory

MD < Name > Enter

Or

MKDIR <Name>

We can make another directory within this directory, but to do that we have to be in the directory we had just created.

C:\IES

To change a directory

CD <name>

The prompt would look like

C: \<IES>

Here we can create another directory using the MD MKDIR command. This directory is called as the sub directory within a directory. For e.g..-

C:\IES > MD ONE

C:\IES > CD ONE

C:\IES\ONE>

Here ONE is a sub directory of IES.

And IES itself is a sub directory of the root directory, denoted by backslash (\)

A subdirectory is also called as the child directory and the directory within which it is present is called as its parent directory.

To change from a subdirectory to its parent directory

CD...

To change from a directory to the root directory

CD\

Note : To change from one directory to another write the whole path name.

To remove a directory

RD < >

Note : To remove a directory, it is necessary that the directory to be removed must be empty i.e. there should be no files or sub directions in that directory. To remove sub directories we have to come to its parent directory and then do the following.

C: \IES\RD ONE

To Delete a File

DEL <filename>

Del [Drive] [path] [filename [\p]

\p – Prompts for confirmation before deleting each file.

ERASE (Drive;] [Path] Filename [\p]

VIEWING the contents of a file

TYPE <filename>

VIEWING the contents of a directory

Online Help With Commands

MS-DOS version 5.0 includes online help for MS-DOS commands. To get help with the syntax, parameters, and switches of any MS-DOS command, type the command name followed by / ? on the command line or type help followed by the command name, for example, for help information about the copy command.

Getting Help

Online help provides a quick way to get information about MS-DOS shell basics, and using menus, Commands dialog boxes, dialog box option., and procedures. You can get help in three ways: by pressing F1 by selecting the help button that appears in most dialog boxes or by using the help menu.

To request Help on a menu:

1. Press ALT.
2. Select the menu you want Help on by using the LEFT ARROW or RIGHT ARROW key.
3. Press F1

   Help window containing information about the selected menu appears.

   To request Help on a command:

Mouse

1. Click the menu that contains the command we want Help on.
2. Select the command we want Help on by using the UP ARROW or DOWN ARROW key.

   #. Press F1.

   A Help window containing information about the selected command appears.

Keyboard

1. Press ALT to select the menu bar.
2. Select the menu that contains the command you want help by using the LEFT ARROW and RIGTH ARROW keys.
3. Select the command you want help on by using the UP ARROW and DOWN ARROW keys.

To request Help on a dialog box option:

1. Open the dialog box you want Help on.
2. Select a command button or option by clicking it, or by using TAB or the arrow keys.
3. Press F1.

if you have selected the Search For box in the Search File dialog box. and you press F1. MS-DOS shell displays the following help window.

Getting Help on a Related Procedure

Often Help refers we to a related procedure. For example, the following Help on the Colour Scheme dialog box contains a reference to the procedure for changing colours.

In Help, related procedures are displayed in colour in reverse video, depending on the color scheme we have selected.

Mouse; Double-click the related procedure.

Help window containing information about the related procedure appears.

Keyboard

1. Press TAB until the related procedure is selected.

2. PRESSES ENTER.

Help window containing information about the related procedure appears.

Using the Help Menu

We can use the commands on the help menu to view an index of help topics ; information on the keys we can use with MS-DOS shell : basic skills for working with MS-DOS Shell commands and procedures' and information about using the help system.

To use the Help menu :

Mouse : From the help menu, choose the Help category you want.

Either information about the subject or a list of topics related to the subject appears.

Keyboard

1. Press ALT, H.

2. Press the highlighted letter for the help category we want.

Or press the UP ARROW or DOWN ARROW key to select the Help category you want, and then press ENTER.

Either information about the subject or a list of topics related to the subject appears.

The following items are on the Help menu

Index provides a list of all MS-DOS shell help topics.

Keyboard Lists and key combinations we can use with MS-Dos shell.

MS-DOS shell provides an introduction of using MS-DOS Basics shell.

Commands explains all MS-DOS shell commands. This information is organized according to the menu in which the command appears. (We can get the same information by selecting a command and then pressing F1.)

Procedures : Provides step-by-step instructions for performing tasks in MS-DOS shell.

Using Help : Provides an introduction to using MS-DOS shell help.

About Shell : Displays copyright and version information of MS-DOS shell.

17.9 Explanation of the DOS Commands

Attrib

Displays or charges file attributes. This command displays, sets or removes the read only, archive, system and hidden attribute assigned to files for an introduction to attrib command.

SYNTAX: ATTRIB [+R-R][+A-A][+S-S][+H-H]

[DRIVE:] [PATH] [FILENAME] [/S]

To display all attributes of all files in the current directory use the following syntax. attrib [drive:] [path] filename

Parameters

Specify the location and name of the file or set files we want to process.

SWITCHES   +R   SETS the read only files attributes.

-R   CLEARS the read only file attributes.

+A   SETS the archive file attributes.

-A   Clears the archive file attributes.

+S   Sets the files as a system file.

-S   Clears the system file attributes.

+H   Sets the files as hidden file.

-H   clears the hidden file attributes.

/S   Possess files in the current directory and all of subdirectories.

CHKDSK

Creates and displays a status report for a disk.

The status report shows logical errors found in the file allocation table (FAT) and file system. If errors exist on the disk, CHKDSK alerts us with a message. You should use CHKDSK occasionally on each disk to check for errors.

The CHKDSK command, available on all versions of DOS, checks the status of selected disk. It is an external DOS command, and displays several important items of information. These include resident program

The general form of the CHKDSK command is

CHKDSK [drive:]

Syntax

CHKDSK [drive:] [path] [filename [/f] [/v]

To display the status of the disk in the current drive, use the following syntax : chkdsk

Drive : Specifies the drive that contains the disk that we want chkdsk to check [path] filename : Specifies the location and name of the file or set of files that we want chkdsk to check for Fragmentation can use wild cards (*,?) to specify multiple files.

Switch

/f Fixes errors on the disk

/v Displays the name of each file in every directory as the disk is checked.

CLS

Starts a new instance of instance of the MS-DOS Command interpreter, COMMAND.COM.

DELTREE

Delete a directory and all of its files and subdirectories, including hidden files. Be careful with DELTREE, as it can be very destructive and we not be able to undo our deletions.

Syntax: -

DELTREE [/y] [drive:] path

/y deletes the directory and its files without prompting for confirmation.

Notes

For safety, do not use the Y option.

You can use wildcards in the path, but be extremely careful because wildcards can match filenames as well as multiple directory names.

DEVICE

DEVICE, used only in CONFIG.SYS, installs for optional devices, such as a mouse, RAM disk extended memory.

Loads into memory devices driver we specify.

Syntax : -device high [drive:][path]filename[parameters].

Option : -[drive:][path]filename, drive, directory location, and filename of device driver parameters.

Command line information required by the device driver.

DISKCOMP

The DISKCOMP command is an external command that compares the contents of two floppy disks to ensure they are identical. DISKCOMP is available on all versions of DOS.

The general form of the DISKCOMP Command is :

DISKCOMP A:B:

DISKCOPY

The DISKCOPY command is an external command that is available with all version of DOS. It makes a copy of one removable disk (the source disk) on another (the target disk). The involved diskettes must be of the same size and format for DISKCOPY to operate property. Never specify a fixed disk with the DISKCOPY command. If the target disk is unformatted, DISKCOPY formats it for you during the copy operation.

The form of the DISKCOPY command is

DISKCOPY A: B:

Where A: is the source disk source drive disk (the disk being copied) and B: is the target disk (the disk to which the copy is transferred).

With the introduction command makes as exact replica of the source disk. If it is single sided or contains data errors, then the resulting copy is also single sided or contains data errors, also. If we want to copy the first side of a disk, we can use the /1 parameter in the form:

DOSKEY

Start the Doskey program, which recalls MS-DOS commands. edits command lines and creates macros.

The Doskey program is a terminate-and-stay-resident program. We can use Doskey occupies about 3 kilobytes or resident memory.

Syntax

Doskey [/reinstall] [/bufsize=size] [/macros] [/history] [/insert/overstrike].

FDISK

The FDISK command is an external DOS command that prepares a fixed (or hard) disk to organize our disk into partitions, which allocates disk space to separate usable areas.

Each partition is assigned a logical drive letter, like C, D, and E when more than one partition is used on a single disk device. Because the maximum amount of disk space addressed by DOS versions released prior to 4.014 was 32 megabytes, it was necessary to be familiar with partitioning strategies offered by the FDISK command in order to organize disk drives having storage capacities in excess of the 32-megabyte barriers. Smaller disks are normally given a single DOS partition.

The FDISK command is used after our fixed disk has received a low-level format. The low-level format process is described briefly in Module 37. You may have to perform a low-level format yourself if you purchase a new fixed disk and controller card directly from the manufacturer or distributor. If you or purchase a new fixed disk and controller card directly from the manufacturer or distributor or if you purchase your computer from a reputable dealer, the fixed disk should be partitioned and formatted for you.

FIND

Beginning with DOS version 2.00, several external commands, called filters, were introduced. These filter commands are used to intercept rearrange, and output selected data. Three filter commands are : SORT, FIND, and MORE.

The find filter is used to search a file for one or more designated character depending upon the form of the FIND command. Each line having the text string is sent to an output device, such as display on the screen a file or the printer. The test string is always typed within quotes. There are three parameters available with the FIND command.

/V Display lines not having the designated text string.

/C Counts and displays the number of lines containing the text string.

/N Display the relative line number in front of each line containing the text string.

/i ignore uppercase or lowercase during the search. A few examples of how the FIND filter is used are shown below. Like SORT piping commands are also available for use with the FIND command.

ECHO

Turns the command-echoing feature on or off, or displays a message.

When we run a batch program, MS-DOS typically display (echoes) the batch program's commands on the screen. We can turn this feature on or off by using the echo command.

SYNTAX ECHO [ON/OFF]

To use the echo command to display a message, use the following syntax:

ECHO [MESSAGE]

Parameters on/off

Specifies whether to turn the command – echoing feature is on or off. To display the current echo setting, use it without parameter.

FORMAT

When you purchase new floppies, they have to be formatted before they can be used. The FORMAT command is executed by FORMAT followed by a space and then the drive you want to format. Don't forget to put: (colon) after the drive letter.

You can format your floppy with the following command:

FORMAT [drive:] format command creates tracks in the new floppy used.

PATH

The path command is an internal DOS command. The PATH command is used to tell DOS, which directories it should search. where it has to look for a program given in the PATH command.

c:\> path=c:\DBASE <-

MS-BACKUP

The MSBACKUP command available in DOS Ver.6 later replaces the backup command. The new command combines improved backup capability with easier of use. The first time you run the MSBACKUP it configures your system.

For performing proper backup, after the command work automatically through a menu driven interpreter.

To start backup type:

C:\MSBACKUP <-

Now follow the steps given below –

1. At the main screen press Alt-B to backup. The next screen is the backup configuration screen.

   (In DOS 6.2 we have the facility to save our setting in the MS backup program in a setup files. If you want to save your own custom setup files then before step 5, press Alt-F, A and then give our setup filename)

   Then the next time we are MSBACKUP press Alt F, o and select setup file from disk or you can start MSBACKUP with the name of a setup file.

   Ex=c:>MSBACKUP MSSETUR

   MSSETUP is the name of setup file.

TIME

This, command is used to set time in current system

Lets we view or charge the system time.

Syntax- Time (hh:mm:ss) (a/b)

hh-hour

mm-minutes

ss-seconds

a/b -A.M./P.M

TREE

Shows graphical display of the names of all directories on a disk. It is an external command.

Tree will also show the names of all files on each directory and subdirectory.

Syntax-TREE (drive:)(path)(/F)(/A)

?F = displays each dir files

/a = displays the dir with text character rather than GRAPHICS.

TYPE

Provides a quick and easy way to look at the contents of a file.

Syntax – Type (drive:)(path) filename

to interrupt the TYPE command press Ctrl + Break (or Ctrl+c)

UNDELETE

Allows you to restore files that were erased with the DEL or ERASE command UNDELETE provides their labels of protection against deletion.

UNFORMAT

You can recover files from an accidental disk format, with the help of this command. Syntax:

UNFORMAT drive: / switches

Switch

/L Lists all files and subdirectories found on the formatted drive

/P Echoes program messages to the standard printing device

/TEST Processes, but does not write any changes to the formatted disk.

VER

The VER command was introduced in DOS version 2.00. It is an internal DOS command that displays the version of DOS we are using. To run the VER program, type VER and press Return.

Because several different version of DOS are available, we may wish to determine which version we are using.

VOL

The volume command is internal DOS Command that display volume label (or name) of the specified disk. The VOL command is used to check the name of volume.

Syntax:

VOL [drive:] (press return)

XCOPY

The XCOPY command is an external command introduced with DOS version 3.20. It is used to selectively copy files from one disk to another, or those files that have been created or modified since the last backup. With the introduction of DSO 6.2, XCOPY prompt you before overwriting an existing file having the same name. The general form of the XCOPY command is

XCOPY A: C:\PATH\FILENAME

This form of the command operates like the copy command. There are a number of options that are added after the target filename to control file selection. The option letter, represented by/X in the following command line example, is quite useful.

XCOPY A: C: \PATH\FILENAME\X

The value of/X controls the way XCOPY operates. Each of the available value are describes in the following list.

/A   Copies files that the archive bit, which is set with the BACKUP and ATTRIB commands, set or a value of one. /D copies all files that are the same or later than a specified data. The data is added to the command as shown:

XCOPY A:C: /D:06-21-88

The data is entered in the format mm-dd-yy, or yy-mm-dd

/E   subdirectories are created on the target disk even if the new subdirectory empty. This happens when the command option used prevent the transfer of files within the directories because they do not meet selection criteria.

/M   Copies files having an archive bit value of one. When copied, the archive bit is reset to zero on the source file. This lets you use XCOPY IN BACKUP operations. An archive bit value of one indicate that the file was created or modified since the last BACKUP or XCOPY /M operation.

/P   Displays a (Y/N)? Prompt before copying a file to allow selection.

/S   files Copies from the source disk that are within and subdirectory to the active (or logged) directory path, as XCOPY searches through the directory tree. This option does not create new directory path on the target disk unless the /E option is also used. If/S is omitted, XCOPY works only within the named directory.

/V This options verify that data is written properly. As in the COPY command, the /V option slows the copy process.

/W Displays the prompt "press any key to being copying files(s)". This option is used to let you insert a diskette.

17.10 Special DOS File

17.10.1 The AUTOEXEC.BAT

The AUTOEXEC.BAT file is the most important batch file located in the root directory. This file is read automatically when you boot your PC. This file is useful because it executes a sequence of commands, like setting the path and prompt, etc as soon as the computer is switched on.

Creating AUTOEXEC.BAT is similar to the creation of any other batch file.

For example, if we want to include the commands for changing the prompt on our screen, setting the path and then clearing the screen, type the following commands:

C:\> COPY CON AUTOEXE.BAT

The cursor will appear on the next line.

TYPE

PROMPT PG

PATH = C:\DOS;C: \LOTUS;C: \DBASE;C: \WE

CLS

After you have finished entering the command, press

^Z

Now each time you switch on your computer, your prompt (C>) will be changed so that it displays the current directory. The PATH command tells DOS to look in the DOS, LOTUS Dbase & WS directories for program files. At the end, your screen will be cleared by the CLS command.

Note : The name of this file must be spelt correctly; otherwise this batch file will not be executed automatically. Also, this file must be present in the root directory.

17.10.2 The CONFIG.SYS

When we start our computer, DOS carries out certain commands. This batch file will not get your hardware and reserve space in memory for information processing. The file, which contains the command, is called CONFIG.SYS. This files helps enhancing your PC's performance. The commands in your CONFIG.SYS determine how your hardware should work.

Now create the CONFIG.SYS file, go to the root directory and type the following commands:

C:\COPY CON CONFIG.SYS ←⌐

FILES = 50

BUFFERS =30

^Z

First line is creates a file named CONFIG.SYS

In the second line, we specify the maximum number of files that can be opend at a time. Here, we specified 50. This number can be increased or decreased, but this is most option setting. The third line specifies how much memory DOS reserves for transferring information form and to the disks.

^Z is pressed to end the file creation.

To execute CONFIG.SYS, reboot the computer.

Various Important Commands Used in These Files

AUTOEXEC.BAT FILE

"A batch file executed automatically whenever the computer is booted up."

AUTOEXEC.BAT is a batch program that's executed automatically when you start your computer.

Simply type C:\autoexec at the command prompt.

A SIMPLE AUTOEXEC.BAT FILE

@ ECHO OFF

C:\DOS\SMARTDRV.EXE

SET DIRCMD=/ON/P

PROMPTpg

PATH C:\DOS;C: \WINDOWS,C: \C: \WP51

C: \DOS\CHKDSK C:

C: \DOS/CHKDSK D:

Set Temp=C: \WINDOWS\TEMP

Set Winpmt=Type 'exit'to return to windows pg

Mode con rate=32 delay=1

C:\DOS/DOSKEY

undelete/load

The command @ECHO OFF prevents DOS from displaying each command as it is executed in the batch program. Most people place an

@echo off – Command at the begning of every batch program.

The Command C:\DOS\MARTDRV.EXE executes the SMART Drive disk caching program.

The Set DIRCMD=/on/p sets the DIRCMD environment variable to specify two automatically switches for the DIR command.

The command PROMPT pg defines the message displayed by the command prompt. This example shows the most widely used prompt command, which displays the current drive and path name followed by the greater than symbol (>). Thus, when we are in the windows directory of drive, C the command prompt will display C:\WINDOW> as it awaits our next instruction. we can use any text (Hello.for example) as well as verity of special character combination in the message following the prompt command. The PATH command tells Dos which drives and directories to search and the order in which to search if a command or program can't be found in memory of in the current directory. To enter several paths on the same line separate them with semicolons (;). Do not include any spaces in the line.

The two CHKDSK command check drives C and D for logical errors.

The command SET TEMP = C:\WINDOWS/TEMP

Associates the directory named C:\WINDOWS/TEMP with the TEMP environment variable. DOS uses the TEMP variable.

TABLE : Character Combinations for the prompt command.

TO DISPLAY THIS.....	USE THIS CHARACTER.
$ (dOLLER SIGN)	$$
< (LESS THEN SIGN)	$L
= (EQUAL SIGN)	$Q
> (GRATER THEN SIGN)	$G
I (PIPE)	$B
ASCII ESCAPE (COAD 27)	$E
BVACKSPACE (for deleting a character written to the command file)	$H
CURRENT TIME	$T
CURRENT DATE	$D
CURRENT DRIVE AND PATH	$P
ENTER LINE FEED (for starting text on the next line)	$_
VERSION OF DOS	$V

CONFIG.SYS COMMAND

As you know the CONFIG.sys file is read whenever you start up your computer and contains special commands used to configure our computer's hardware components A CONFIG.SYS can include any of the commands listed in Table below.

Table 17.1 Config.sys file command.

FUNCTION	CON.SYS. COMMAND
To specify where DOS should look for keyboard interrupts.	BREAK
To specify the number of buffers and caches	BUFFERS
To designate the time, data decimal separators and other conventions used in a particular country	COUNTRY
To tell DOS which drives to load	DEVICE
To load drives into upper memory	DIVICEHCH
To specify were to load dos	DOS
To define block device parameters	DRIVPAKM
To specify how many file control blocks (FCBS) can be open at the same time.	FCBS
To include the contents of a configuration block for a specify menu block	INCLIDE
To load memory resident programs	INSTALL
To specify the number of drives	LAST DRIVE
To set the startup menu colours	MENUCOLOUR
To specify the default item in the startup menu	MENUDEFAULT
To set the number key	ON/FF NUMLOCK
To include comments or remarks	REM
To display set or remove environment variable	SET
To specify name and location.	SHELL
To use data stacks for hard ware interrupts	STACKS
To define a set of menu item under a Startup menu item.	SUBMEN
To provides special device options	SWITCHES
To verify accuracy of a file written to a disk	VERIFY

17.11   Unix Operating System

17.11.1   What is UNIX?

UNIX is an operating system which was first developed in the 1960s, and has been under constant development ever since. By operating system, we mean the suite of programs, which make the computer work. It is a stable multi-user, multi-tasking system for servers, desktops and laptops

UNIX systems also have a graphical user interface (GUI) similar to Microsoft Windows, which provides an easy to use environment. However, knowledge of UNIX is required for operations, which aren't covered by a graphical program, or for when there are no windows interface available, for example, in a telnet session.

They are many different versions of Unix, although they share common similarities. The most popular varieties of Unix are Sun Solaris, GNU/Linux and Marcos X.

The UNIX operating system

The UNIX operating system is made up of three parts; the kernel, the shell and the programs.

The Kernel

The kernel is the hub of the operating system: it allocates time and memory to programs and handles the file store and communication in response to system calls.

As an illustration of the way that the shell and the kernel work together, suppose a user types **rm m yfile** (which has the effect of removing the file **my file**). The shell searches the filestore for the file containing the program **rm**, and then requests the kernel, through system calls, to execute the program **rm** on **myfile**. When the process **rm myfile** has finished running, the shell then returns the UNIX prompt % to the user, indicating that it is waiting for further Commands.

The Shell

The shell acts as an interface between the user and kernel, when a user logs in, the login program checks the username and password, and then starts another program called the shell. The shell is a command line interpreter (CLI). It interprets the commands the user types in and arranges for them to be carried out. The commands are themselves programs: when they terminate, the shell gives the user another prompt.

The adept user can customize own shell, and users can use different shell on the same machine. Staff and students in the school have the trash shell by default. The trash shell has certain features to help the user inputting commands.

Filename Completion

By typing part of the name of a command, filename or directory and pressing the **[Tab]** key, the tics shell will complete the rest of the name automatically. If the shell finds more than one name beginning with those letters you have typed, it will Beep, prompting you to type a few more letters before pressing the tab key again.

History shell keeps a list of the commands you have typed in. If you need ton repeat a command, use the cursor keys to scroll up and down the list or type history for a list of previous commands.

Files and process

Everything in Unix is either a file or a process. A process is an execution program identified by a unique PID.

A file is a collection of data. Users using text editors, running compilers etc, create them.

Examples of files :

- A document (report, essay etc.) –
- The text of a program written in some high-level programming language.
- Instruction comprehensible directly to the machine and incomprehensible to a casual user, for example, a collection of binary digits (an executable or binary file).
- A directory, containing information about its contents, which may be a mixture of other directories and ordinary files.

The directory structure

All the files are grouped together in directory structure. The file system is arranged in a hierarchical structure, like an inverted tree. The top of the hierarchy is traditionally called **root.**

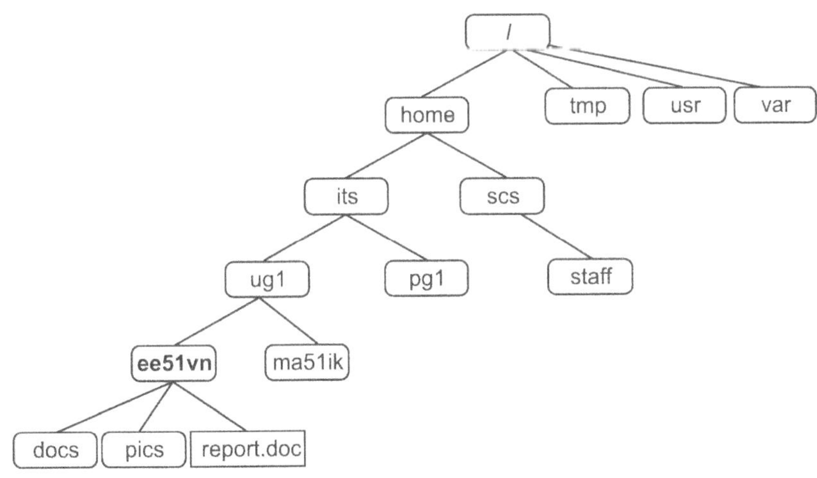

The Directory Structure

CHAPTER 18

Computer Languages

18.1   Introduction

A language is a system of communication. With a natural language such as Hindi, we can communicate with one another our ideas and emotions. Similarly, a computer language is a means of communication. With the help of a computer language, a programmer tells a computer what he wants it to do. A Computer Programming Languages is a set of rules that tells the computer what operations to perform. All Natural languages (Hindi, French, German etc.) use a standard set of symbols for the purpose of communication. Everyone using those languages understands these symbols. We normally call this set of symbols the vocabulary of that particular language. All computer languages have a vocabulary of their own. Each symbol of the vocabulary has a definite, unambiguous meaning, which can be looked up in the manual of that language. Hence, each symbol of a computer language is used to tell the computer to do a particular job. The main difference between a natural language and a computer language is that computer language uses a very limited or restricted vocabulary. This is mainly because a programming language by its very nature and purpose does not need to say too much. Each and every problem to be solved by a computer has to be broken down into discrete (simple and separate), logical steps which basically comprise four fundamental operations – input and output operations, arithmetic operations, movement of information within the CPU, and logical or comparison operations.

The symbols of a particular computer language must also be used as per prescribed rules, which are known as the syntax rules of the language. Computers, being machines, are receptive only to exact vocabulary used correctly as per syntax rules of the language. Thus, in case of a computer language, we must stick by the exact rules of the language if we want to be understood by the computer. As yet, no computer is capable of correcting and deducing meaning from incorrect instructions. Computer languages are smaller and simpler than natural languages but they have to be used with great precision. Unless a programmer adheres exactly to the syntax rules of a programming language, even down to the correct punctuation marks, the computer will not understand his commands.

18.2 Characteristics of Programming Language

A programming language should possess the following characteristics to be considered as a good high-level language:

(a) The language should be relatively independent of a given computer system. That is, instead of being machine based, it should be oriented more towards the problem to be solved.

(b) Each statement of the language should be a macroinstruction that gets translated into many machine language instructions.

(c) The language should enable the programmers to write instructions using familiar words and mathematical symbols. It should be natural and should use abbreviations and words used in everyday communication.

(d) The language should be independent of machine language instructions and other pieces of system software except for the compiler or the interpreter.

(e) The language should not be experimental in nature and should exist on more than one computer system.

18.3 Types of Programming Languages

Programming languages have improved just as computer hardware improved. They have progressed from machine-oriented languages that use strings of binary 1's and 0's to problem-oriented languages that use common mathematical and/or English terms. However, all computer languages can be classified into the following five broad categories:

Machine languages (First Generation Languages – 1945)

Assembly languages (Second Generation Languages – mid 1950s)

High-level languages (Third Generation Languages – early 1960s)

Fourth Generation languages (Very High Level Languages or SQL – early 1970s)

Fifth Generation languages (Natural Languages – early 1980s).

18.3.1   Machine Languages

The set of instruction codes, whether in binary or decimal, which can be directly understood by the CPU of a computer without the help of a translating program, is called a machine code or machine language. This is the basic language of the computer, representing data as 1s and 0s. Machine language programs vary from computer to computer. i.e. they are Machine Dependent.

Advantages and Limitations of Machine Languages

Machine Language is the fundamental language of a computer and is normally written as strings of binary 1s and 0s. The circuitry of a computer is wired in such a way that it immediately recognizes the machine language and converts it into electrical signals needed to run the computer. An instruction prepared in any machine language has two parts. The first part is the command or operation, and it tells the computer what function to perform. The second part of the instruction is the operand, and it tells the computer where to find or store that data or other instructions that are to be manipulated. Thus, the data field is involved in the operation. Typical operations involve reading, adding, subtracting, writing, and so on.

As all computers use binary digit (0s and 1s) for performing Internal operations, most computers' machine language consists of strings of binary numbers and this is the only number system the CPU directly understands. When stored inside the computer, the symbols, which comprise the machine language program, are made up of 1s and 0s. For example, a typical program instruction to print out a number on the printer might be look like.

     101100111111010001100011000

The program to add two numbers in memory and print the result might look something like the following

     001100111110001110001001

     1100010000111100001100011

     00011000010000000100001000

     1000010000010000010000100

This is obviously not a very easy language to learn, because it is difficult to read and understand and it is written in a number system with which we are not familiar.

Programs written in machine language can be executed very fast by the computer. This is mainly because machine instructions are directly understood by the CPU and no translation of the program is required. However, writing a program in machine language has several disadvantages, which are discussed below.

Machine Dependent : The internal design of every type of computer is different from every other type of computer and needs different electrical signals to operate; the machine language differs from computer to computer.

Difficult to Program : Although easily used by the computer, machine language is difficult to program. It is necessary for the programmer either to memorize the dozens of code numbers for the commands in the machine's instruction set or to constantly refer to a reference card.

Error Prone : For writing program in machine language, since a programmer has to remember the opcodes and he must also keep track of the storage location of data and instructions, it becomes very difficult for him to concentrate fully on the logic of the problem. This frequently results in program errors. Hence, there is a large likelihood to make errors while using machine code.

Difficult to Modify : It is difficult to correct or modify machine language programs. Checking machine instructions to locate errors is as tedious as writing them initially. Similarly, modifying a machine language program at a later data is so difficult that many programmers would prefer to code the new logic afresh instead of incorporating the necessary modifications in the old program.

18.3.2 Assembly Languages

Assembly languages are one step ahead of machine languages. Assembly language (also called Low Level Language) is a language that allows a programmer to use abbreviations or easily remembered words instead of binary numbers. Each assembly language statement is translated into one-machine instructions by the assembler program. To program in an assembly language, we have to be well versed in the computer's architecture. Unless well-documented, assembly language programs can be extremely difficult to maintain.

Assembly languages are hardware dependent; there is a different assembly language for each CPU series, and their language statements are quite different. In the past, systems software (operating systems, database managers, etc.) was written in assembly language to maximize the machine's performance.

Advantages of Assembly Languages over Machine Languages

Assembly languages have the following advantages over machine languages:

Easier to Understand and Use : Assembly languages are easier to understand and use because mnemonics are used instead of numeric op-codes and suitable names are used for data. The use of mnemonics means that comments are usually not needed; the program itself is understandable. Symbolic programming also saves a lot of time and effort of the programmer because it is easier to write as compared to machine language programs.

Easy to Locate and Correct Errors : While writing programs in an assembly language, fewer errors are made, and those that are made are easier to find and correct because of the use of mnemonics and symbolic field names. Furthermore, assemblers are so designed that they automatically catch errors. If we use an invalid mnemonic or a name that has never been defined, the assembler will print out an error indication. For example, suppose one instruction in the symbolic program reads ADD SUM, and we forget to define what SUM is, the assembler will look through its table to find whether SUM is earlier defined or not. If not, it will indicate the error.

Easier to Modify : Assembly language programs are easier for people to modify than machine-language programs. This is mainly because they are easier to understand and hence it is easier to locate, correct, and modify instructions as and when desired. Moreover, insertion or removal of certain instructions from the program does not require change in the address part of the instructions following that part of the program. This is required in case of machine languages.

No Need to Track Addressee : One of the greatest advantages of assembly language is that it relieves us of worrying about addresses for instructions and data. This is more important than it seems at first glance. Suppose we have written a long machine language program involving many steps and many reference to itself within the program, such as looping, and address modifications, and so on. At the very end we may suddenly discover that we have left out an instruction in the middle. If we insert that entire program to check any reference to other steps. This is a tedious job. But if we write the same program in symbolic language, we merely add the extra instruction at their right place, and the assembler will take care of step numbering automatically.

Easily Relocatable : Suppose that an assembly language program starts at address 2000 and we suddenly find that we have another program to be used with this program and this program also starts at location 2000. Obviously, one of the two programs will have to be rewritten to be moved somewhere else. In machine language, this can be a complicated job. But in case of assembly language, we merely have to change the first statements: for example instead of:

    START PROGRAM AT 2000 AND START DATA AT 3000

We merely change this first statement to :

    START PROGRAM AT 3000 AND START DATA AT 4000

and run the symbolic program once more through the assembler.

Efficiency : In addition to the above-mentioned advantages, an assembly language program also enjoys the efficiency of its corresponding machine code because there is one-to-one correspondence between the instructions of an assembly language program and its corresponding machine language program. There is one-to-one relationship between symbolic and machine codes.

Limitations of Assembly Languages

Machine Dependent : Because each instruction in the symbolic language is translated into exactly one machine language instruction, assembly languages of the processor being used.

Knowledge of Hardware required : Since assembly languages are machine dependent, so the programmer has to be aware of particular machines' characteristics and requirements as the program is written. An assembly language programmer must known how his machine works and should have a good knowledge of the logical structure of his computer in order to write a good assembly language program.

Machine Level Coding : In case of an assembly language, instructions are still written at the machine-code level i.e. one assembler instruction is substituted for one machine-code instruction.

Machine and assembly languages being machine dependent, are referred to as low-level language. In general, assembly languages are termed one-for-one in nature, i.e. each assembly language instruction will result in one machine language instruction.

A language in which each statement is directly translated into a single machine code is known as a low-level language. Examples of low-level languages are assembly languages of various processors.

18.3.3 High–Level Languages

To overcome the difficulties associated with assembly languages, high-level or procedure-oriented languages have been developed. High–level languages permit programmers to describe tasks in a form, which is problem oriented rather than computer oriented. One can formulate problems more efficiently in a high-level language. The programmer does not need to have a precise knowledge of the architecture of the computer he is using.

The instructions written in high-level languages are called statements. The statements more clearly resemble English and mathematics as compared to mnemonics in assembly languages. Examples of high-level languages are BASIC, PASCAL, FORTRAN, COBOL, ALGOL, PL-II, PROLOG, LISP, ADA, SNOBOL, etc.

Advantages of High–Level Languages

High-level languages enjoy the following advantages over assembly and machine languages:

Machine Independence : High-Level languages are machine independent. This is a very valuable advantage. Thus a program written in a high-level language can be run on many different types of computers with very little or practically no modification.

Easy to Learn and Use : These languages are very similar to the languages normally used by us in our day-to-day life. Hence they are easy to learn and use. The programmer need not learn much about the computer he is using. The programmer does not have to necessarily know the machine instructions, the data format, and so on.

Few Errors : In case of high-level languages, since the programmer need not write the entire small steps carried out by the computer, he is much less likely to make errors. The computer takes care of all the little details, and will not introduce any error of its own unless something breaks down. Furthermore, compilers are so designed that they automatically catch and point out the errors made by the programmer. Hence, diagnostic errors, if any, can be easily located and corrected by the programmer.

Lower Preparation Cost : Writing programs in high-level language requires less time and effort, which ultimately leads to lower program preparation cost. Generally, the cost of all phases of program preparation (coding, debugging, testing, etc.) is lower with a high-level language than with an assembly language or with a machine language.

Better Documentation : A high-level language is designed in such a way that its instructions may be written more like the language of the problem. Thus a person familiar with the problem can easily understand the statements of a program written in a high-level language. For the documentation of such programs, very few or practically no separate comment statements are required.

Easier to Maintain : Programs written in high-level languages are easier to maintain than those in assembly languages or machine languages. This is mainly because high-level language programmes are easier to understand and hence it is easier to locate, correct, and modify instructions as and when desired. Insertion or removal of certain instructions from a program is also possible without any complication. Thus, major changes can be incorporated with very little effort.

Limitations of High-Level Languages

Two disadvantages of high-level languages are:

Lower Efficiency : Generally, a program written in an assembly language of machine language is more efficient than the one written in a high-level language. That is, the programs written in high-level languages take more time to run and require more main memory.

Lack of Flexibility : Because the automatic features of high-level languages always occur and are not under the control of the programmer, they are less flexible than assembly languages. An assembly language provides programmers access to all the special features of the machine they are using. This lack of flexibility means that some tasks cannot be done in a high-level language, or can be done only with great difficulty.

In most cases, the advantages of high-level languages far outweigh the disadvantages. Most computer installations use a high-level language for most programs and use an assembly language for doing special tasks that cannot be easily done otherwise.

Difference between Assembly Languages and High-Level Language

One statement of a high-level language corresponds to many instructions of the assembly language program. Hence, a high-level program is much shorter compared to an assembly language program.

Many high-level languages have been developed; some are for general purpose and some for special purposes. For example, PASCAL, PL-II and ADA are general-purpose languages. FORTRAN and APL are for scientists and engineers. They are designed to solve mathematical problems. COBOL is for business applications. BASIC is for newcomers to programming. PROLOG is based on logical reasoning and used for artificial intelligence (i.e. expert system). SNOBOL is suitable for text processing. APT is used in manufacturing applications to control machine tools.

Brief Description of some popular High-Level Languages

BASIC : It is an abbreviation for Beginners All-purpose symbolic Instruction Code. It is a very simple and easy language. It is suitable for scientific computations. But it is not as powerful as FORTRAN. It was introduced in 1965 by Dartmouth College, UK. It is a widely - used language for simple computations and analysis. It is the most popular high-level language used in personal computers. To translate BASIC instructions into machine language codes interpreters are frequently used in PC systems. But BASIC language compliers are also available for these systems.

FORTRAN : It is an abbreviation for Formula Translation. IBM introduced it in 1957. It is a very useful language for scientific and engineering computations as it contains many functions for complex mathematical operations. It is a compact programming language. Huge libraries of engineering and scientific programs written in FORTAN are available to users. It is not suitable for processing large business files are COBOL is. It has a number of versions. Earlier, FORTRAN IV was very popular. In 1977 the American National Standard Institute (ANSI) published a standard for FORTRAN called FORTRAN 77 so that all manufacturers could use the same form of the language. The latest version is in known as FORTRAN 90.

C Language : A high-level programming developed by Dennis Ritchie and Brian Kernighan at Bell Labs in the mid - 1970s. Although originally designed as a systems programming language, C has proved to be a powerful and flexible language that can be used for a variety of applications, from business programs to engineering. It is a popular language for personal computer programmers because it is relatively small – it requires less memory than other languages.

The first major program written in C was the UNIX operating system, and for many years C was considered to be interlinked with UNIX. However, C is important independent language of UNIX.

Although it is a high-level language, C is much closer to assembly languages than other high-level languages. This closeness to the underlying machine language allows C programmers to write very efficient code. The low-level nature of C, however, can make the language difficult to use for some types of applications.

C++ : A high-level programming language developed by Bjarne Stroustrup at Bell Labs. C++ adds object-oriented features to its predecessor; C. C++ is one of the most popular programming languages for graphical applications, such as those that run in Windows and Macintosh environments.

JAVA : A high-level programming language developed by Sun Microsystems. Java was originally called OAK, and was designed for handheld devices and set-top boxes. OAK was unsuccessful. So in 1995 Sun changed the name to Java and modified the language to take advantage of the World Wide Web.

Java is an object-oriented language similar to C++, but simplified to eliminate language features that cause common programming errors. Java source code files (files with a java extension) are compiled into a format called byte code (files with a class extension), which can then be executed by a Java interpreter. Compiled Java code can run on most computers because Java interpreters and runtime environments, known as Java Virtual Machines (VMs), exist for most operating systems, including UNIX, the Macintosh OS, and Windows. Byte code can also be converted directly into machine language instructions by a just in time compiler (JIT). Java is a general purpose programming languages with a number of features that make the language well suited for use on the World Wide Web. Small Java applications are called Java applets and can be downloaded from a Web server and run on your computer by a Java-compatible Web browser, such as Netscape Navigator or Microsoft Internet Explorer.

18.3.4   Fourth Generation Languages (4GLS)

A very high-level language is often a 4GL (4th generation language). 4GLs are much more user-oriented and allow programmers to develop programs with fewer commands compared with third-generation languages. 4GLs are called nonprocedural because programmers cannot write the programs that need only tell the computer what they want, not all the procedures for doing it. That is, they do not have to specify all the programming logic or otherwise tell the computer how the task should be carried out. This saves programmers a lot of time because they do not need to write as many lines of code as they do with procedural languages.

Fourth generation languages consist of report generations, query languages, application generators, and interactive database management system (DBMS) programs. Some 4GLs tools are applicable for end-users and some for programmers.

Difference between 4GLs and High-Level languages

1. The 4GLs are often easier to use than high-level languages.
2. The 4GLs are not supported by the industry standards. They offer less control over output results than do high-level languages.
3. 4GLs do not use hardware resources as efficiently as do the high-level languages. Therefore, most application programs are written in high level languages only.

4GLs will probably not replace third-generation language because they are usually focused on specific tasks, hence offer options, Still, they improve productivity because programs are easy to write.

18.3.5   Fifth Generation: Natural Languages

Natural languages of two types: The first are ordinary human languages : Hindi, English, German, French, Spanish, and so on. The second are programming languages that use human language to give people a more natural connection with computers. Some of the query languages mentioned above under 4GLs might seem pretty close to human communication, but natural languages-which are still in their infancy-try to be even closer.

With 4GLs, you can type in some rather reutilized inquires. An example of a request in FOCUS, for example, might be:

SUM SALES BY STATE BY DATE:

Natural languages allow questions or commands to be framed in a more conversational way or in alternative forms. For example, with a natural language, you might be able to state:

"I want the sales of personal computers for Madhya Pradesh and Chhatisgarh broken down by city for January and February. Also, I need January and February sales list by cities for laser printers sales in Keral and Madhya Pradesh".

Natural languages are part of the field of study known as artificial intelligence. Artificial intelligence (AI) is a group of related technologies that attempt to develop machines to emulate human like qualities, such a learning, reasoning, communicating, seeing and hearing.

CHAPTER 19

Concept of Programming

19.1 Flowcharts

From writing algorithm to solving problems, we take the help of flow charts. A flow-chart is a diagrammatic representation of the various steps involved in the solution of a problem. Flow-chart is a diagrammatic representation of the logic paths contained within a solution to the given problem. Flow-charts are drawn up as a pictorial guide for assisting in writing of an algorithm.

The flow-chart indicates the direction of flow of a process, relevant operations and computations, points of decisions and other information which are a part of the solution. Once developed and properly checked, flow-chart provides an excellent guide for writing the program.

Flowcharts are of two types :

- System flowcharts.
- Program flowcharts.

A system flowchart describes the data flow and operations for a data processing system. The flowchart shows how the data processing is to be accomplished. A program flowchart describes the sequence of operations and decisions for a particular program. Program flowcharts are sometimes referred to as block or logic diagrams.

After the program has been defined and the processing system designed, the first step in the programming for the application is the preparation of a description of the computer procedures required performing the required processing. Program flow-chart are usually the most convenient methods of preparing this description. Program flowcharts are prepared in the same way as for lower-level language programs, except that less detail is required for describing higher-program steps.

19.1.1   Flowchart Symbols

A flowchart is a drawing giving a suitable step-by-step solution of a problem, using suitable annotated geometric figures (having predefined meanings) connected by flow lines. The flowcharts are used for designing and documenting a process of a program. They represent the program logic and the sequence of steps to be performed for writing the program.

Each symbol in the flowchart has a well-defined shape, meaning and expresses operation or flow of data. Sufficient annotation is incorporated within the symbols to make a flowchart self-explanatory. Templates are available for drawing the flowchart symbols. Flowcharts are helpful in devising algorithms for solving problems.

There is sufficient creativity and flexibility in the design of flowcharts, so much, so that no two people will draw them exactly alike.

Flowcharts go by many other names like the diagram, system chart, run diagram, process chart, procedure chart, and logic chart. As a programming aid, flowcharts are often prepared by systems analysts and designers to describe systems and to specify the work to be accomplished by programs. Programmers use flowcharts as a basis for writing programs and as a means of communication among each other, particularly when the programming is done as a team effort. Programmers as well as systems analysts also use flowchart as a source of information for maintenance work on program and systems.

Flow chart is more widely used than decision tables, publication languages, or abstract notations. This popularity is due to their advantages.

The flowchart provides an excellent means for depicting the flow of program logic. In this diagram different types of boxes represent the different steps. These boxes and other symbols used in flowchart are shown in Table along with there use/ meaning.

In flow-charting, it is customary to label each box to show the action performed by it. For example, the followinh symbols indicate the start of a process or procedure and its end.

Symbol	Name	Meaning / Use
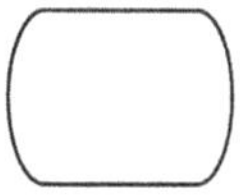	Terminal Box	A flattened oval box. It denotes 'start' and 'stop' of a program. A flowchart starts from it and ends into it.
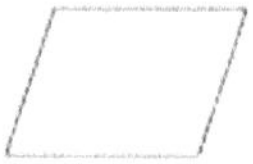	Input / Output Box	A parallelogram shaped box, showing the location where data is required to be input into the program and the point where the results are output by the program.
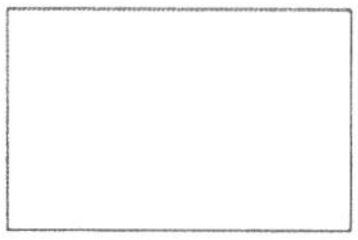	Processing Symbol	A rectangular box, used for indicating the types of process or action which result in singular outcome. They indicate arithmetic processes, assignment statements, macro instructions. It can also be a command for moving data from one place of storage to another.
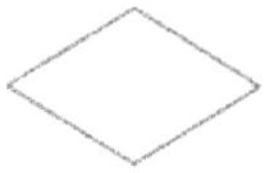	Decision Box	It is a diamond (rhombus) shaped box. It contains a logical question with a Yes or No (True of False). The branch followed by the program depends on the outcome of the questions.
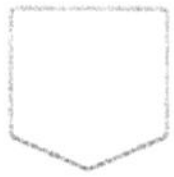	Connector	Long flow charts spanning more than a sheet of paper can be terminated at the bottom of the sheet and labeled with a number. The activity can begin at another connector with the same number on the next sheet. Exit connectors and entry connectors are depicted as shown.
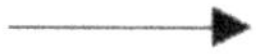	Flow lines and	Flow lines connect symbols to show the sequence of logical steps. An arrowhead indicates the direction of flow. Usually the direction of flow is indicated but in the absence of an arrow head flow is assumed from top to bottom and from left to right.
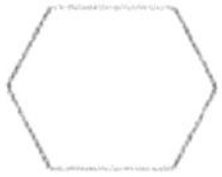	Preparation Symbols	The symbol indicates the preparation for some procedure like initializing certain variables. Some programmers indicate a preparation by the process symbol (3) – a rectangular box.

In flowchart where the program branches into more than one direction – one along the "yes" path and the other along the "no" path. Decision is possible as the computer is able to tell whether the values stored in two fields of its main memory are equal or not. In case they are not equal it can also tell which one contains the higher value.

19.1.2 Rules for making a Flowchart

1. Only those symbols should be used which are discussed above. Using conventional symbol the flowcharts are easy to understand.

2. The arrows in flow-chart represent the direction of flow or data in the problem.

3. The logic of a program flowchart should flow from top to bottom and from left to right. This follows Standard English convention and imposes consistency upon the drawing.

4. Normally flow lines should not cross each other.

5. Horizontal arrow inside the box indicates that the terms on both sides of the arrow are synonyms. It can be taken as symbol for the words "Let the term on left hand side represent the expression on right hand side" or let the number be incremented by one".

6. Each symbol (except decision box) used in program flowchart should have one entry point and one exit point. A computer thinks linearly- i.e., one step at a time in a sequential fashion. This rule forbids multiple exits form processing symbols or input / output symbols. The one exception to this rule is the decision symbol, which, by definition, is a branching symbol with more than one exit.

7. As far as possible, the instructions within the symbols of a program should be independent of any particular programming languages. Sometimes , it is not known what computer language will be used to write a particular program. At other times, a program will be written in one language and then, rewritten in another language. This rule keeps the flowchart at the logic level rather at the language-coding level that follows.

8. All decision branches should be labeled. Decisions usually ask questions that require labels like "Yes" and "No" or "True" or "False". Without labels, the different logic paths that data processing can take remain undefined.

19.1.3   Examples of Flowcharts

***Example* 1**

Flowchart for finding the sum S, the average A, and the product P of three numbers X, Y, and Z.

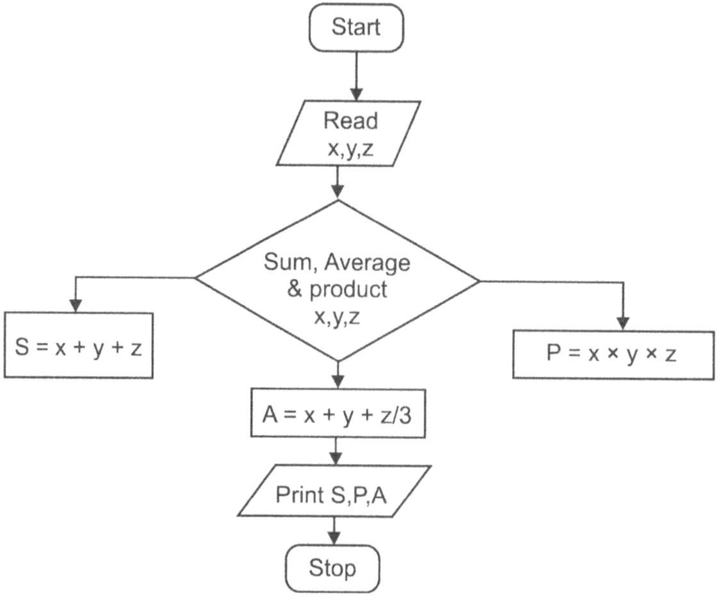

Fig. 19.1 Flowchart for sum, average & product.

Example 2

Fig 19.2 shows a flowchart which reads two numbers, A and B and prints them in decreasing order, after assigning the larger number to BIG and the smaller number to SMALL. Observe the two arrows leaving the decision "Is A > B ?" One labeled "No" and the other labeled "YES".

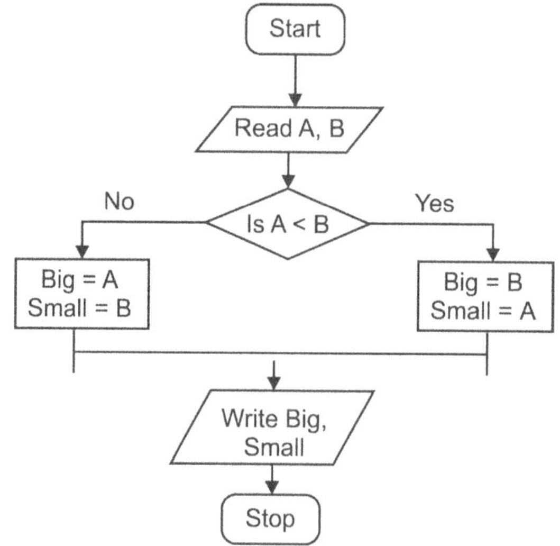

Fig. 19.2 Flowchart for finding BIG and SMALL.

Example 3

(Solution of Quadratic Equation) : Recall that the solution of the quadratic equation

$$ax^2 + bx + c = 0$$

Where a # 0, are given by the formula $X = \left(-b \pm b^2 - 4ac / 2a\right)$

The quantity $D = D = \sqrt{\left(b^2 - 4ac\right)}$ is called the discriminate of the equation. If D is negative, then there are no real solutions. If D = 0, then there is only one (double) real solution, x = b/2a. If D is positive, than we gate two distinct real solutions, Fig. 19.3, is a flowchart. Which inputs the coefficients a,b,c of a quadratic equation, and outputs the real solutions, if any. Observe how the three alternate routes have been implemented with two decision symbols. It is not possible to do so in single decisions as three outputs cannot be taken form a single decision diamond.

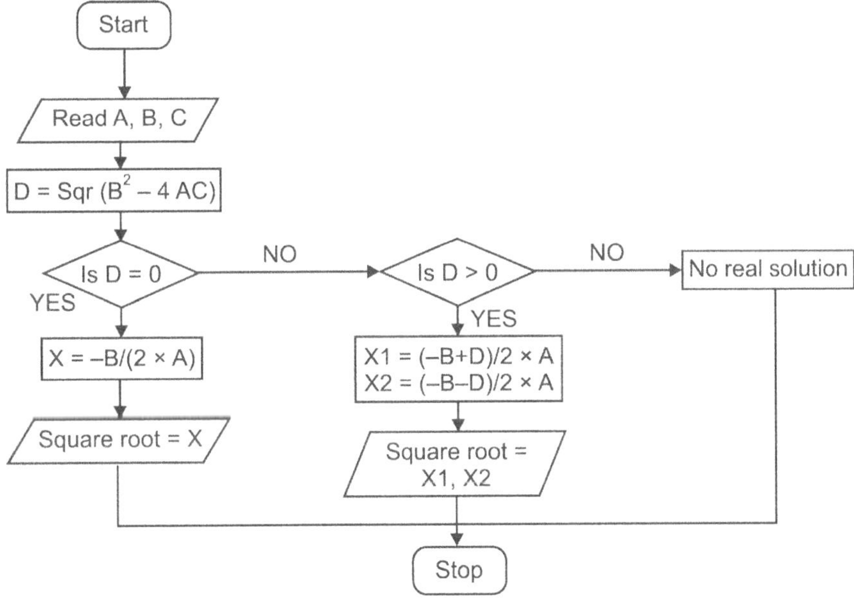

Fig. 19.3 Flowchart for Mathematical functions.

19.1.4   Advantages of using Flowcharts

Flowcharts are used for a broad variety of applications in different types of work. For example, they are as convenient to use in administrative file handing as in scientific or engineering computation. This popularity, born out of wide applicability, generates further so much so that flow-charting is a lingua among persons of various disciplines working with computers.

- Flowcharts give a clear graphical/ pictorial representation of the various paths that must be followed to perform the acts to accomplish the goals of the program.

- Flowcharts are invaluable at the time when modifications must be made to the original program to perform additional services not planned originally. It help to locate the exact sports in the program where the changes should be made. A good flow chart enables the programmer to visualize whether or not such changes might upset program features.

- Flowcharts are languages independent. Knowledge of a programming language is not normally necessary to be able to use them or to create them. This is always true for the pictorial part of flowcharts, and ideally should be true for the wording inside the symbols in a flowchart.

- Flowcharts are constraining and precise in ways that the useful to programmers and analysts. These are a limited means of description that force the user to give attention to many significant matters while suppressing attention to a host to less important details.

- Flowcharts are a visual representation, and hence provide a convenient alternative to the usual narration description for a program or system. This enables a more rapid scan or search of a flowchart than is possible with a description when particular items of information are sought. The graphic format enables a user to comprehend a lot in a single glance.

- Flowcharts offer a controllable level of details. They are usable from the most summary systems level to the most detailed programming level. The wide range of detail options greatly enhances the communication value of the flowchart. It is generally concluded that the flowchart is more valuable to the summary than what is provided by the programming language (for flow diagrams) or in the English language narrative (for system charts). For this reason, arranged from very summary to quite detailed, so that the user may choose the level for detail most convenient for his particular purposes. In this regard it should be noted that the system chart variety of flowchart inherently provides a more summary view than does the flow diagram variety of flowchart.

19.1.5   Disadvantages of Flowcharts

- On the disadvantages side, some programmers and analysts complain that flowcharts are a waste of time, since people do not think in graphic terms. In their view, a flowchart an unnatural means of communication.

- Flow charts are something new and strange to work with for beginners. They are reluctant to accept term.

- When modifications are made in the original program corresponding changes must be made in the flow charts of the program in the documentation. If the programmer is too busy, or other wise, forgets to up-data the flow harts each time.

- It is often difficult to draw the line as to the extent of details of the program to be incorporated in the flowchart. When too many details are included in the flowchart it may become obscure to other programmer.

- Flow charts may not reveal significant steps to be followed in actual coding. Also, they do not guide the programmer, how to code a step as given by the flow chart.

- Flowcharts are often cumbersome to use and costly to produce. Because of their graphic format, flowcharts may devote more than a page of space to present what may requires form a few lines to less than a half-page of equally detailed description in some other format. Manual preparation of flowcharts is slow, although detailed flow diagrams can be preparation by computer if the program to be flow-charted exists in source form.

- Flowcharts do not constitute programming languages. They are person-to-person means of communication, not person-to-computer. No translators exist for accepting program systems described in flowchart form.

- The flow diagram variety of flowchart does not fit well with all programming languages. Although flow diagrams go well with Cobol, Algol, PL/1, and Basic. They seem less compatible with Snobol, Comit, Lisp, and IPL-V.

- Flowcharts may not highlight what is important. Each operation commonly receives as much attention in a flowchart as any other, given the level of detail at which the flowchart is prepared. Yet, intuitively, people feel that some operations are more significant than others. The flowchart does not possess any convenient, automatic way to highlight these.

- Flowcharts are difficult to Produce at a summary level. No consistent logical rules have yet been developed to aid the process of producing meaningful summary flowcharts.

19.1.6 Types of Flowcharts

Presently two major varieties of flowcharts are used in practice :

- System chart
- Program flow diagram.

The flow diagram in figure connects rates on part of what a system chart shows. The unit of data transformation for the two is thus very different. For a flow diagram, the unit of data translation is usually an operation or short sequence of operations that a computer can perform (such as an instruction or a series of instructions that comprise a subroutine). An example is testing for the presence of leading zeros in a number.

By contrast, in a system chart the unit of data transformation is usually the work done by an entire computer program. Example are : sorting a file of data, inverting a matrix, or producing a report. Flow diagrams commonly have an algorithmic orientation, stressing how data is transformed, whereas systems charts primarily identify inputs and outputs to algorithms, stressing what data is used or produced at various point in a sequence of operations.

19.1.7   Uses of Flowcharts

Flowcharts are the most widely used graphic method for describing computer operations. They are adaptable to wide from the early days of the computer programming.

The major use of flowcharts is in documentation and programming. As a documentation device, the flowchart is a way of communicating, from one person to another, the nature of the operation to be performed and of the data upon which it is to be performed, regardless of the programming language or computer used. Since a flowchart is a graphic means of communication, this feature makes it a good choice for use the usual programming languages and English language.

All the flow charts we have drawn, which give details of each step of a process or procedure. But these are more common in the flowcharts of large engineering project Micro-level flowcharting is seldom used in computer programming.

19.2 Algorithm

In our daily life we encounter with a number of problems, which can be solved by two methods.

- Algorithms

- Heuristic

In algorithm, there is set procedure to solve the problem in such a manner that solution is definitely obtained. Heuristic is the method of obtaining optimum solution of the problem intuitively by experienced guess.

For solving a problem by computer, we have to be very clear in writing the instructions for the computer. The set of instructions is known as program. The solution is obtained by breaking the contents of the problem and given data in such a manner, that all instructions are given in sequence. This procedure is known as algorithm and has to be devised prior to the actual coding of the computer program. Actual computer program is written in coded languages, known as programming language. Algorithm is thus a design or plan of obtaining a solution to the problem. It is logical process of analyzing a mathematical problem and data step by step so as to make it easier to understand and implement solution to the problem. Certain operations must be performed on data for producing the required results. In order that a computer can perform an operation, it must be converted into a form that the computer is able to execute. Moreover the operations must be carried out in a specific sequence. In our day-to-day work, the brain automatically performs the algorithms by experience but not in a systematic and error-free way. But for processing on computer, one has to be systematic and to the point, as computer does not know alternatives. For example we must read a record before using its content in calculations. Sometimes it is necessary to perform an operation only if the data satisfies a particular condition. For example, income tax must be deducted from the salary of an employee only if income exceeds a certain limit.

Writing algorithm for solution of a problem is a method of successive iterations. Algorithm is first roughly estimated and written. Then it is carefully gone through a number of times and refined each time. The final form of an algorithm emerges through a number of stepwise refinements carried out successively, till the detailed steps become precisely clear to the person or machine, which is going to execute the steps. In an algorithm, all items of instructions are listed in the order in which they are to be carried out. This is done with the help of flowcharts.

However complex the problems may be (numeric, or non-numeric), they can always be broken into a set of smaller sequence of steps and procedures. We can always think it to be solved with the help of a systematic step problem solving procedure, which if following meticulously, will lead us to a definite solution. This step-by-step procedure is technically known as algorithm. In contract to this, there are heuristic procedures, which most of the time may offer a person some optimum solution to correct solution or any solution at all will be achieved all the time. Algorithm may constitute of sequence, selections and repetitions. Therefore, it is necessary that all these terms be understood.

19.2.1 Efficient Algorithms

The following points must be born in mind before writing an efficient algorithm.

- Every procedure should carefully specify the input and output variable.
- The meaning of all variables should be defined.
- The flow of the program should generally be forward except for normal looping and unavoidable instances.
- Indentation rules should be established and followed, so that computation units of program text can more easily be identified.
- Documentation should be short, but meaningful. Avoid commands like "J is increased by one."
- Use subroutines, where appropriate.

Let us see method of evolving by writing the steps for solving certain day to day problems.

It is not sufficient that only the method of solving a problem is written and solution is obtained through computer. But we expect that computer also prints results in a systematic manner such that the user is able to identify the set of results. Suppose in a problem we want to calculate the value of three variables A,B and C and get the results printed. Now computer will print 3 values, but it may not be easy for user to identify which is the value of A out of these 3 results. So for this purpose remarks such as "Answer A=", or "Answer: Temp in Celsius is" are also printed.

Example

Develop an algorithm for converting given temperature in Celsius scale into Fahrenheit scale.

From our knowledge of physics, we know the relationship between temperature in the two given scales i.e. temperatures in Fahrenheit and Centigrade. This is

$$C / 5 = (F - 32) / 9$$

First, we have to write this formula in such a way so that values of temperature in degree Fahrenheit are equated to value in centigrade, namely,

$$F = 1.8 \times C + 32$$

No we can write down steps for writing the algorithm for solving this in such a manner that any person with average intelligence can go on follow the procedure and come to definite solution. The algorithm shall be similar to following algorithm:

1. Read (obtain) the given values of C i.e. temperature in Celsius.
2. Multiply this value with 1.8 and equate it equal of F i.e. F-1 8*C.
3. Now replace this value of F by F+32.
4. Write the Answer.
5. STOP.

Explanation

1. For deriving or obtaining any value from the given problem, we have written "Read" because in most of the computer programming languages, "Read" is a statement which causes the computer to read the given value of a data item. We have to feed this value in computer's memory and computer will read this value in the program automatically as and when necessary.

2. The value of F is in two parts which are 1.8*C and + 32. In computer applications it is customary to calculate the value in part and equate them equal to the required parameter and store this part value in memory. This part value is further added with remaining part and replaced with original value.

3. It is customary to write stop at the end, otherwise sometimes due to mistake in designing the algorithm the computer may continue to work infinitely. Now we will define the algorithm by writing.

Refined Algorithm

1. Read value of C
2. F = 1.8 × C
3. F = F + 32
4. Print "Answer: The value of F is = ; followed by the calculated value of F.
5. STOP

Explanation

1. In second step of the algorithm we have written F = 1.8 C instead of F = 1.8 × C to indicate that computer is to replace value in storage location F by 1.8 × C which is its part value. In next step it replaces this part value of F i.e. F = 1.8*C by any value of F which is equal to F = 1.8 C + 32 in the same location.
2. The calculated value i.e. result obtained, if printed simply numerically will not make any sense on the paper unless we write the words "The answer is equal to"; and fill in the blanks with the answered value. For making the computer to print these words' it is necessary that they are written under the quotes "..." because computer understands either the numeric values written without quotation marks or the strings of words written under quotation marks. This is one of the rules of BASIC Programming language.
3. Observe carefully that we have placed semi-colon, symbol immediately after quote marks. This is necessary according to rules of the programming languages like BASIC that allow the answered value to be printed immediately after the result after a space. Here the computer will not print the quote marks, or the semicolon. Actually these two symbols are a part of the instruction.

CHAPTER 20

Computer Networks

20.1 Introduction

All computers, which are connected via a transmission media, are known as Computer Networks. Suppose a server, which is kept in office where all computers are connected together, means they can share their data and file. Fig. 20.1 shows the data transmission over the network in the office. We can say all interconnected collection of autonomous computer is termed as computer network. Two computer are said to be interconnected is they are able to exchange the information. Computer network started its journey by Telegraph Network & Telephone network

Some simple definitions of network are:

- A *computer network* is computers and devices connected together.
- A single computer is limited to its own hardware and software.
- The capabilities of a computer are increased when connected with other devices to form a computer network

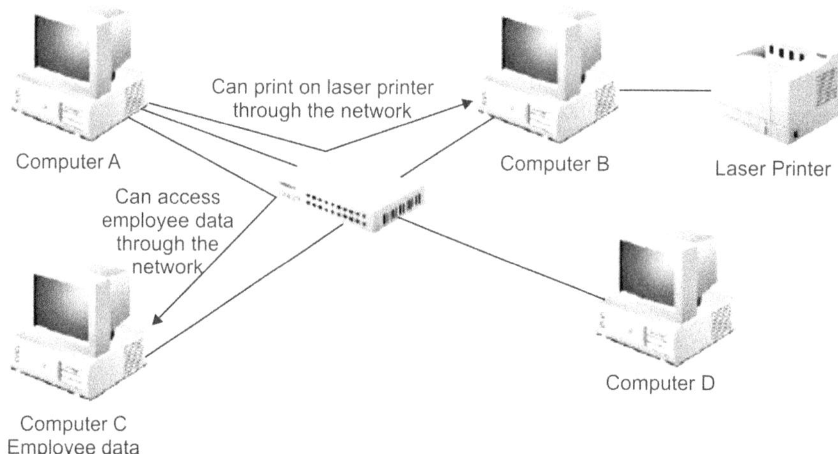

Fig. 20.1 Data Transmission over the Network in the Office.

In 1851 the first submarine cable was established between London and Paris. Eventually, networks of telegraph stations were established covering all the continents. In these networks a message or telegram would arrive at a telegraph station, and an operator would make a routing decision based on the destination address.

In 1875 Alexander Graham Bell invented **Telephone network,** which transmit voice signal. Nowadays this is known as modern telephone service. It is connection oriented service because they require setting up of connection before the actual transfer of information can take place.

The first Computer Network was the Semi-Automatic Ground Environment **(SAGE)** system developed between 1950 and 1956 for air defense system [Green 1984]. The system consisted of 23 computer networks, each network connecting radar sites, ground to air data links and other locations to a central computer. In the 1960s tree topology terminal oriented networks were developed to allow user terminals to connect to a single central shared computer.

The **ARPANET (**Advanced Project Research Network) was the first major effort at developing a network to interconnect computers over a wide geographical area. At the end of 1967 ARPA initiated a small contract with the Stanford Research Institute for the development of specifications for the necessary communications system. Elmer Shapiro was to be the key person on this study the first sites of the ARPANET were picked to provide either network support services or unique resources.

Advantages of Computer Networks :

- Sharing computers
- Networked computers can share resources such as Printers, fax modems, scanners, hard disk, CD-ROMs, and DVDs (Resource Sharing).
- Networks also make computer management easier.
- Maximum utilization of resources.
- This reduces costs and the work of support staff.
- Computer networks can help in improved communications through groupware.
- E-mail, electronic calendars, collaborative writing, and video conferencing are available.
- Computer networks allow computers to be managed from one central location.

20.2 Types of Network

According to the capacity of network is divided into following categories:

- Server-Based Network
- Local Area Network (LAN)
- Wide Area Network (WAN)
- Metropolitan Area Network (MAN)
- Wireless Network
- Internet
- Internet work

20.2.1   Server-Based Network

This type of the network belongs to Client Server Model . It consist of one powerful machine which is known as server & rest are known as Clients . This is commonly used TCP/IP protocol to transfer their data.

- The network has special high-powered server controls.
- The server is dedicated to running the network.
- Print and file servers, application servers, communication servers, and directory service servers are common.

20.2.2   Local Area Network (LAN)

A local area network (LAN) is a group of computers and associated devices that share a common communications line or wireless link and typically share the resources of a single processor or server within a small geographic area (for example, within an office building). Usually, the server has applications and data storage that are shared in common by multiple computer users. A local area network may serve as few as (for example, in a home network) or as many as thousands of users (for example, in FDDI network).

- Network computers are located relatively close to each other.
- They are generally limited to buildings owned by one organization.
- They operate at high speeds.
- They are low-cost networks.

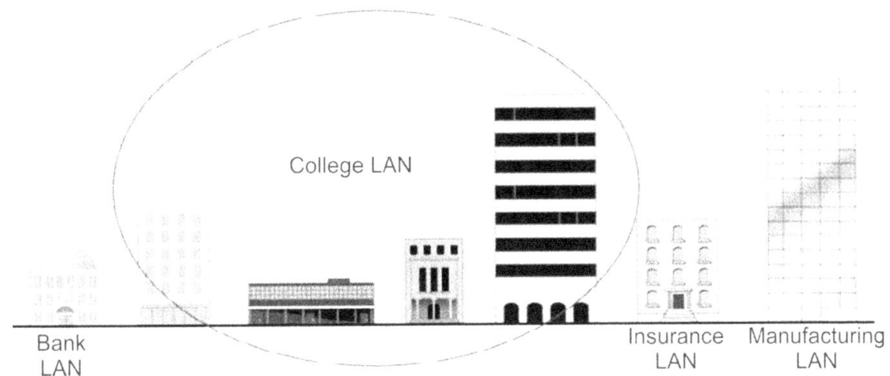

Fig. 20.2 Showing diagram of (LAN).

FDDI

Ethernet is by far the most commonly used LAN technology. A number of corporations use the Token Ring technology. FDDI is sometimes used as a backbone LAN interconnecting Ethernet or Token Ring LANs. Another LAN technology, ARCNET once the most commonly installed LAN technology, is still used in the industrial automation industry.

Typically, a suite of application programs can be kept on the LAN server. Users who need an application frequently can download it once and then run it from their local hard disk. Users can order printing and other services as needed through applications run on the LAN server. A LAN server may also be used as a Web server if safeguards are taken to secure internal applications and data from outside access.

In some situations, a wireless LAN may be preferable to a wired LAN because it is cheaper to install and maintain.

20.2.3 Wide Area Network (WAN)

A *WAN* is a data communications network that covers a relatively broad geographic area and that often uses transmission facilities provided by common carriers, such as telephone companies. Typically, a WAN consists of two or more local-area networks (LANs). WAN technologies generally function at the lower three layers of the OSI reference model: the physical layer, the data link layer, and the network layer It connects computers and LANs over a larger geographical area. It crosses public thoroughfares such as roads, railroads, and water.

- Network computers are spread out over a larger area.

- They generally cross public thoroughfares.

- Public carriers often manage them.

- They operate at lower speeds.

- They are a higher-cost network

20.2.4   Metropolitan Area Network (MAN)

These networks serve an area of 3 to 30 miles, approximately the area of a typical city. MAN support high-speed disaster recovery systems, real-time transaction backup systems, interconnections between corporate data centers Internet service providers, and government, business, medicine, and education.

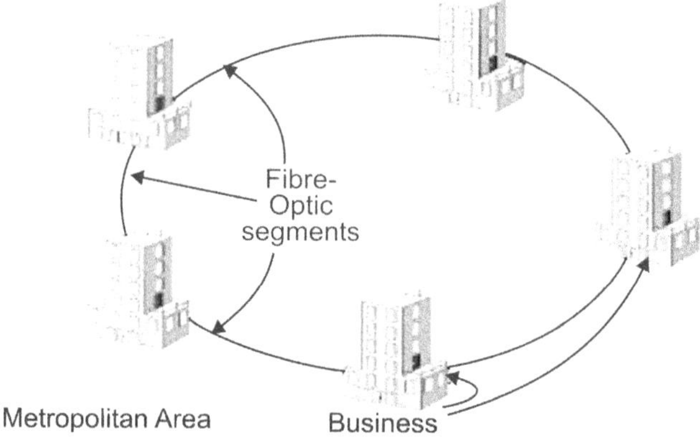

Fig. 20.3 Metropolitan Area Network (MAN).

20.2.5   Wireless Network

The term wireless networking refers to technology that enables two or more computers to communicate using standard network protocols, but without network cabling. A wireless network can also use an access point, or base station. In this type of network the access point acts like a hub, providing connectivity for the wireless computers. It can connect (or "bridge") the wireless LAN to a wired LAN, allowing wireless computer access to LAN resources, such as file servers or existing Internet Connectivity. An ad-hoc, or peer-to-peer wireless network consists of a number of computers each equipped with a wireless networking interface card. Each computer can communicate directly with all of the other wireless enabled computers. They can share files and printers this way, but may not be able to access wired LAN resources. Following diagram shows a wireless network, which can access from H/W access point.

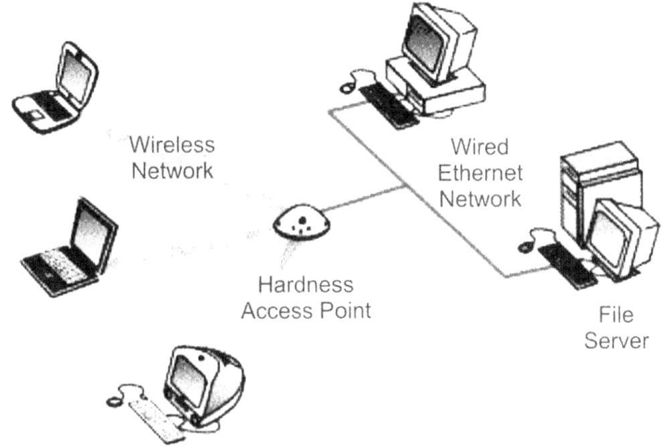

Fig. 20.4 showing Wireless Network.

20.2.6   Internet

The Internet uses high-speed data lines, called backbones, to carry data. Smaller networks connect to the backbone, enabling any user on any network to exchange data with any other user. Every computer and network on the Internet uses the same protocols (rules and procedures) to control timing and data format.

- The World Wide Web is a part of the Internet, which supports hypertext documents, allowing users to view and navigate different types of data.

- A Web page is a document encoded with hypertext markup language (HTML) tags. HTML allows designers to link content together via hyperlinks.

- Every Web page has an address, a Uniform Resource Locator (URL).

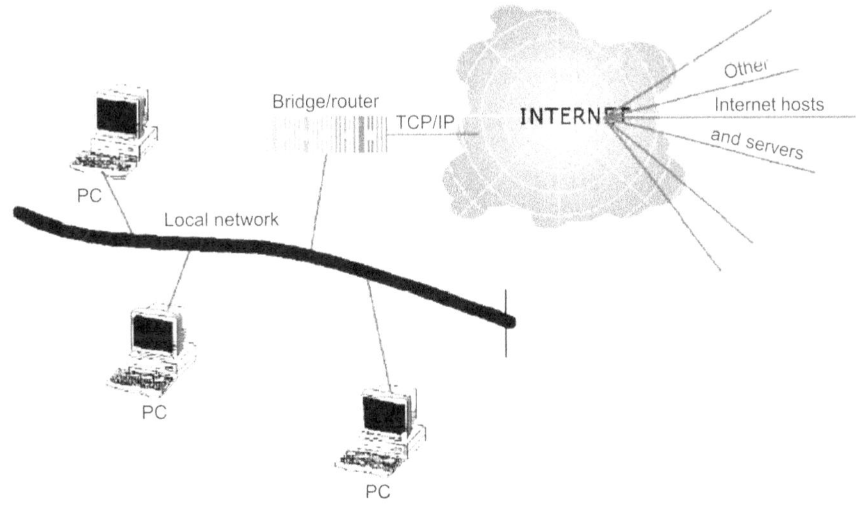

Fig. 20.5 Diagram of Internet.

20.2.7   Intranet

A network connected within university, college or any organization to transfer data between those organizations is known as Intranet. It is usually a connected collection of LANs.   It is also known as Internet work. An *Internet work* is a collection of individual networks, connected by intermediate networking devices, which function as a single large network. Internet working refers to the industry, products, and procedures that meet the challenge of creating and administering Internet works. For example a University having 4 computer Lab, i.e. Computer Lab, Physics Lab, Electronics Lab, Chemistry Lab and if they are connected from the LAN, that is known as intranet.

Some Features of Networking

Hosts : A computer system that is accessed by a user working at a remote location. Typically, the terms are used when there are two computer systems connected by modems and telephone lines. The system that contains the data is called the host, while the computer at which the user sits is called the remote terminal.

Node : In networks, it is a processing location. A node can be a computer or some other device, such as a printer. Every node has a unique network address, sometimes called a Data Link Control (DLC) address or Media Access Control (MAC) address.

Download : To copy data (usually an entire file) from a main source to a peripheral device. The term is often used to describe the process of copying a file from an online service or bulletin board service (BBS) to one's own computer. Downloading can also refer to copying a file from a network file server to a computer on the network.

Upload : To transmit data from a computer to a bulletin board service, mainframe, or network. For example, if you use a personal computer to log on to a network and you want to send files across the network, you must upload the files from your PC to the network.

20.3 Advantages of Networks

The following advantages are particularly true for LANs, although they apply to MANs and WANs as well.

Sharing of peripheral devices : Laser printers, disk drives, and scanners are examples of peripheral devices. As you'll recall,, a peripheral device is any piece of hardware that is connected to a computer. Any newly introduced piece of hardware is often quite expensive, as was the case with laser or color printers. To justify their purchase, companies want them to be shared by many users. Usually the best way to do this is to connect the peripheral device to a network serving several computer users.

Sharing of programs and data : In most organizations, people use the same software and need access to the same information. It could be expensive for a company to buy one copy of, say, a word processing program for each employee. The company will usually buy a network version of that program that will serve many employees.

Organistions also save a great deal of money by letting all employees have access to the same data on a shared storage device. This way the organization avoids such problems as some employees updating customer addresses on their own separate machines, while other employees remain ignorant of such changes.

Finally, network-linked employees can, using workgroup software, work together online one-shared projects.

Better communications : One of the greatest features of networks is electronic mail, as we have seen. With e-mail everyone on a network can easily keep others posted about important information. Thus, the company eliminates the delays encountered with standard interoffice mail delivery or telephone tag.

Security of information : Before networks became commonplace, an individual employee might be the only one with particular information, stored in his or her desktop computer. If the employee was dismissed–or if a fire or flood demolished the office-no one else in the company might have any knowledge of that information. Today such data would be backed up or duplicated on a networked storage device shared by others.

Access to databases : Networks also enable users to tap into numerous databases, whether the private databases of a company or the public databases of online services.

20.4 Local Area Networks (LANs)

A computer network that spans a relatively small area. Most LANs are confined to a single building or group of building. However, one LAN can be connected to other LANs over any distance via telephone lines and radio waves. A system of LANs connected in this way is called a wide-area network (WAN).

Most LANs connect workstations and personal computer. Each node (individual computer) in LAN has its own CPU with which it executes programs, but it is also able to access data and devices anywhere on the LAN. This means that many users can share expensive devices, such as laser printers, as well as data. Users can also use the LAN to communicate with each other, by sending e-mail or engaging in chat sessions.

There are many different types of LANs, Ethernets being the most common for PCs. Apple Macintosh networks are based on Apple's Talk network system, which is built into Macintosh computers.

The following characteristics differentiate one LAN to another :

Topology : The geometric arrangement of devices on the network. For example, devices can be arranged in a ring or in a straight line.

Protocols : The rules and encoding specifications for sending data. The protocols also determine whether the network users a peer-to-peer or client/server architecture.

Media : Twisted-pair wire, coaxial cables, or fiber optic cables can connect devices. Some networks do without connecting media altogether, communicating instead via radio waves.

LANs are capable of transmitting data at very fast rates, much faster than data transmitted over a telephone line; but the distances are limited, and there is also a limit on the number of computers that can be attached to a single LAN.

LANs may be client-server or peer-to-peer and include components such as cabling, network interface cards, operating system, other shared devices, bridges and gateways. The topology, or shape, of a network may take five forms: star, ring, bus, hybrid, FDDL

Although large networks are useful, many organizations need to have a local network an in-house network-to tie together their own equipment. Here let's consider the following aspects of local area networks:

- Types of LANs
- Components of a LAN
- Topology
- Impact of LANs

20.4.1   Types of LAN

Client / Service architecture : A network architecture in which each computer of process on the network is either a client or a server. Servers are powerful computer or processors dedicated to managing disk drives (file servers), printers (print servers), or network traffic (network servers). Clients are PCs or workstations on which users run applications.

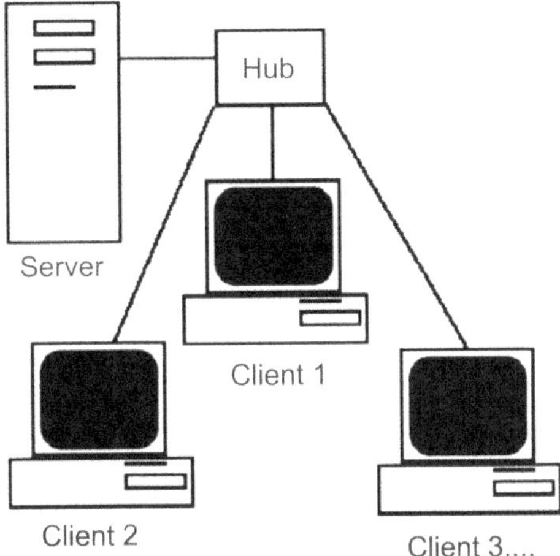

Fig. 20.6 Client / Server architecture.

Peer-to-peer architecture, In each workstation has equivalent capabilities and responsibilities. This differs from client/server architectures, in which some computers are dedicated to serving the others. Peer-to-peer networks are generally simpler and less expensive, but they usually do not offer the same performance under heavy loads.

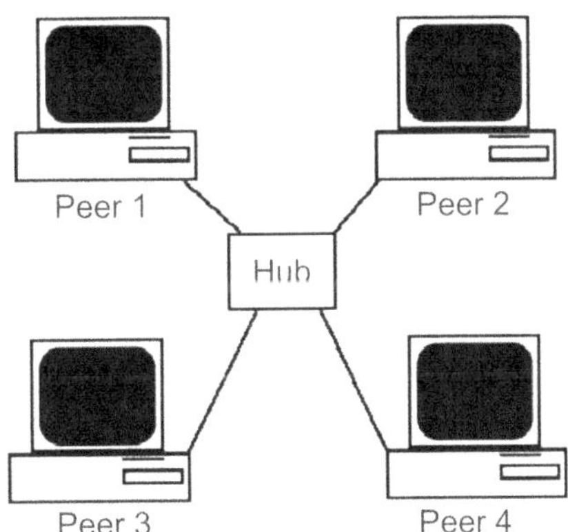

Fig. 20.7 Peer-to-peer architecture.

20.4.2   Components of LAN

Media or cabling system : In computer networks, media refer to the cables linking workstations together. There are many different types of transmission media, the most popular being twisted-pair wire, coaxial cable (the type of cable used for cable television), and fiber optic cable (cables based on higher propagation).

Computer with Network Interface card : More than one computer are required to make a network interface card often abbreviated as NIC, an expansion board you insert into a computer so the computer can be connected to a network. Most NICs are designed for a particular type of network, protocol, and media, although some can serve multiple networks. The most popular NIC protocol is Ethernet.

Ethernet : A local-area network (LAN) protocol developed by Xerox Corporation in co-operation with DEC and Intel in 1976. Ethernet uses a bus or star topology and supports data transfer rates of 10 Mbps. The Ethernet specification served as the basis for the IEEE 802.3 standard, which specifies the physical and lower software layers. Ethernet uses the CSMA/ICD access method to handle simultaneous demands. It is one of the most widely implemented LAN standards.

A newer version of Ethernet, called 100Base-T (Fast Ethernet), supports data transfer rates of 100 Mbps. And the newest version, Gigabit Ethernet supports, data rates of 1 gigabit (1,000 megabits) per second.

Network Operating System (NOS) : An operating system that includes special functions for connecting computers and devices into a local-area network (LAN). Some operating system, such as UNIX have networking functions built in. The term network operating system, however, is generally reserved for software that enhances a basic operating system by adding networking features. For example, some popular NOS's for DOS and Windows systems include Novell Netware, Artisoft's LAN testic, Microsoft LAN Manager, and Windows NT.

Bridges : A device that connects two local-area networks (LANs), or two segments of the same LAN. The two LANs being connected can be alike or dissimilar. For example, a bridge can connect an Ethernet with a Token-Ring network.

Unlike routers, bridges are protocol-independent. They simply forward packets without analyzing and re-routing messages. Consequently, they're faster than routers, but also less versatile.

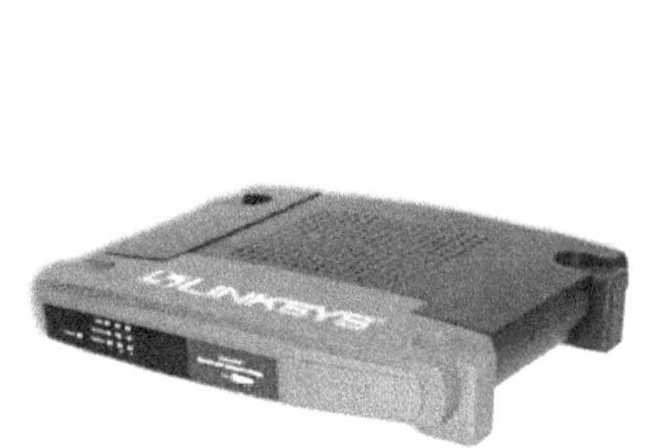

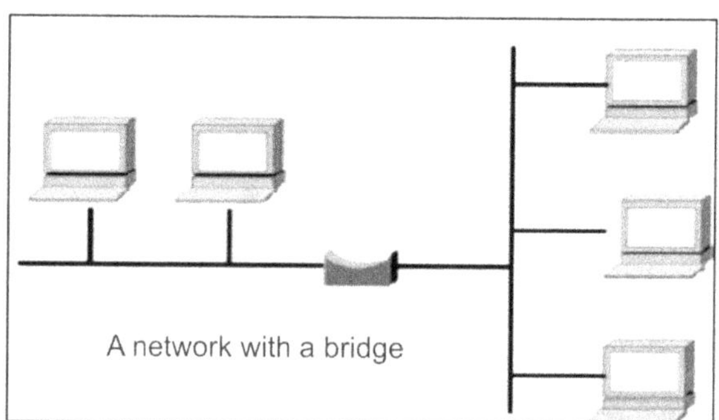

Fig. 20.8 Bridge.

HUB *:* A common connection point for devices in a network. Hubs are commonly used to connect segments of a LAN. A hub contains multiple ports. When a packet arrives at one port, it is copied to the other ports so that all segments of the LAN can see all packets.

A passive hub serves simply as a conduit for the data, enabling it to go from one device (or segment) to another. Intelligent hubs include additional features that enable an administrator to monitor the traffic passing through the hub and to configure each port in the hub. Intelligent hubs are also called manageable hubs.

A third type of hub, called a switching hub, actually reads the destination address of each packet and then forwards the packet to the correct port.

Router *:* A device that connects two LANs. Routers are similar to bridges, but provide for additional functions, such as the ability to filter messages and forward them to different places based on various criteria.

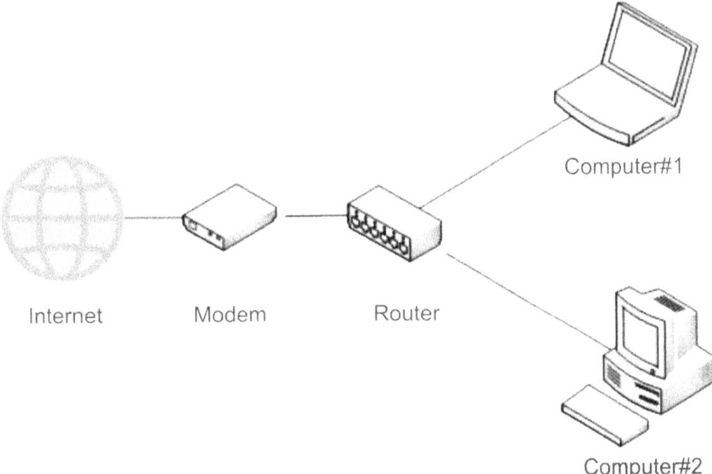

Fig. 20.9 Components of LAN.

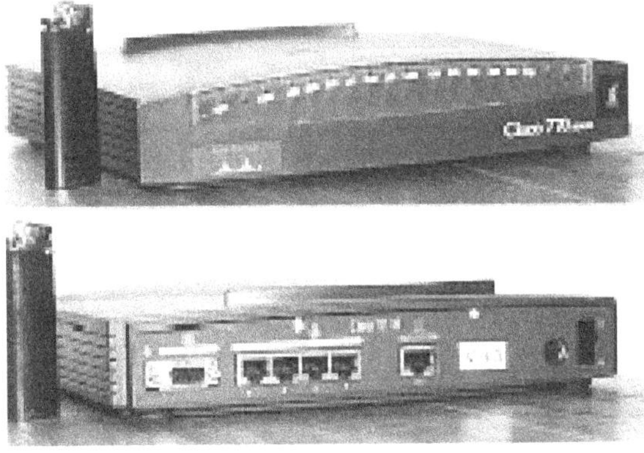

Router

Repeater *:* A network device used to regenerate or replicate a signal. Repeaters are used in transmission systems to regenerate analog or digital signals distorted by transmission loss. Analog repeaters frequently can only amplify the signal while digital repeaters can reconstruct a signal to near its original quality.

In a data network, a repeater can relay messages between sub-networks that use different protocols or cable types. Hubs can operate as repeaters by relaying messages to all connected computers. A repeater cannot do the intelligent routing performed by bridges and routers.

Gateway *:* In networking, a combination or hardware and software that links two different types of networks. Gateways between e-mail systems, for example, allow users on different e-mail systems to exchanges messages.

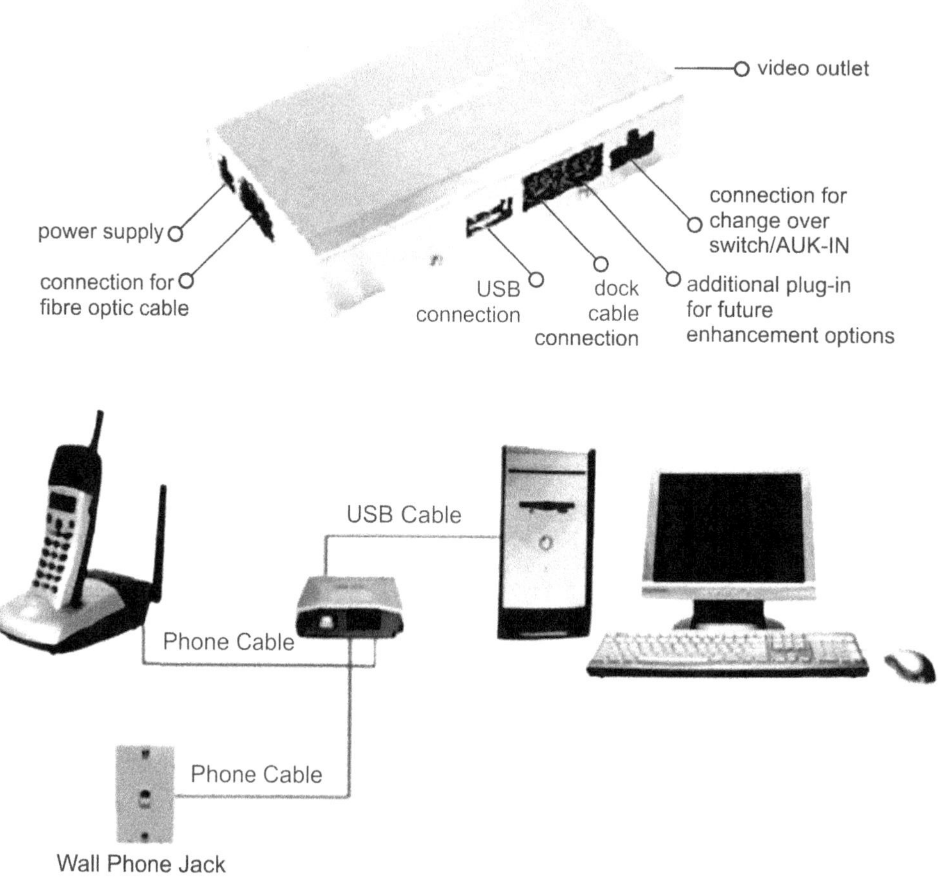

Fig. 20.10 Gateway.

20.4.3   Topology of LAN

The geometric arrangement of a computer system or the shape of a local-area network (LAN) or other communications systems is called topology. There are three principal topologies used in LANs.

Bus topology *:* In bus topology all devices are connected to a central cable, called the bus or backbone. Bus networks are relatively inexpensive and easy to install for small networks. Ethernet systems use a bus topology.

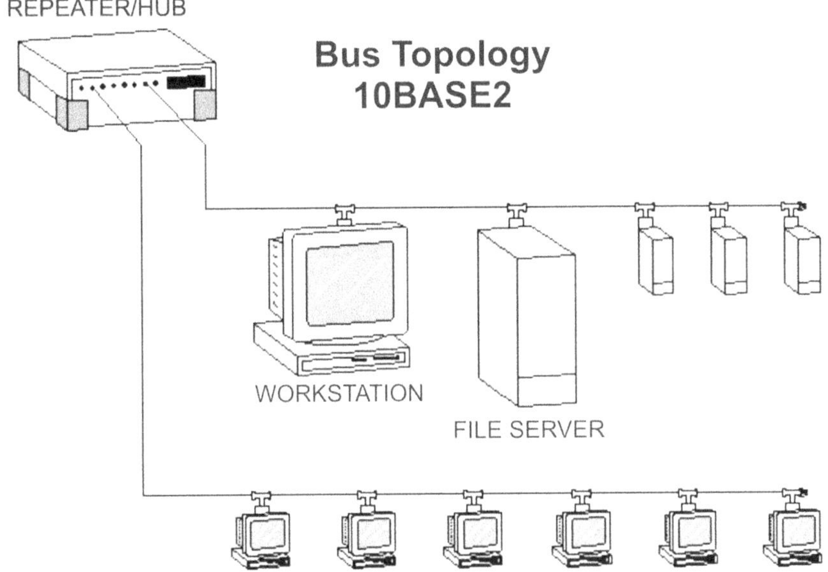

Fig. 20.11 Bus Topology.

Advantages of Bus Topology

- ***Short cable length and simple layout*** *:* Because there is a single common data path connecting all nodes, the bus topology allows a very short cable length to be used. This decreases the installation cost, and also leads to a simple, easy-to-maintain, wiring layout.

- ***Easy to extend*** *:* Additional nodes can be connected to an existing bus network at any point along its length. More extensive additions can be achieved by adding extra segments connected by a type of signal amplifier known as a repeater.

- ***Resilient architecture*** *:* The bus architecture has an inherent simplicity that makes it very reliable from a hardware point of view. There is a single cable through which all data passes and to which all nodes are connected.

Disadvantages

Fault diagnosis is difficult : Although the simplicity of the bus topology means that there is very little that can go wrong, fault detection is not a simple matter. In most LANs based on a bus, control of the network is not centralized in any particular node. This means that detection of a fault may be performed from many points in the networks.

- ***Fault isolation is difficult:*** In the star topology, a defective node is easily be isolated from the network by removing its connection at the center. If a node is faulty on a bus, it must be rectified at the point where the node is connected to the network. Once the fault has been located, the node can simply be removed. In the case where the fault Is in the network medium it self, an entire segment of the bus must be disconnected.

- ***Nodes must be intelligent:*** Each node on the network is directly connected to the central bus. This means that some way of deciding who can use the network at any given time must be performed in each node. It tends to increase the cost of the nodes irrespective of whether this performed in hardware or software.

- ***Repeater configuration:*** When a bus-type network has its backbone extended using repeaters, reconfiguration may be necessary. This may involve tailoring cable lengths, adjusting terminators etc.

Ring topology : In ring topology all devices are connected to one another in the shape of a closed loop, so that each device is connected directly to two other devices, one on either side of it. Ring topologies are relatively expensive and difficult to install, but they offer high bandwidth and can span large distances.

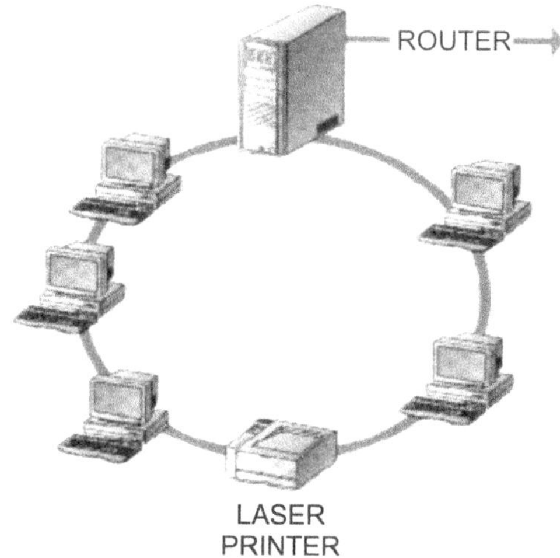

Fig. 20.11 Ring topology.

Advantages

Short cable length : The amount of cabling involved in a ring topology is comparable to that of a bus and is small relative to that of a star. This means that fewer connections will be needed, which will in turn increase network reliability.

- ***No wiring closet space required :*** Since there is only one cable connecting each node to its immediate neighbors, it is not necessary to allocate space in the building for wiring closes.

- ***Suitable for optical fibers :*** Optical fibers offer the possibility of very high-speed transmission. Because traffic on a ring travels in one direction, it is easy to use optical fibers as a medium of transmission. Also, since a ring is made up of nodes connected by short segments of transmission medium, there is a possibility of mixing the types used for different parts of the network.

Disadvantages

Node failure causes network failure : The transmission of data on a ring goes through every connected node on the ring before returning to the sender. If one node fails to pass data through it, the entire network fails and no traffic can flow until the defective node has been removed from the ring.

- ***Difficult to diagnose faults :*** The facts the failure one node will affect all others has serious implications for fault diagnosis. It may be necessary to examine a series of adjacent nodes to determine the faulty one. This operation may also require diagnostic facilities to be built into each node.

- ***Network reconfiguration is difficult :*** The all or nothing nature of the ring topology can cause problems when one decides to extend or modify the geographical scope of the network. It is not possible to shut down a small section of the ring while keeping the majority of it working normally.

- ***Topology affects the access protocol :*** Each node on a ring has a responsibility to pass on data that is received. This means that the access protocol must take this into account. Before a node can transmit its own data, it must ensure that the medium is available for use.

Star topology : In a star topology several devices are connected to one centralized computer. In this topology none of the other computer can communicate with each other if the central computer breaks down. All the transmission between with each other of the network is through the central computer. This topology is used in the case where centralized record keeping is necessary, like in banking sector.

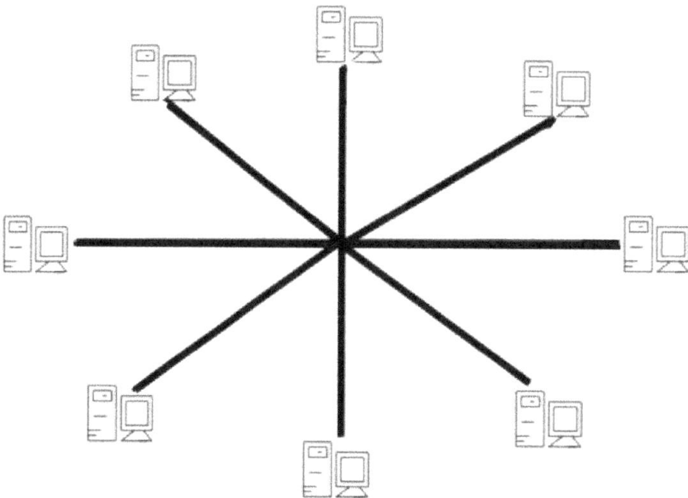

Fig. 20.12 Star Topology.

The star topology has found extensive application in areas where intelligence in the network is concentrated at the central node. The tendency in latest computer systems is away from host-based computing power, and the advent of microprocessor-based systems where all nodes possess a high level of processing power have led to a fall off in the use of this topology. Nevertheless, the technology Is well understood and because It is currently the dominant configuration in traditional data communication, it Is likely to be with us for many years to come.

Advantages

Ease of service : That star topology has a number of concentration points, i.e. at the central node or at intermediate wiring closets. These provide easy access for service of reconfiguration of the network.

- ***One device per connection :*** Connection points in any network are inherently prone to failure. In the star topology, failure of a single connection typically involves dis-connecting one node from an otherwise fully functional network.

- ***Simple access protocols :*** Any given connection in a star network involves only the central node and one peripheral node. In this situation, concentration for who has control of the medium for transmission purposes is easily solved.

- ***Centralised control/problem diagnosis :*** The fact that the central node is connected directly to every other node in the network means that faults are easily detected and isolated. It is a simple matter to disconnect failing nodes from the system.

Disadvantages

Long cable length : Because each node is directly connected to the center, the star topology necessitates a large quantity of cable. While the cost of the cable is often small, congestion in cable ducts and maintenance and installation problems can increase costs considerably.

- *Difficult to expand:* The addition of a new node to a star network involves a connection all the way to the central node. Providing large numbers of redundant cables during the initial wiring usually caters for expansion. However, problems can arise if a longer cable length is needed or an unanticipated connect ration of nodes is required.

- *Central node dependency :* If the central node in a star network fails, the entire network is rendered inoperable. This introduces heavy reliability and redundancy constraints on this node.

Tree topology : In tree topology all devices are linked in a hierarchical fashion. This topology is also known as hierarchical topology. This topology is commonly used in the organisation where the headquarter communicate with regional officers and they communicated with branch officers and district officers, and so on.

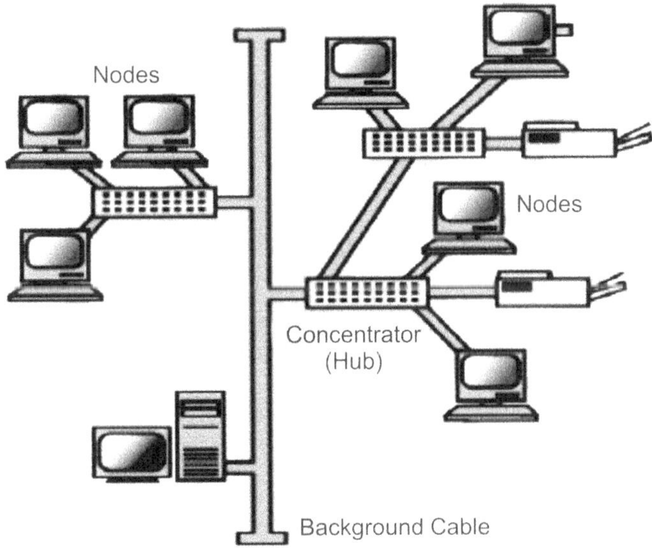

Fig. 20.13 Tree Topology.

Advantages

Easy to extend : Because the tree is, of its very nature. divided into subunits, it is easier to add new nodes or branches to it.

- ***Fault isolation :*** It is possible to disconnect whole branches of the network from the main structure. This makes it easier to isolate a defective node.

Disadvantages

Dependent on the root : If the 'head end' device fails to operate, the entire network is rendered inoperable. In this respect the tree suffers form the same reliability problems as the star.

Mesh Topology : In mesh topology point-to-point connections have between every device in the network. Each device requires an interface for every on the network, mesh topologies are not usually considered practical. In addition, unless each station frequently sends signals to all the other stations, an excessive amount of network bandwidth is wasted. However, mesh networks are extremely fault–tolerant, and each link provides guaranteed capacity.

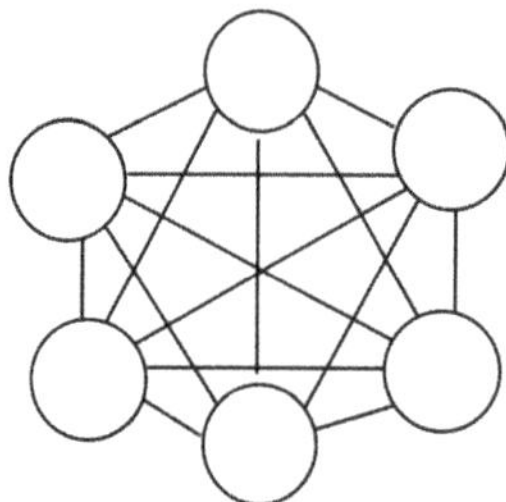

Fig. 20.14 Mesh Topology

Generally mesh topologies used in a hybrid network with just the largest or most important sites interconnected. For example, suppose your organization operates a WAN with 4 or 5 main sites and a large number of remote officers. Each main site has a mainframe and all or the mainframes must communicate to maintain a distributed main site to ensure continuous communications between the mainframes.

Advantages and Disadvantages of the Mesh Topology

- ***Units Affected by Media Failure :*** Mesh topologies resist media failure better than other topologies Implementations that include more than two devices will always have multiple paths to send signals from one device to another. If one path fails, the transmission signals can be routed around the failed link.

- ***Ease of Troubleshooting:*** Mesh topologies are easy to troubleshoot because each medium link is independent of all others. You can easily identify faults and can isolate the affected link.

Disadvantages

- ***Ease to install*** *:* Mesh networks are relatively difficult to install because each device must be linked directly to all other devices. As the number of devices increase, the difficulty of installation increases geometrically.

- ***Ease of Reconfiguration:*** Mesh topologies are difficult to reconfigure for the same reasons that they are difficult to install.

20.5 Wide Area Network (WAN)

As the name suggest, WAN spread across countries and continents, satellite being the transmission media. A wide area network is a network that links separate geographical locations. A WAN can be public system or can also use most other types of circuit including satellite networks, value added networks (VANS/VADS).

The network can be a private system made up from a network of circuits leased from the local telephone company or setup public system as virtual private networks. A virtual private network is our which operates in the same way as a private network but which uses public switched services for the transmission of information. The main distinguishing feature between a WAN and LAN is that the LAN is under the complete control of the owner, where as the WAN needs the involvement of another authority. LAN are also able to handle very high data transfer rates at low cost because of the limited area covered, LAN's have a lower error rate than WAN's.

20.5.1 Types of Wide Area Networks

The essential purpose of WAN, regardless of the size or technology used is to link separate locations in order to move data around. A WAN allows these locations the access shared computer resources and provides the essential infrastructure for developing widespread distributed computing systems. The different types of WAN are:

Public Networks *:* Public networks are those networks, which are installed and run by the telecommunications authorities and are made available to any organisation or individual who subscribe it.

Public Switched Telephone Network (PSTN) *:* The feature of the PSTN are it low speed, the analog nature of transmission, a restricted bandwidth and its widespread availability. The PSTN is most useful in wide area data communication systems as an adjusted to other mechanism.

Public Switched Data Network's (PSDN) *:* The term PSDN refers to a number of technologies, although currently it is limited to public packet switched network available to the public. The main feature of all PSDN's are their high level of reliability and the high quality of the connections provided. PSDN is very popular for connecting public and private mail system to implement electronic mail services with other companies.

Value Added Services (VANS/VADS) : In value added services the provider of such services must process, store and manipulate the data carried onto the network, that is, add value to it. The technique can be used in specific type of business in which it is advantageous to be able to share information with other companies in the secure line. Electronic data interchange (EDI) is one area for value added services in which two trading partners exchange trading documents.

Integrated Service Digital Network (ISDN) : The ISDN is a networking concept providing for integration of voice, video and data services using digital transmission media and combining both circuit and packet switching techniques. The motivating force behind ISDN is that telephone networks around the world have been making a transition towards utilizing digital transmission facilities for many years.

Private Network : The basic technique used in all forms of private WAN is to use private circuits to link the locations to be served by the network. Between these fixed points the owner of the network has complete freedom to use the circuits in anyway they want. They can use the circuits to carry large quantities of data or high-speed transmission.

20.6 Transmission Media

Magnetic Media

One of the most common way to transport data from one computer to another is to write them onto magnetic tape or floppy disks, physically transport the tape or disks to the destination machine. While this methods is not as sophisticated as using a geo synchroms communication satellite it is after much more cost effective, especially for applications in which high bandwidth or cast per bit transported is the key factor.

A simple calculation makes this point clear. An industry slandard 6250 bpi magnetic tape can hold 180 megabytes. A station wagon or light truck can easily transport 200 tapes at one time. Suppose the source and destination machines are an hour's due apart. The effective data rate between these two machines is then 288000 megabits in 3600 sec or 80 Mbps. No wide area network transfer in this order of magnitude of this bandwidth. Few local networks can even match it for a bank with gigabytes of data to be backed up daily an a second machine it is likely that no other transmission technology can even begin to approach magnetic tape for performance or cost–effectiveness.

Twisted Pair

Although the bandwidth characteristics of magnetic tape are excellent, the delay characteristics are poor. Transmission time is measured in minutes or hours not milliseconds. For many application an online connection is needed. The oldest and still most common transmission medium is twisted pair.

UTP Cable (4-pair)

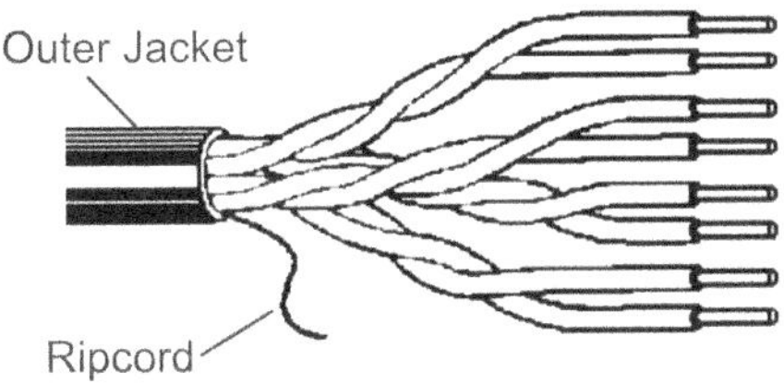

Fig. 20.18 Twisted Pair

A twisted pair consists of two insulated copper wires, typically about 1 mm thick. The wires are twisted together in a helical form, just as in a DNA molecule the twisted from is used to reduce electrical interference to similar pairs close by. The most commonly used application of twisted pair is telephone system.

Coaxial Cable

Another common transmission medium is the co-axial cable (known to its many funds as just "Core"). Two kinds of coaxial cables are widely used. One kind 50-ohm cable is used for analog transmission.

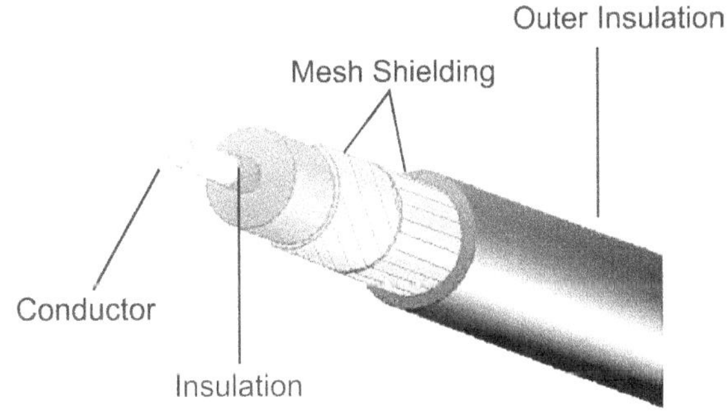

Fig. 20.19 Coaxial Cable.

The construction of the coaxial cable gives it a good combination of high bandwidth and excellent noise immunity. The bandwidth possibly depends on the cable length. For 1 km cables a data rate of 10 Mbps is feasible. Coaxial cables are used for local area networks and for long distance transmission within the telephone system.

There are two ways to connect computers to a coaxial cable. The first way is to the cable cleanly and insert a T junction a connector that reconnects the cable but also provide a third wire leading off to the computer. The second way is to use a vampire tap, which is a hole of exceedingly prices depth and width drilled into due cable, terminating in the core. Into this hole is secured a special connector that achieves the same goal as a T-junction, but without the need to cut the cable in two.

Inserting a T-junction requires cutting the cable; if the hole is drilled too deep it may break the core into unconnected pieces. If it is not deep enough the connection may give inter milder errors.

The cable used for empire tops are the thickest and more expensive than the cable used width T-junctions.

The other kind of coaxial cable system uses analog transmission in slandard cable television cabling. It is called broadband. Through the term broad comes from the telephone world, where it refers to anything wider than 4 Khz in the computer networking used "broadband" means any cable network using analog transmission.

Since broadband networks use standard cable television technology, the cables can be used up to 300 MHz and can run for nearly 100 km due to the analog signaling which is much critical than digital signaling. Thus transmits digital signals and analog network, each interface must contain electronics to convert the outgoing bit stream to an analog signal, and the incoming analog signal to a bit stream.

Broadband systems are normally decided into multiple channels frequently the 6-MHz channels used for television broadcasting. Each channel can be used for analog televisions, high quality audio, or a digital bit stream at, say 3 Mbps, independent of other channels. Television and data can be mixed on the some cable.

One key difference between base band and broadband is that broadband systems need analog amplifiers to strengthen the signal periodically. This amplifier only transits signals in one direction. so a computer outputting a packet will not be able to reach computer " from it if an amplifier lies between them. To get around this problem two types of broadband systems have been developed–cable and single cable systems.

Fiber Optics

Recent developments in optical technology have mode it possible to transmit data by pulse of light. A light pulse can be used to signal a 1 bit. The absence of a pulse signals a 0 bit. Visible light has a frequency of about 10 MHz, so the bandwidth of an optical transmission system is potentially enormous.

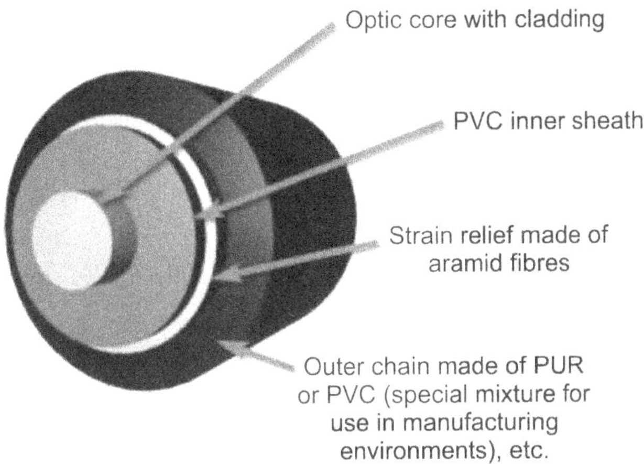

Fig. 20.20 Fiber Optics.

An optical transmission system has three components : The transmission medium the light source, and the detector. The transmission medium is an ultra thin fiber of glass or fused silica. The light source is either an LED (Light Emitting Diode) or a laser diode, which unit light pulses when an electrical current is applied. The detector is a photodiode, which generates an electrical pulse when light falls on it. By attaching an LED or lesser diode to one and of an optical fiber and a photodiode to the other, we have a unidirectional data transmission system that accepts an electrical signal, concerts and transmits it by light pulses and then reconverts the output to an electrical signal at the receiving ends.

This transmission system is based on an uninteresting principle of physics. When a light way passes from one medium to another, for example, from fused silica to air, It is refracted at the silica air boundary. Here we see a light ray incident on the boundary at an angle $\alpha1$ emerging at one angle $\beta1$. The amount of refraction depends on endurance properties of the two media. For angles of incidence above a certain critical value, the light is reflected back into the silica. Name of it escapes into the air. Thus a light ray incident at or above the critical angle is trapped inside the fiber and can propagate for many kilometers with virtually no loss.

Fiber optics links are being installed for long distance telephone lines in many countries. Fibers can also form the basis for lanes although the technology is more complex. The basic problem is that which ampire taps can be made on fiber LAN's by fusing the incoming fiber from the computer with the LAN fiber, the process of making a tap is very tricky and substantial light is lost.

Two types of interfaces are used. A passive interface consists of two fused onto the main fiber. One tap has an LED or laser diode at the end of it and other has a photodiode. The tap itself is completely passive and is thus extremely reliable because a broken LED or photodiode does not break the ring. If one computer does not break the ring, it just takes one computer offline.

Two other interface type is the active repeater. The incoming light is corrected to an electrical signal, regenerated to full strength if it has been weakened, and retransmitted as light. The interface width the computer is an ordinary copper wire that comes into the signal regenerator.

In this design each interface has a fiber running from its transmitter to a silica cylinder, with due incoming fibers fused to one end of the cylinder.

Similarly fibers fused to the other end of the cylinder are run to each of the receivers whenever an interface a light pulse, it is diffused inside the passive to star illuminate all the receivers, thus achieving broad cost. In effect the passive star performs a Boolean OR of all the incoming signals and transmits the result out on all lines.

Since the incoming energy is decided among all the outgoing lines the number of nodes in the network is limited by the sensitivity of the photodiodes. It is instructive to compare coaxial cable to fiber optics. Fiber provides externally high bandwidth with little power loss; it can run for long distances between repeaters.

CHAPTER 21

Database Management

21.1 Spreadsheets

The prime objective of using spreadsheets or worksheets is its facility of performing automatic calculations. These calculations in a spreadsheet can be performed by two methods :

1. Ready-made built-in functions
2. Specifying formulas to perform calculations.

In MS–Excel you can perform powerful calculations in mathematical, logical, statistical, financial, trigonometric etc. The basic arithmetic operator is used in spreadsheets.

21.2 Calculation by Using Formulas

In MS-Excel a formula always begins with an equal to Sign C=S. In a simplest formula of Excel the Excel Sign is followed by a set of values separated by +, -, *, or / for example :

$$= 21 + 6 + 5$$

The above said formula when entered in any blank cell of Excel worksheet gives the result 31.

Table 1

	A	B	C	D	E	F	G
	NAME	MATHS	HINDI	SCIENCE	ENGLISH	SUM	%
1	RAM	89	68	95	92	=B2+C2+D2+E2	=F2/4
2	NAIVEDYA	92	70	92	88	=B3+C3+D3+E3	= F3/4
3	NEETA	86	90	91	66	=B4+C4+D4+E4	=F4/4
4	NISHTHA	72	89	86	72	=B5+C5+D5+E5	F5/4

The above worksheet is a sample worksheet to calculate the total marks obtained by the four students of a class. The marks of four subjects Maths, Hindi, Science, English are given. Formulas are used in column E and column F to calculate the total marks obtained by each student and their percentage.

21.3 Calculation by Using Functions

The spreadsheet softwares provides built in functions to perform the simple mathematical functions. Functions provided by MS-Excel are as shown in the Table :

Table 2

S.No.	Function Name	Operation
1.	Average	Find Average
2.	Max	Find the maximum Value
3.	Min	Find the Minimum Value
4.	Round	Convert the integer with decimal places into whole number
5.	Sum	Find the sum of given numbers
6.	IF	Check for given condition
7	Count	Counts the number
8	Vlookup	Look up the value in vertical coloumn

There are a lot of functions besides the above listed functions.

SUM

The function SUM is used to find the sum of given numbers. In this function entered the ranged of cells specified within the function.

Syntax :

= SUM (First cell, Last cell)

e.g. (In Table 1)

= SUM (B2, E2) = 334

21.4 Copying Cell

In MS-Excel the cell entries made in one cell or range of cells can be easily copied to another cell or another range of cells. The user can copy an entry or group of entries any where with in the same worksheet or another worksheet. The copy operation includes the use of two commands :-

1. COPY   2. PASTE

These commands are present as buttons in the standard toolbar just below the menu bar. These commands are available in the Edit menu.

Steps are:

- Select the cell or range of cells.
- Click on the copy button / select the copy command
- Select the new cell
- Click the paste button/Select the paste command.

21.5 Moving Cell

In MS-Excel the cell entries made in a cell or range of cells can be moved from one place to another cell or range of cells. You can move an entry or group of entries any where within the same worksheet or another worksheet, mere operation include cut and paste command.

Steps are :

- Select the first cell or range of cells
- Click the cut Button/Select the cut command
- Select new cell
- Click the Paste button/Select the paste command

21.6 Formatting the Cell

A variety of formatting facilities are provided to enhance and beautify the cell entries in a worksheet. It helps to display data in different ways and emphasize specific portion of a worksheet. The few basic facilities used for formatting cells are discussed below:

*Formatting character styles

The character styles are used to distinguish different categories of information. These styles change the appearance of the characters in the worksheet. The basic styles used in character formatting are :

Bold : The character appears darker than normal colour when it is made bold. To do this follow the steps.

- Select any cell that contains some text
- Click the bold button (IB) in the standard tool bar.

*Formatting character alignment

By default the cell entries are having some pre defined alignments as :

Text is Left Aligned.

Number/Value is Right Aligned.

These cell entries can be aligned in three way within a cell. Steps involved in character alignment are :

- Select the cell entry

- Click the Align (Centre/Right/Left) Button.

21.7 Graphs Creation

In MS-Excel charts and graphs are made to represent the data in pictorial methods. These graphs are plotted very easily using the chart wizard available as a button on the tool bar. A varity of charts or graphs can be plotted by using the data stored in the worksheet. The various types of charts are : Line, Pie, Bar, Area, Doughnut, 3-D etc.

Steps for plotting Graphs :

- Select the range of cells.
- Click the next button to confirm your selection.
- Select the type of chart and click next.
- Tables of the chart, chart title and other information to be added to your chart.
- Finally the preview comes in front of you.
- Click the finish button.

CHAPTER 22

C Programming Language

22.1 Introduction

C is general purpose, structural programming language which can be used to write very concise source codes for commercial and scientific applications. It is an outgrowth of two earlier language called Basic Combined Programming Language (BCPL) and B. It was originally developed by Dennis Ritchie Bell Laboratories.

C is charaterised by the ability to write very concise source program, due in part to the large number of operators included within the language. It has a relatively small instruction set. The compiler combines the capability of an assembly language with the feature of a high level language and therefore it is well suited for both system software and application software. Program written in C are efficient and fast. It is many times faster than BASIC.

The important characteristic of C is that it is highly portable. It is well suited for structured programming, thus requiring the user to think of a problem in term of function modules or blocks.

Proper collection of these modules would make a complete program. This modular structure makes program debugging, testing and maintenance earlier.

22.2 Structure of a 'C' Program

A C program can be viewed as a group of function. A function is a subroutine that may include one or more statement designed to perform a particular task.

The following structure usually followed to write a C program :

- C Program consists of one or more functions.
- A function contains
  - Heading of the function, which consist of the function name, followed by optional list of arrangement enclosed in parenthesis.
- A list of arrangement declaration.

- A compound statement, which comprises the reminder of program.
- The program is to be typed in lower case.
- First line of the program contains a reference to a special file (Stdio.h) which contain information that must be included in the program when it is compiled.
- Second line contains a comment about the program. This may be in Upper case.
- Third line is the heading of the function.
- Next line starting coading bracket ('{') which indicate the starting of compound statements.
- The first line of compound program is a variable decleation.
- Next one for the logic of the program.
- Each statement of compound statement ends with a semi-colon except of compiler directives like define and include.
- The program ended by a closing curly brackets ('}')

22.3   The C Character Set

C uses the uppercase letters A to Z the lower case letter a to z, the digits form 0 to 9 and certain special characters as building blocks to form words, numbers and expression in a program. The characters in C are grouped in to following types :

- Letters   A - Z, a – z
- Digits   0 – 9
- Special characters
- White spaces

Special characters

,	Comma
.	Period
;	Semicolon
&	Ampersand
^	Caret
*	Asterisk
:	Colon
?	Question marks
"	Quotation
!	Exclamation
/	Slash
\	Backslash
~	Tilde
_	Under score
%	Percentage sign
#	Heber sign
!	Verticle bar

White spaces

- Blank space
- Horizontal tab
- Carriage return
- New line
- Form feed

C also uses certain combination of the character set like \b, \n and \t to represent special combinations such as back space, new line or horizontal tabs etc.

22.4 Constants

Constants are those value which remains stationary throughout the execution of the program. The value may be a digit or a character.

Classification & Constants

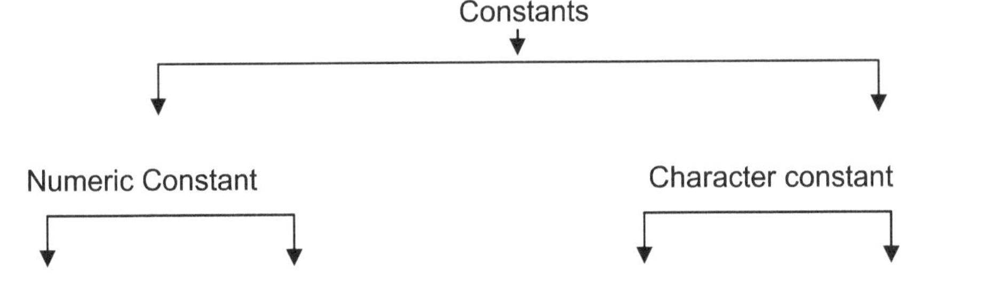

Integer Constant

An integer constant refer to an integer valued number. They are the sequence of a digits. An integer constant may be written in decimal.

Valid decimal integer constant are   101,   14675,   -12345

Embedded spaces, commas and non digit characters are not permitted. Some invalid decimal integers are :

15,750   -   Invalid character ',' used

15 750   -   Space not allowed

15.750   -   . is not allowed

Floating Point Constant

Floating point constants are those numetic values that may contain a decimal point or an exponential notation of the form (e^x), or both to accurately represent certain values that very continuously like distance, weight, temperature, percentage, average etc.

Valid Floating Point Constant are :

2.01,   0.2247,   22.467   2E + 3,   0.45E-2

Invalid Floating Point Constants are :

26   - decimal point or exponent must required

2,576,2.03 - , is not allowed

Floating point constants have much greater range than integer constants. Typically the range from $3.4E - 38$ to $34E + 38$

Character Constant

Character constants are a single character or a string of characters enclosed in single quotation mark. Even if a number is written between the quotation mark, then it is treated as character constant.

Single character constant

A single character constant is a single character enclosed within single quotation mark. Some examples are 'a', 'y' etc.

String Constant

A string constant is a sequence of characters enclosed within single quotation marks. The characters may be letters, spaces, number, special characters. For example :

'Good bye',   'See you',   '2007'

22.5 Variables

A variable is a data name that may be used to store a data value. This variable may take different values at different stages of executions. The data item must be assigned to the variable at some point in the program and it is then accessed or modified later in the program simply by referring to the variable name.

The variable name may consist of letters, digits, underscores (_) or a combination of all these. Usually the maximum width of a variable name is eight character, lower case and upper case variables are treated separately.

Examples for valid variables are :

Next, deep, total, rest

Examples of invalid variables are :

148,   area-of-cone,   printf,   Name1

22.6 Arithmetic Expressions

We can use various type of data in a single expression but C converts all of them in a single form before evaluating the expression. The lower data types converts into higher data types.

In case of floating point operands the low precession operand and the result is the higher precession operands.

If one operand is floating point and another is an integer then the integer converted into floating point and result will be a floating point.

Some times we have to present the data in form, different from the usual form, for example the finding of area of cylinder :

$$A = \frac{3}{4}\pi r^2 h \,,$$

where π is equal to 3.14

Now if we have define   r and h an integer variable, the formula always gives output in the integer form which is not correct all the time. So we have modify the formula as:

$$A = \pi \; Float \; (r^2) \; Float \; (h)$$

This will locally convert value of r and h into a floating form and the result will be in floating form. The original value of r and h remain unchanged.

The type conversion generally takes the form as

Type (name) expression

Where (Type-name) is any valid C data type and expression is the value or expression whom.........

Some changes most occur when convert one type into another. The list below shows the response of some of the type conversion activities.

Activity.	Response
X = (int) 7.6	7.6 converted into integer by truncation
Y = (float) a + b	a is converted into float and then is added into b.

22.7 Functions

All programmers need data to work on. Data is provided either by the keyboard or it is automatically read by the program from some predefined data files. This data may be single character or a character string or any type of numeric value. This data processed by the program and then out passed on screen or on a printer. C, like many other languages, does not have any in built command for data input or output executes this work by some functions, called s/o functions. All such functions included is the stdio, (In file of c library). This file is called a header file and the include is done via = include statement.

C provides 6 main functions for input/output of single character, string or number values. They are getchar ( ), putchar ( ), scanf ( ), Print ( ), gets ( ) and puts ( ). These functions are very useful in writing, many simple programs.

When include the header file at the top of the program, the program begins with statement. # include stdio.h. The command will cause consent of the header file to be included within the program.

These commands are also compiled with the proper block.

Single character input. The Getchar ( ) Function: This is the simplest of the function which accepts a single character from the user. Its standard form is

> Character variable = getchar ( ),

where character variable is c variable name which is defined as character.

> Examples　　　Char name ;
>
> -
>
> -
>
> -
>
> name = getchar ( );

More than one character can be entered using getchar ( ) function with one character at a time but we have to use some looping structure.

Single character output : The put char ( ) function: *Single character can be output by using putchar ( ) function. The return value of this function is a character type data. Its standard form is*

> Putchar (character variable),

where character variable is any variable name which is previously defined as a character type and which has some predefined value.

For Ex.

    Char C.

    C = getchr ( );

    Putchar (c);

The last function will display the value of the variable on the screen. The statement putchar (in); will cause the cusor on the screen to move to the next line. The putchar ( ) function can also be used to display a string of the characters by using some looping statement.

22.8   The scanf ( ) Function

The scanf ( ) function is the most commonly used function used to input from the keyboard. This can be used to enter any type of data including the numeric data; single character data or character string. Its standard form

    Scanf ("control string." arg1, marg2 .... argn).

The central string comprises individual group of character with one character group for each input data. Each character group must starts with a percent (%) sign followed by the formatting group character.

With the control string comprises, more than are formatting. Character group can be written either continuously or separated by white spaces.

The argment are written as variable started with an ampersand (&), however the array name should not begin with ampersand.

    int value;

    scanf ("%n".&value);

22.9 printf ( ) Function

The printf ( ) function is the counter part of the scanf ( ) function by which all the input data items or some calculated results can be printed on the screen. The printf () function can be used to print a single character or a character string or any numeric data. Its standard form

    printf ("control string", arg', arg2, arg3.... Argn)

where control string is some formatting string which will decide the type of data to be printed and is similar as used with scanf( ) function, and arg1, arg2....... Argn are variables whose values are to be printed.

i.e.

printf ("%d" , Principal);

In this example Printf function will Print the value of the variable value which should be of inleger type.

printf ("%d", 2467) will Print 2467

printf ("%bd", 2467) will Print with one heading blank

22.10   The gets ( ) Function

The gETS ( )functions used to accept the string and puts ( ) is used to print the character string. Its standard form

gets (Character variable);

gets (name);

puts (character variable);

puts (value);

22.11   Repetition Statements (Loops)

Looping is an important way associated with decision making in which a particular process is repeated for a certain times. A variable is initialized and the process is repeated until the variable reaches to a certain value. These looping facility enables to develop concise programs containing repetitive modules without using the goto statement.

Depending on the control statement a loop may enter controlled loop or may be an exit controlled loop.

The C language provides three lopping structures to perform these operations. They are :

1. The while statement
2. The do statement
3. The for statement

while statement

It is the most simplest and commonly used looping structure in which a loop is performed until the defined condition is true. The general form of this structure is :

while (condition)

{

Body of loop

}

The start and end of loop are marked by opening and closing curly brackets.

Example - Find the factorial of given number

```
# include < stdio.h >
main ( )
{
int n, n , fact = 1 ;
clrser ( );
printf ("enter the number") ;
scanf ("%d", & n);
n = n;
While (n > = 1 )
{
 fact = fact*n
n = n – 1 ;
}
printf ("Factorial of % d is % d", n1, sact ) ;
getch ( );
}
```

do – while loop

This loop is an exit controlled loop in which the control entered into the loop without testing any condition is evaluated. If the condition is found true then the body of loop is executed once again. The process is continuous till the condition is true. As soon as condition becomes false, the control exists from the loop and executes the statement Just below the while statement. Its standard form :

```
do
{
body of the loop
}
while (test – conditions)
```

Ex B Factorial of given number.

```
# include <stdio.h>
main ( )
int n, n1 ;
clrscr ( );
printf (" Enter the number :") ;
```

```
scanf ("/ d", & n) ;
printf (" Reverse is : " ;
do
{
n1 = n% 10 j
n = n/10 j
Printf ("%d" , n1) j
}
while (n > 9) j
printf ("%d" , n) j
getch (  ) j
}
```

for statement

The for loop is the most effective and commonly used loop structure, used for repeating the execution of a group of statements. It is an entry controlled loop structure. Its standard form :

```
for (initialization j test condition ; increment )
{
body of loop
}
```

The execution of a for loop consists of following steps :

- Intilization of control variable
- Comparing the value of test variable with test condition.
- If the test condition is true, excute the loop once and increment the test variable as continued with the loop.
- If the test condition is false then exit from the loop and execute the statement just below the for- loop.

```
for (i=0;i<=9;i=i+1)
{
    Boddy of loop
}
```

Example: Sum of n numbers

```
# include <stdio.h>
main ( )
{

int i=1 ; sum =0
for(i=0;i<=n;i=i+1)
{
sum =sum=I;
printf ("%d"\n , i)
}
printf ("sum is:%d" , Sum) ;
}
```

Nesting of loop

The for loop can be nested successfully.The ineer and outer loop may or may not be generated by same control variable. A MAXIMUM OF 15 for LOOPS CAN BE PLACED ONE BELOW ANOTHER. The nesting of for loop takes the following structure.

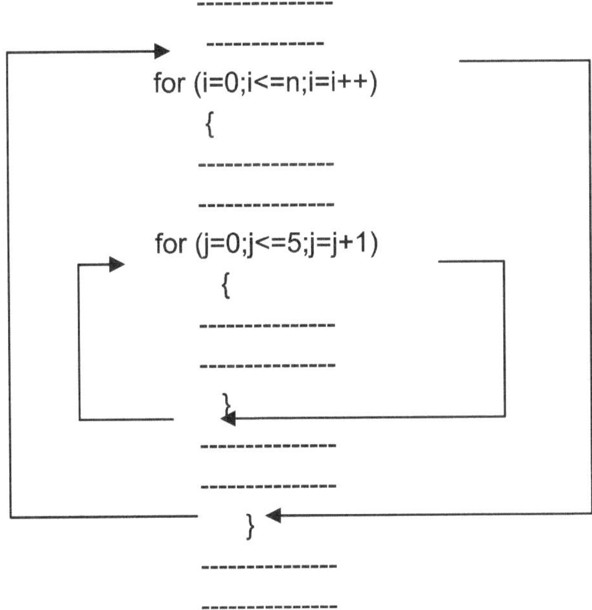

22.12   Structure

The keyboard struct is used to define a structure. The general form of a structure definition is

        struct tag;

{

data type number1;

data type number2;

data type number3;

----

data type numbern;

}

Example : Employee data base consisting of account name, card no, basic salary
          Struct employee;

{

char name [30];

char cardno[10];

ch ar section[20];

float salary;

}

22.13   Array

It is often required to handle a number of data of same nature in a program. For example, in a program for marksheets of students, we may have to use a thousand of names. We can not assign separate variables for each value nor we can retain all values within single variable name because the techniques we studied so far does not facilitate to do so because whenever we assign a value to a variable, the previous value of the variable automatically disappears. So we can use only the last value entered.

C, like many other programming language provides an excellent way to store many variables under a single variable name. This is known as array. An array is a group of related data items that share a common variable name. The elements of the array are of the form of x1, x2, x3….. xn where x is the common variable name and n is the maximum number of element in that array.

Each array element is reffered to by specifying the array name followed by one or more subscript with each subscript is enclosed within a square bracket. We can understand an array as a column which is divided into several parts.

X

1

2

3

--

--

n

where x is the common variable name and 1,2,3....n are the elements of that array.

Defining an Array :

Array are much similar to the ordinary variables except that the elements are subscripted within it. The general form of an array is:

type variable-name (size);

where type is the data-type which the array is going to held, variable-name is the name of array and size is the maximum number of elements in the array. For ex. :

Int marks (10);

will define an array with its type as integer, name as marks and maximum number of elements as 10. The individual element of array will be defined as.

marks (0);

marks (1);

marks (2);

...

...

...

marks (9);

The subscripts of the variables i.e. 0,1,2,...n can be controlled through some looping structure.

Whenever we define an array, the computer reserves the specified locations for the data to be entered.

If we have 10 values as 60, 65, 67, 68, 80, 79, 52, 59, 60, 70 then computer will assign 60 to marks (0), 65 to marks (1), 67 to marks (2), and so on.

marks (0) = 60

marks (1) = 65

marks (2) = 67

...

...

...

marks (9) = 70

These elements i.e. marks (0), marks (1), marks (2) etc. can be used any where in the program as any other variable.

The subscript of an array can be a numeric constant or a predefined numeric variable whose value is keep on changing.

The type of the array may be an integer, float or character. We have seen the example of an integer array earlier in this chapter.

Float average (50);

will define an array of 50 real numbers with the array name as average.

The C language treats all the character string in the form of array only.

char name (60);

declares the name as array name whose type is character and the string contains 60 character. The program will treat each character of the string as an element of the array. If we read following string constant into the string variable name

"INDIA",

then each character will become one element of the array and will be stored separately as bellow

Name (0) = 'I'

Name (1) = 'N'

Name (2) = 'D'

Name (3) = 'I'

Name (4) = 'A'

Name (5) = '\O'

when the compiler sees a character string it adds a null character at the end of the string which indicates the end of the string. So whole declaring arrays of character type, we have to make provision for one extra character.

Data are most often read into an array through some looping structure and then each element of array is also processed through the looping structure. We can use any looping command to store and output the data into and from the array.

Now we will see one simple example that will accept 5 numbers and store them in an array and then print them.

```
#include <stdio.h>
main ()
{
int no [5];
```

```
int I = 0 ;
clrscr () ;
for (i =1 ; i <= 5 ; i++)
{
scanf("%d" ,&no [i]) ;
}
I = 0 ;
for (i=0 ; I <=5 ; i++)
{
printf ("%d\n" , no[i] ) ;
}
getch () ;
}
```

The program defines the array of 5 integer number. Then through a for loop, 5 digits are read using scanf command. The subscript of array are defined through the control variable i. When loop starts, then the value of i. is zero. So the program reads the first value and store it as sum[0]. Then it will store another variable as sum [1], sum [2], sum [3], sum [4].

After reading the value it will print all the subscripts in the same way. Notice that reading and printing of the integer array is same as that of other integer variables.

Now here is an example that will accept a character string of 10 character and then print each character of that string.

```
#include <stdio.h>
main ()
{
char name [10] ;
int i ;
clrscr () ;
printf ("Enter string of 10 character \n") ;
for (i=1;I <=10 ; i++)
{
scanf ("%C" , %name [i]) ;
}
for (i=1 ; i<=10 ; i++)
{
printf ("%C\n" ,name [i]) ;
}
getch () ;
}
```

Initialization of Array :

The array can be provided an initial value similar to that of other ordinary variables. The general form of an array initialization is:

static type array name [size]={list of values};

For example,

static int code [5] = {101, 102, 103, 104, 105}

will define an array code with size five and will assign 101 to code [0], 102 to code [1], 103 to code [2], 104 to code [3], 105 to code [5].

If the number of values are less then the number of element, then only that many element will be initialized. The remaining element will be set to zero automatically.

For example,

static int code [5] = {101, 102, 103}

will assign 101, 102 and 103 to code [0], code [1] and code [2]. The value of code [3] and code [4] will be zero.

The size of array can be omitted while initialization of array. This will allocate the same space as the number of elements. For example,

static int code [ ] = {101, 102, 103, 104}

will define the array code which will contain four element (size is 3). Character array can also be defined in a similar way.

For example,

char colour [3] = {'R', "E", "D"};

This will assign "R" to color [0], "E" to color [1], "D" to color [2]. While the value of color [3] will '\O'

It is to be noted that the word 'static' is used before the type declaration. The 'automatic' type of array cannot be initialized.

Now we will see some examples which use the feature of array.

Prog. Write a prog to enter 10 integers and then print the number, the biggest number among them. Also print the sum and average of the numbers.

```
#include <stdio.h>
main ()
{
int I = 1;
float no [10], small, big ;
float tot = 0.0 ,avg ;
clrscr () ;
printf ("Enter 10 numbers :\n") :
```

```c
for (i = 0; i< = 9; i++)
{
scanf ( "%f" ,&no [i] ;
tot = tot+no[i];
}
avg = tot/10;
big = no[1];
small = no[1] ;
for (i=0;i<9;i++)
{
if (no[i]>big)
{
big = no [i] ;
}
if (no[i] < small)
{
small = no [i] ;
}
}
printf ("Biggest Number is : %f\n" ,big) ;
printf ("Smallest Number is : %f\n" ,small);
printf ("Total is : %f\n" ,tot);
printf ("Average is : %f\n", avg);
getch ();
}
```

This is a typical use of array. An array is defined with its maximum size as 10 and then ten numbers are entered which are assigned to various subscript of array. After this, the first element is assigned to available big and then subsequent value is campaired with this variable. If the value is less than the value of variable then it is skipped and next element is read, otherwise the value of variable big is replaced with the value of element and then the next element is read. The process of adding continuous simultaneously with each step.

Now we will see an example which will deal with the character array. Recall that each character including the blanck character of the string are considered as the element of the array.

Prog. Write a program to accept a string of five character and then print it in reverse order.

```c
#include <stdio.h>
main()
{
```

```
char str [5] ;
int i ;
clrscr () ;
printf ("Enter the string of 5 characters") ;
for (i=0 ;i<5;i++)
{
scant("%c" ,&str[i]) ;
}
i = 5 ;
printf ("Reverse is : " );
for (i = 5 ; i < 1 ; i -- )
{
printf ("%c" ,str [i]) ;
}
getch () ;
}
```

Two Dimensional Array :

All the arrays seen so for are single dimension arrays in which there is only a single column. C allows the elements to arrange in double dimension also in which the array has more then one row and column. This takes the general form as.

type array-name [i],[j] ;

where type is type of array, array-name is the name of array and i is the number of rows and j is the number of column in that array. Note that no. of rows and columns are indicated in two different brackets. The total number of element in the array is equal to the multiplication of the number of rows and columns.

Two-dimensional array are stored in the memory as shown in the figure.

When we issue data to a double dimension array, it is accepted there row-wise. The first data is placed at first row first columns, 2nd data is placed at first row second column. 3rd data at first-row third column. When first row is completed then it starts to occupy the second row in the same manner (second row first column, second row second column, second row third column etc.).

For example, if we have defined an array of 2 rows and 3 columns and data provided is 5,6,8,10,2,20 then the position of data in the array will be:

first row - first column	5		
first row - second column		6	
first row - third column			8
second row - first column	10		
second row - second column		2	
second row - third column			20

This can be represented as:

5	6	8
10	2	20

Initializing a two dimension array : The two dimensional arrays are initialized in the same way as the single dimension array. The initialization starts with the static command.

For example,

static int count [2] [3] = {1, 1, 1, 2, 2, 3}

This command will initializes all the element of first row as 1 and second row as 2. It is obvious that initialization done row by row. The above statement can also be written as static int count [2] [3] = {{1,1,1}, {2,2,}};

Two-dimensional array can be initialized in a form of matrix.

static int count [2] [3] = {
{1, 1, 1},
{2,2,2}
};

As stated earlier that total number of elements in an array is equal to the multiplication of number of rows and columns. If the values are less in the initialize then they are automatically set to zero.

For example,

static int count [2] [3] = {1,1,2,2};

This will assign following values to the elements.

count [1] [1] = 1
count [1] [2] = 1
count [1] [3] = 2
count [2] [1] = 2
count [2] [2] = 0
count [2] [3] = 0

It is obvious from the above discussion that the two dimension arrays are of the form of a matrix. We perform several matrix operations by using a double dimension array.

Now we will see a program, which will accept integers for 2x2 matrixes and then add the elements of array and print it in a form of third matrix.

```c
#include ,stdio.h.
main ()
{
int a [2] [2] ,b [2] [2], c[2] [2] ;
int I, j;
clrscr () ;
printf ( "Enter numbers for first array \n") ;
for (i = 1 ; i,=2 ; i++)
{
for (j=1; j<=2 ;j++)
{
scanf ("%d" ,&a [i] [j] ) ;
}
printf ("\n") ;
}
printf (Enter numbers for second array\n") ;
for (i = 1 ; i<=2 ; i++)
{
for (j=1 ;j<=2 ; j++)
{
scanf ("%d" ,&b [i] [j] ) ;
c [i] [j] = a [i] [j] + b [i] [j] ;
}
printf ("\n") ;
}
printf ("Addition of array is \n") ;
for (i=1 ; I ,=2 ; i++)
{
for (j=1 ; j<=2 ; j++)
{
printf ("%d/t" ,c[i] [j] ) ;
}
printf ("\n") ;
}
getch () ;
}
```

If first matrix is A and second matrix is B then their sum can be shown in the third matrix C as :

$$C[i] \; [j] = A[i] \; [j]$$

The element of first row-first column of first matrix is added with the element at first row-first column of second matrix and placed at first row first column of the resultant matrix. Similarly the other elements are also added. Note that two matrix can be added only if they are of same order.

Here is one more example of using a double dimension array.

Write a program to Transpose the elements of a two dimensional array. Transpose means interchange the elements of rows and columns.

```
#include<stdio.h.
#include<conio.h>
main ()
{
int x [3] [3] ,i , j ;
clrscr () ;
printf ("ENTER THE ELEMENTS OF MATRIX \n") ;
for (i = 0 ; i<3; i++)
{
for (j=0;j<3; j++)
{
scanf ("%d" ,& x [i] [j] ) ;
}
}
printf ("MATRIX IS \n") ;
for (I = 0; I < 3 ; i++ )
{
for (j = 0 ; j<3; j++)
{
printf ("%d\t" ,x [i][j]) ;
}
printf ("\n") ;
}
printf ("THE TRANSPOSE OF MATRIX IS \n" ;
for (i = 0 ; i< 3 ; i++)
{
for (j = 0 ; j < 3 ; j++)
{
printf ("%d\t", x [j] [i] ) ;
}
printf ("\n") ;
}
getch () ;
}
```

We will see one more example of double dimensional array.

Prog. The annual examination of 50 students is shown in the table.

Roll No.   Marks 1   Marks2   Marks3

Write a program to determine

Total marks obtained by each students.

```c
#include <stdio.h>
main ()
{
int roll, marks;
int class [2] [3] ;
int tot ;
int i, j ;
clrscr () ;
for (i = 1 ; i<=2; i++)
{
printf ("Enter marks for student %d\n", i) ;
for (j=1 ; j < = 3 ; j++)
{
scanf ("%d", & marks) ;
class [i] [j] = marks ;
}
}
for (i = 0 ; i< = 1 ; i++)
{
for (j = 0 ; j< = 2 ; j++)
{
tot = tot + class [i] [j] ;
}
printf ("Total marks of student %d = %d\n " , i, tot);
}
tot = 0 ;
getch () ;
}
```

Multidimensional arrays :

Three of more dimensional arrays can be defined and used in the same way as a double dimensional array. The general form is

type array-name [S1] [S2] [S3] ……….. [Sn]

Where type is the data type, array-name is a valid array-name and S1, S2, S3...Sn are positive valued integer expressions that indicates the number of array elements associated with each subscript.

For example,

```
int score [3] [5] [10];
float marks [5] [3] [2] [5]
```

The score array is a three dimensional array with 150 integer elements while marks is a four dimensional array with 150 float elements.

Remember that a three-dimensional array can be represented as a series of two-dimensional array as shown below.

The initialization of multidimensional array can be made as any other array.

For example,

```
Int p(10) (20) (30) = {
{
{ 1 , 2 , 3 , 4 }
{ 5 , 6 , 7 , 8 }
{ 9 , 10 , 11 , 12 )
},
{
{ 22 , 22, 23, 24 }
{25 , 26, 27, 28 }
{29, 30, 31, 32 }
}
} ;
```

This table can be understood as 10 tables each having 20 rows and 30 columns.

Prog. Now here is one example which uses single dimension array and do the following.

1. Read 10 number into an array.
2. Sort the item in increasing order
3. Find the median of the number.

We will explain each aspect of this program in detail.

```
#include <stdio.h>
#include <conio.h>
main ( )
{
int i, j ;
float median , a [10] , t ;
clrscr ( ) ;
printf ( "Enter 10 numbers \") ;
for ( I = 1 ; i < = 10 ; i++)
scanf ("%f\n", &a [i] ;
```

```
for (i = 1 ; I < = 9 ; i++)
{
for (j = 1 ; j < = 9 – I ; j ++)
{
if (a[j] < = a [j+1])
{
t = a [j] ;
a [j] = a [j + 1] ;
a [j + 1] = t ;
}
else
continue ;
}
}
median = (a [5] + a [6]}/2 :
for (i = 0 ; I < = 10 ; I ++)
{
printf ("%f \n", a [i]) ;
}
printf ("Median = %f", median) ;
getch ( ) ;
}
```

Prog. A test consisting of 25 multiple-choice items is held from 5 students. Correct answers and the responses are tabulated in array. Write a program to

- Read correct answer into an array
- Read the response of a student and count the correct ones.
- Repeat the above step for each statement
- Print the results.

```
/*PROGRAM TO CHECH THE ANSWERS OF FIVE STUDENTS AND DISPLAY THE NUMBER OF
CORRECT AND WRONG ANSWERS*/
#include<stdio.h>
#include<conio.h>
main ( )
{
int i, a = 0, b = 0 , k = 0;
char x [25] , y [25] ;
clrscr ( ) ;
printf (" ENTER THE ANSWER OF 25 MULTIPLE CHOICE QUESTION");
```

```c
for (I = 0; i < 25; i++)
{
scanf ("%s" , &x [i]) ;
}
while (k < 5)
{
printf ("\n ENTER THE ANSWER GIVEN BY STUDENT ");
for (I = 0 ; i < 25 ; I ++)
{
scanf ("%s" , &x [i]) ;
}
while (k<5)
{
printf("\n ENTER THE ANSWER GIVEN BY STUDENT " ) ;
for (i = 0 ; I < 25 ; i++)
{
scanf ("%s" ,&y [i]) ;
if (x[i] == y [i])
{
a++;
}
else
{
b++;
)
b++;
}
}
printf ("\n NUMBER OF CORRECT ANSWERS ARE ") ;
printf ("%D" , A) ;
printf ("\n NUMBER OF WRONG ANSWERS ARE") ;
printf ("%d" ,b) ;
k++;
a=0;
b=0
}
getch ( );
}
```

Three arrays are defined at the beginning of the program.

Array 1 to store correct answers. Array 2 to store responses of the student. Array 3 to store correct results to prepare the result. Then the correct answers are stored in first array through a for loop. After storing correct answers the evolution starts. A for loop is executed to count the number of students and within this loop one more loop is executed to accept the answer of each student. After keying the answer, each answer is compared with the correct answer in the form of subscripted values and at the end, the result for first student is printed. The process is continued for all the students.

22.14   File

Concept of Files

In computer jargon a file is an orderly, self-contained collection of information. Any type of information may be included. Hence a file may contain C programs, or it may be consist of data values. Later one is called data file. Data files offer a convenient means of storing data sets, since data files can easily be read and updated.

A file may also be assigned a name, let us call this Std-File. In practice, we come across several types of files such as inventory files, hospital patient file, payroll file, employment detail files etc.

Records are organized sequentially in file as shown here :

Std-Record-1			

Records of a file may be reach either sequentially or vertically. The mode of access depends on the type of storage media that is sequential or direct access type. Records on magnetic taps are always accessed sequentially however the access method may be sequential or direct for records on magnetic disks.

Based on the mode of record organization, we can define the following types of files

- Sequential file
- Direct or random access file
- Indirect sequential file

In sequential file, records are accessed one after another in sequence. If it is designed to reach the 20th record in a file, then the earlier 19 records must be transferred. Records are identified by an identification field, called key field. Key field may be numeric or alphabetic. Sequential files may be a magnetic tapes, cassettes, disks etc. The output you see on a printer is also an example of a sequential file.

Sequential files use relatively inexpensive storage devices and are easy to design and understand. They are also efficient and economical to use to the proportion of file records to be processed is high, i.e. activity rate is high. However when the activity rate is low, they are very inefficient. Storage space is also better utilized by the sequential file. Software needed to manipulate such files is also forward. Sequential files are used in the batch processing.

Direct access file (also called random files) are those in which records may be accessed at random. Each record is independently accessible without reading intermediate records. Every record is assigned an address. Whenever a particular record is to be read, altered or deleted, this is done by using its address and performing other relevant operations. The location of address of record in a file is automatically taken care of by the computer. Direct access file organization required, direct access devices for access the records.

Direct access files are much more efficient for fast and immediate access to records for inquiry and process. They are extensively used for a line applications and whose activity role may not be very high. Random files are less efficient in the use of storage spaces than sequential files and also need more software and hardware for their implementation and manipulation.

CHAPTER 23

Applications of Computers in Pharmaceutical and Clinical Studies

23.1 Introduction

Now-a-days computers are used in pharmaceutical industries, hospitals and in various departments for drug information, education, evaluation, analysis, and medication history and for maintenance of financial records etc. They have become indispensable in the development of clinical pharmacy, hospital pharmacy and in pharmaceutical research. They co-ordinate effective communication and support clinical and financial management functions.

Effective functioning of any organization largely depends upon continuous flow or information, i.e., receiving the information, storing it, processing it and disseminating it. An effective management information system always provides the needed information in the right form, at the right time and at the right place. Actually each information of organization is connected with other informations, through communication channels, thus making organizational entity a decision–making point. Computers play an effective role for retrieval of information. In hospitals, data management involves creating, modifying, adding and deleting data in patient files to generate reports. Now many doctors for further investigation as they are connected through various personal computers share these reports. Some popular Data Base Management System (DBMS) packages for personal Computer are: Dbase III+ and Fox Base +. Hence, computer help in maintaining overall health care system and this can be best illustrated by enlisting its applications.

23.2 Patient Monitoring

Patients monitoring includes monitoring of physiological processes in patients such as blood pressure, pulse rate, temperature, etc. This information plays special role in detection and prevention of critical conditions in patients. It helps in giving warning of critical conditions for immediate nursing attention and enables medical staff to make accurate judgments of patients' progress. It further provides data for research purpose to monitor patients under intensive care.

Hence computers play an important role in communication by acquiring the data about patient's metabolism and then communicating the same to medical staff by displaying graphs. Detecting critical conditions and generating alarms involve both numerical and logical data processing. This processing helps in giving warning of critical conditions, enabling the medical staff for proper judgment of patients progress, and in the long-term provides data for medical research.

Actually computers controls number of equipments simultaneously to obtain samples of body fluids and then get them analyzed through auto-analyser for their physical and chemical parameters.

After analysis of parameters "AND or OR" statements indicate logical relationship where as IF...THEN mark a conditional computation. This combination of logical and conditional data processing enables the patient monitoring system as a decision making instrument for interpretation of results.

23.3 Medication Monitoring

To meet the goal of optimum drug therapy, medication is very essential. In this case, prescription of the patient received over a period of time is entered into the computer data which serves as a chronological drug file of the patient. It helps in suggesting number of drugs along with their dosage schedule. Computers provide two types of information.

(a) Pharmacokinetic   (b)   Non-Pharmacokinetic

Pharmacokinetic Information :

"NONLIN" is a computer program which can predict pharmacokinetic parameters very easily. These parameters include volume of distribution, bioavailability, rate of clearance etc. It helps in maintaining dosage schedule of various drugs like antibiotics, aminoglysosides etc.

Non-Pharmacokinetic Information

It includes various allergic reactions, drug interactions, adverse drug reactions etc. For such information two computer programmes are available.

1. MEDIPHOR (Monitoring and evaluation of drug interactions by a pharmacy oriented reporting)
2. PAD (Pharmacy Automated drug interaction screening)

23.4 Maintenance of Records

Various records like patient's medication history, current treatment and financial records etc., are maintained in computers by feeding accurate data as 'DATA' is a collection of facts and computer works as a 'DATA BASE' manager. MEDLINE is a data base package used for such purpose. It gives the current information of patients regarding their name, age, sex, room number, weight, allergic reaction etc. These records are stored in a 'FILE' like "Physician name" file, "Direction" file, "Drug Interaction" file etc. Now these files contain specific information like physician's name, registration number, phone number, address, etc. and provide such information whenever required.

23.5 Materials Management

Computers play vital role in material planning, purchasing, inventory control and forecasting prices. Inventory control is very essential because it maintains the balance between stock-in-hand and excessive capital investment. Techniques such as ABC analysis and EOQ can be easily programmed. It will eliminate the tedious and time-consuming task of calculations. Computers are used to detect the items, which had attained minimum order level. It then prepares a list and purchase orders for further supplies. Generally there are two systems for inventory control.

(a)   Periodic inventory control

(b)   Perpetual system

(a)   ***Periodic Inventory Control System :*** In this system stock levels are checked manually and the amount of inventory in hand is compared with minimum and maximum stock maintained in the computers. Computers help in placement of order to different suppliers after checking their terms and conditions because all the entries of stocks are present in it.

(b)   ***Perpetual System :*** In this system computer tells about the present position of all the drugs because when they are received, they are entered in the initial stocks to get the current stocks. When the drugs are delivered to various departments the quantities are subtracted accordingly. Such type of additions and deletions from inventory balance is done with the help of "data base" package.

The information as output from the computer may be obtained in various forms like,

- Planning of material
- Drugs formulary
- Vendor detail for procurement
- Tender rate and analysis
- Determination of EOQ

- Pending supply orders
- Inventory analysis
- Records points
- Safety stocks
- Ledger for narcotics
- Over/under stocking
- Slow moving/Fast moving items
- Expired drugs

23.6 Data Storage and Retrieval

Hospital administration computer helps in rapid data storage and retrieval, particularly when the data stored is subjected to frequent changes and when group of items based on the stored data need to be retrieved. Admission of in-patients and their discharge from a hospital require data, which gets changed every minute, e.g., admission of in-patient ties up resources like clinical and nursing staff, a bed, operation theatre, Intensive care unit, pharmacy department, radiological services etc.

Hence decision to admit a new patient is not a simple one. Even the availability of a suitable bed is difficult to determine in male and female ward, isolation ward etc. A prediction must be made that a suitable bed will be available at future date because if the estimation is over optimistic, then patients who are called in, may be turned away at the last minute. If the prediction is over pessimistic expensive resources lie idle and the waiting period for treatment is extended.

Once the patient gets admitted, computer records and stores information like clinical information, catering information, diagnosis, sex, medication etc. It helps in providing detailed information about medical and paramedical staff including their duty chart. It helps the senior personnel to keep a check on ward-by-ward loading of nursing staff and to allocate additional help whenever required.

23.7 Diagnostic Laboratories

Computers meet the growing demand for testing laboratories as manual procedures were lengthy and time consuming whereas automated computerized instruments perform a number of tasks with accuracy in diagnostic laboratories. Generally LIS (Laboratory Information System) is used to manage large amount of data. In this, instruments contain preprocessors, which convert raw data into digital format and help in transmitting numerical values for report generation. LIS also performs administrative and managerial function, including specimen tracking, product analysis and quality control. Similarly many instruments have microprocessors that facilitate all phases of testing processes, including calibration of instrument till reporting of results.

The developments of powerful computers offer opportunity for improved viewing and interpretation in radiology department. In this many of the latest imaging techniques such as Computerized Tomography (CT) and Magnetic Resonance Imaging (MRI) are inherently digital. In this, computer creates a "functional image" by performing complex calculations on measured data.

23.8 Pharmaceutical Education

Computer-aided instructions help in improving the shortcomings of traditional teaching methods. They provide a medium for interactive learning offer immediate student-specific feedback. Support individuals tailored instructions finally form a basis for objective testing.

23.9 Hospital Pharmacy and Retail Pharmacy

Computers are used in pharmacies to maintain accessible, legible and up-to-date medication records. They help in keeping overall patient care by maintaining their records, consumption of drugs, registration numbers and detailed records of accounts and purchase section. Even for retail pharmacist, computers have been of valuable assistance in the prescription processing. It includes display of computer information about patient and drug, its adverse drug reaction, causation, duplication of orders, labeling conditions etc.

Following are the other applications in hospital and retail pharmacy :

- Calculation of monthly gross income
- Generating pay slips
- Updating the employee information
- Placement of supply order
- Keeping track of total payment and amount due to supplier
- Checking the quality and quantity of hospital supplies recorded and identifying any discrepancies.
- Recording purchases for accounting purposes.

A number of computer programs have been developed to assist physicians in dosing and scheduling drug. But there are certain drugs, which are extremely sensitive to certain patients. For such patient's physicians use computer programs to forecast drug levels and to choose the amounts and schedule of drug doses that will achieve target level. Similarly 'HELP' is a system, which identifies abnormal chemistry levels, concurrent diseases and other related patient conditions.

23.10   Hospital Setting

Duties of the pharmacist have been changing tremendously and hence it has become impossible to remember and to recheck everything. Therefore, computer manages the hospital systems and allows the pharmacists to check the work. Software is available for the pharmacist to provide professional services and to automate the technical staff. This will ultimately result in efficient and cost effective operation and will further maximize clinical and patient oriented functions of pharmacists.

23.11 Patient Counselling

Computers play an important role in in-patient counseling. Sophisticated software is available to educate patients by giving patient education leaflets. These leaflets provide information about name of medication, its uses, side-effects, precautions, drug interactions, missed dose, storage, how to take the medication etc.

It should always be kept in mind that computer program should be an intelligent one so that it should not affect adversely by giving too much or too less of the information to patient.

23.12 Drug Interactions

Pharmacists cannot remember each and every medication, its therapeutic usage, its effects and drug interactions. Therefore computers offer knowledge base systems to extend our professional services. Computerized pharmacy can alert physician/ pharmacist for serious drug-drug, drug-food and drug-disease interactions, which are likely to occur in prescription. Examples of such database and online services are MEDLINE, IDIS and pharmline.

23.13 Community Pharmacy

Computers help in streamlining refilling of prescriptions. It has terminated the long standing problem and waiting in a queue for refilling of prescription. It has been becoming popular because it reminds the patient for refilling and compliance of medication. These systems not only help in filling of individual prescriptions but in processing the prescription in a right manner. It also enables to manage inventory, sales, accounts, etc., in community pharmacy.

23.14 Drug Information Services

Various software, Internet, Intranet and online services are available for the pharmacist to provide drug information service to medical, paramedical professional and patients. Computer–aided drug design helps the chemist to formulate a new drug molecule possessing desired therapeutic action. These new drug entities can be generated through graphics and by changing molecular configuration: CD-ROM technology has helped a lot in the evolution of compact electronic libraries. Various software programs of different companies are listed here.

23.15   Important Pharmacy Websites

1. www.aaps.org - American Association of Pharmaceutical Scientists
2. www.abpi.org.uk/- Association of the British Pharmaceutical Industry.
3. www.wizard.pharm.wayne.edu - American Chemical Society Division of Medicinal Chemistry.
4. www.who.int/dap/Word Health Organization program
5. www.accp.com American Clinical pharmacy.
6. www.bpsweb.org Board of Pharmaceutical Specialties.
7. www.fda.gov:80/default.htm Food and Drug Administration
8. www.pharmweb.net - Guide to pharmacy and related resources on the internet
9. www_sci.lib.uci.edu~martindale/pharmacy.html-   Hugesite   with pharmacy, pharmacology, clinical pharmacology and toxicology information.
10. www.aegis.com- Largest AIDS/HIV database in the world
11. www.merek.com/pubs/manual-Manual of diagnosis and therapy
12. http://www.pharmweb.net/- Extensive directory of most aspects of pharmacology
13. www.medmarket.com/tenants/.-Covers regulated product industries
14. community.net/~neils-Pharmaceutical drug directory, links
15. www.bio.com/.-Directory of pharmaceutical and biotechnology companies.
16. www.lilly.com Eli Lilly and Company
17. www.glaxowellcome.co.uk/-Glaxo wellcome
18. www.hmri.com - Hoechst Marion Roussel USA
19. www.hoechst.com/-Hoechst
20. www.jnj.com/-Johnson & Johnson
21. www.nerck.com - Merck & co.
22. www.novartis.com -Novartis
23. www.oncor.com -Organon
24. www.pg.com-P & G Global Community
25. www.parke-davis.com/varsions_1/index.html-Parke-Davis
26. www.pfizer.com/main.html-Pfizer
27. www.pnu.com/ns4index.html-Pharmacia & Upjohn
28. www.rpr.rpna.com-Rhone-Poulence Rorer
29. www.roche.com-Roche

30. www.searlehealthnet.com/searle -Searle

31. www.sb.com -Smithkline Beecham

32. www.arcwebserv.com/pharm-weekly pharmacy articles by registered pharmacist

33. http//157.142.72.143./gaps/pkbio/pkbio.html- Online course pharmacokinetics and biopharmaceutics

34. www.hmri.com/managingyourhealth/guides/tym.html-Instructions about dose, route and taking of medication-www.rxlist.com/top200.htm -List of the 200 most popular US pharmaceuticals

35. www.henryschein.com/medical.htm-Henry Schein Medical products – Online Ordering

9 789352 300723